HOSPICE HANDBOOK

A Guide for Managers and Planners

Contributors

David M. Bass
John D. Blum
Nancy Burns
Kim Carney
David M. Dush
T. Neal Garland
Catherine M. Lamb
Kenneth H. Lazarus
Joanne Lynn
Karen H. May McArdle
Greg Owen
Linda Proffitt
Michael P. Rosen
Paul T. Werner

HOSPICE HANDBOOK

A Guide for Managers and Planners

Edited by

Lenora Finn Paradis, Ph.D.
Medical Center
Allied Health Education
and Research
University of Kentucky

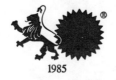

AN ASPEN PUBLICATION®
Aspen Systems Corporation

1985

Rockville, Maryland
Royal Tunbridge Wells

Library of Congress Cataloging in Publication Data
Main entry under title:

Hospice handbook.

Includes bibliographies and index.
1. Hospices (Terminal care) — Administration. 2. Hospices (Terminal
care) — Finance. I. Paradis, Lenora Finn.
R726.8.H669   1985   362.1'75   85-6195
ISBN: 0-87189-104-2

Editorial Services: Martha Sasser

Library of Congress Catalog Card Number: 85-6195
ISBN: 0-87189-104-2

Printed in the United States of America

1   2   3   4   5

This book is dedicated to my grandmother,
Sophie Rudner 1889–1963,
who died of intestinal cancer, and my father,
William Finn 1912–1969,
who died of lung cancer.

Table of Contents

Foreword

As a sociologist who teaches courses in both health administration and planning, often I am asked to recommend a state-of-the-art book on hospice management. While several fine volumes have been written on the clinical application of hospice care to the terminally ill, the actual management of hospice programs at the organizational level has received little systematic attention. This book is the first volume to address the critical issues and problems of managing a hospice program in today's complex health care environment. It provides administrators with a philosophical overview of hospice, discusses the components necessary for effective programming, planning, and evaluation, and suggests a set of organizational strategies to guide hospice personnel in providing high-quality, cost-effective hospice care. Each chapter is written from the perspective that hospice is a dynamic process that fails when reduced to mere recipe. Drawing upon a contingency approach to management, the authors emphasize the design of efficient administrative systems in which the rich values of hospice are preserved. For these reasons, the book is highly useful to researchers, health planners, clinicians, and administrators in providing efficient and personalized hospice care.

My own interest in hospice administration developed out of my research during the seventies on the emergence of hospice as a social movement. Although the hospice at New Haven already had begun operations, activities were just getting underway in the neighborhoods and suburbs of my own city, Chicago. This was an exciting time, filled with hope and fueled by the belief that hospice could make health care more responsive to the needs of dying patients and their families. The movement was sparked by people of diverse backgrounds who came together with one common goal: to create supportive environments where the terminally ill could die with dignity and without pain.

During this early period, movement activities took a variety of structural forms. A hospice might be as small as three people meeting regularly at a kitchen table, as institutionally autonomous as a community-based support program, or as formal as a demonstration project planned for a suburban hospital. These early groups later developed into the organizational models that have become the focus of this volume. Their history, programmatic variation, and ideological diversity form a framework through which the authors analyze current managerial problems.

Looking back from this vantage point, one observes that the 1970s for the hospice movement was a decade devoted to the formation of organizational identity and survival. By contrast, the 1980s is an era when hospices are struggling with success. Government recognition and financial support through Medicare signify formal institutionalization and public acceptance for the concept. If the past proves predictive, nonprofit and for-profit insurers will follow suit. Indeed, hospice has become a burgeoning social service network of organizations spanning the country. Each state has at least one advisory association and the National Hospice Organization functions as a visible and effective lobby in shaping social policy. Yet such institutionalization and popularity raises an important question: Can quality hospice services be integrated into mainstream health care without compromising the movement's values or losing sight of its ideals? *Hospice Handbook* is timely in that it addresses the critical issues central to this concern.

We know from the social movement literature that as social movements grow, they develop a more complex and specialized division of labor. Vertical levels of hierarchy emerge and authority for decision making becomes centralized. In social movements like hospice where membership is built upon egalitarian principles, the need develops for new staffing practices and protocols that define work boundaries while respecting personal rights. The benefits derived through unity of command must be tempered by programmatic policies that recognize participatory decision making at all organizational levels.

Any increase in organizational complexity also coincides with a demand for higher levels of education and training. The first hospice programs were administered and staffed by men and women instrumental in building the movement. As high-level volunteer and salaried jobs became available, these positions were filled by candidates from within the movement. This custom is changing, and many hospice programs now look outside the movement for professionals with experience in managing large social service agencies. As a result, hospices typically have two types of staff: grass-roots workers (including those with professional degrees) who joined the movement during the charismatic years and managerial or medical professionals recruited at a later date to operate the bureaucracy or oversee clinical services. Informational resources and in-service training must address both groups. Newcomers require a grounding in hospice history, movement philosophy, and methods of service delivery. Meanwhile, those who have risen from the ranks often need more training in financial management, program planning, evaluation, and other formal administrative skills.

In contrast to the past where social movements were financed solely by contributions from their members, today's successful social movements typically draw upon business, foundations, and the government for their resources. As a result, most social movement organizations must operate according to the same accounting and financial procedures common to business or public agencies. The danger with this mode of movement financing is that it easily leads to organizational goal displacement. With hospice, for example, qualifying for and maintaining the right to third-party reimbursement takes considerable know-how and carries steep ideological risk. Such payment structures require hospice personnel to supply detailed records, follow complex legal regulations, and be ready to defend the treatment they deliver. Under intense pressure to comply, programs may become caught up in the very bureaucratic paperwork and "people processing" that hospice was designed to ameliorate. The temptation also exists for programs to redefine their goals and objectives to fit funding priorities or reimbursement guidelines.

Four organizational requisites must be met to avoid this scenario. First, hospice programs need sound advice in financial planning, cost assessment, and basic accounting techniques. Second, with health care as one of the nation's most regulated industries, programmatic policies must address issues of individual and organizational liability, respond to a complex web of health care regulations, utilize sound methods of risk management, and reflect an awareness of the criminal-law implications of delivering hospice services. Third, periodic reexamination of movement goals, values, and both organizational and personal ethics are necessary to clarify issues and keep the program on track. Finally, careful measurement and evaluation techniques must be used to judge whether or not the program has met its objectives.

If hospice follows the typical course of a social movement, successful institutionalization will lead to membership complacency. Feeling that things have improved, both members and the general public disengage and turn their energies to other concerns. With its initial energy channeled elsewhere, the movement dwindles or dies. Social movements that survive this stage expand their base and turn their attention to new challenges.

With hospice, the possibilities for extending the movement are many. Nursing homes and other long-term care institutions stand to benefit greatly from adopting hospice methods. In addition, the advent of Medicare reimbursement for hospice services has opened the way for hospice programs to serve new patient populations. When the movement began, many programs were reluctant to admit children because staff lacked the experience necessary to treat young people. With organizational maturity, however, an increasing number of programs now are ready to serve the young. Bereavement programs, comprised of follow-up services for the family of the deceased, also have emerged as an important aid to helping families adjust to death and personal loss.

Perhaps the greatest challenge to the hospice concept lies with medicine itself. Over the last fifty years, the medical order has been remarkably resistant to attempts to limit its power or to change its patterns of service delivery. Where conflict has failed to eliminate a challenger, co-optation has been used to neutralize its power. The absorption of the once-independent system of homeopathy into mainstream medicine serves as a case in point. The future of hospice may well lie with its practitioners' ability to recognize and successfully avoid the pitfalls of operating within a system where accommodation may prove more threatening than overt hostility.

Hospice administrators and staff will find *Hospice Handbook* a valuable guide for negotiating such difficult terrain. Taken as a whole, the chapters provide the conceptual framework, identify the key issues, and suggest the managerial strategies needed to implement the hospice concept in home, community, or institutional settings. I heartily recommend the volume to anyone with an interest in designing human service organizations that efficiently address the complex problems of medicine without sacrificing either the dignity or the values of human life.

Judith A. Levy

Preface

The chapters of *Hospice Handbook* provide hospice program developers and policymakers with a comprehensive, realistic, and pragmatic assessment of how, when, where, why, and in what fashion hospice programs are created and sustained. All information is practical, easy to understand and use. The authors raise salient issues and address a myriad of concerns expressed by hospice staff, administrators, and patients.

Part I provides an overview of the hospice concept, describes divergent models of hospice care, and examines critical management information. My own chapter on the hospice movement, in conjunction with Michael Rosen's in Part III, provides the single most comprehensive description of the formation and expansion of the American hospice movement. Chapter 1 addresses the growth and change of hospice development philosophically and programmatically as it progressed from small, community-sponsored programs staffed predominately by volunteers, to large, institutionally affiliated programs employing paid personnel. Chapter 8 covers major issues in hospice reimbursement and costs. Rosen artfully details the trials and tribulations of organizers as they labored for passage of Medicare standards and exhaustively explains the new hospice certification rules, regulations, and reimbursement requirements.

Catherine Lamb's chapter provides a detailed analysis of hospice programming, planning, and management. Chapter 2 describes the regulatory, organizational, and fiscal intricacies of developing hospices of diverse programmatic origin (freestanding, home health agency-based, or hospital-based) and provides administrators with a checklist for designing all aspects of hospice care.

Neal Garland and David Bass have taken great pains to instruct program administrators in the "how tos" of patient satisfaction research. As hospice administrators seek increased levels of third-party funding, they will have to justify their requests for reimbursement and also define a mechanism for assessing quality of care. Patient satisfaction indices are one mechanism for assessing quality of care. In Chapter 3 Garland and Bass illustrate how hospice staff and organizers can obtain essential information about program improvement and also future funding requests.

Application is the foundation of this book. Parts II and III provide explicit information regarding the planning, design, costs, and benefits of varied organizational structures for delivering hospice care. In Part II, Greg Owen's chapter on long-term care facilities illustrates how administrators and policymakers can estimate the potential value of implementing hospice practices in the long-term care environment. Chapter 4 describes critical staffing, training, and cost factors.

Using an approach similar to that of Owen, Karen McCardle, in Chapter 5, advises hospital planners about the practical considerations they will face as they design hospice programming for hospitals. McCardle identifies the strengths and weaknesses of several organizational approaches to providing hospice care, including scattered-bed and single-unit arrangements. Her chapter focuses on a myriad of administrative issues, from staff selection, training and recruitment to medical and nursing roles and budgetary considerations.

Since its inception, the hospice movement has focused its attention on caring for the dying adult. As the movement spread, providers realized the importance of addressing another group of patients, those 18 years of age and younger. While it is hard to think of anyone so young as having a terminal illness, the number of children dying from cancer is escalating. Ken Lazarus, in Chapter 6 on pediatric hospice care, provides one of the few detailed descriptions of designs for pediatric hospice care. Analyzing the differences between adult and pediatric programming concerns, Lazarus identifies the needs of pediatric patients and their families and discusses ways to train staff to cope with and describe death to children.

The cost of hospice care is a consistent theme throughout *Hospice Handbook*, as it is in the minds of planners and administrators. Because hospice organizers must be concerned with their financial base, cost considerations are of utmost importance. In the chapters by Linda Proffitt and Kim Carney and Nancy Burns, the focus is on costs of care. In Chapter 7, Proffitt examines the costs of using a home-based hospice program model along with the varied organizational dimensions planners and managers should know before they begin developing a program for home care. Proffitt's work complements that of Kim Carney and Nancy Burns in Part III. In Chapter 10 Burns and Carney use a case study to explore the economic and nursing elements of hospice care. Considering that the majority of care received by hospice patients is nursing oriented, the authors identify the distinct elements of quality care and also describe the arrangement in which services are delivered to hospice patients. Their following chapter (Carney and Burns) uses a macro approach to develop an economic model for viewing the interface between hospice supply and demand. Costs, related to supply and demand, are delineated using an economic approach and described so that planners and managers can use the model to predict service needs in their area. Part III focuses on general cost issues as well as financing and reimbursement for hospice providers. Chapter 9, John Blum's chapter on legal issues facing hospice providers, includes an in-depth review of those legal areas that potentially impact individual and corporate liability faced by hospice practitioners. Individual staff liability, informed consent, withdrawal of life support systems, and criminal implications of hospice care are discussed. It is often difficult to separate legal from ethical concerns. Joanne Lynn's chapter on ethics expands on many concerns described by Blum. Chapter 12 deals with distinctions between terminally ill and curative care patients, defines standards of care, and addresses potential ethical conflicts for hospice program providers.

Bereavement programming is a central concern for hospice programmers. Care of the family after death of a loved one is considered preventive medicine. The objectives of bereavement, methods of interventions, and identification of effective bereavement counseling are examined by David Dush in Chapter 13 of Part IV. His chapter deals with strategies for assessing divergent client needs as well as staffing and professional back-up requirements.

In all phases of hospice care, the physician plays a crucial role in patient care planning and delivery. The physician, as gatekeeper to the medical care system, determines not only which patients receive hospice care but also how much and what type of care they will receive. Paul Werner, in Chapter 14 on the changing role and status of the physician, examines the way in which the physician-patient relationship is altered by the hospice concept. The patient, family, and staff have different expectations for the physician. Werner provides suggestions for hospice physicians to use in working with patients and their families. He also identifies characteristics that hospice managers should look for when selecting a physician to work with a hospice program.

Finally, the future for hospice is analyzed in the concluding chapter. Will it survive in the face of increased government regulation and institutional control? Can hospice continue its unique and individualized form of patient care? Can the National Hospice Organization decrease the growing fragmentation among hospice providers—particularly between small, volunteer-dominated programs and those that are institutionally affiliated? These and related concerns are discussed in detail in Chapter 15.

The issues presented in *Hospice Handbook* cover a wide range of hospice patient and provider concerns. The material is current and provocative. The authors do more than merely point to potential problem areas, they provide solutions. This book is *critical* for anyone working in the hospice setting, whether planning a new program, developing additional services, or revising existing ones. It is a crucial guide for policymakers who need a mechanism to assess, evaluate, and address changes occurring in the hospice movement. Practical, critical, and applicable, *Hospice Handbook* gives readers much-needed planning, management, policy, and administrative information.

Lenora Finn Paradis

Part I

Hospice Overview

Chapter 1

The Development of Hospice in America: A Social Movement Organizes

Lenora Finn Paradis

THE CONCEPT OF HOSPICE

Hospice is a recent form of health care delivery that has taken a prominent place on the stage of the American health care industry. The word "hospice" connotes a calm vision of death where the dying spend their final days in the comfort of their home surrounded by friends and relatives.

The upsurge in hospice programs throughout the United States can be viewed as an organized reaction to a social problem: the depersonalization of care for the terminally ill. Attracting attention in the early 1960s, the hospice concept is considered by some to be a human rights movement focusing not only on the terminally ill patient's rights, but also on the failure of the existing medical care system to meet the needs of the dying.

As defined by Flexner, hospice is a "medically directed, nurse-coordinated program providing a continuum of home and inpatient care for the terminally ill patient and family. It employs an interdisciplinary team acting under the direction of an autonomous hospice administrator."[1]

The chief objective of the hospice program is to provide supportive care for the dying person. The program emphasizes keeping the patient at home. The principal products of the hospice program are nursing, palliative care, and counseling services to the dying; its central concern is the comfort of the dying patient.

The hospital, on the other hand, is most concerned with the treatment of illness within the limits of present-day technical-medical knowledge.[2] The principal products of the hospital are medical, surgical, and nursing services to the patient and its central concern is the life of the patient.

In its pristine, ideal form, hospice care welcomes "guests" into a "high-person, low-technology" setting, unsegregated from sights, sounds, persons, and activities of the world of wellness. Patients surrounded by staff, volunteers, family members, and friends receive "holistic" care from individuals who spend nonmedical as well as medical time with them. The major objectives are to dispel psychic pain and suffering, reduce anxiety and fear of death, and control physical pain and discomfort.

According to Fox, "Attending to the emotional, social, spiritual and physical needs of the terminally ill and their families is considered essential to the hospice's commitment and to its capacity to transform the process of dying into a tolerable, meaning-filled experience for all those who participate in it."[3]

Senator Jennings Randolph, in establishing National Hospice Week (S.J. Resolution 170, March 18, 1982), stated, "Hospice is a place, people, and a philosophy. It is a system of care that seeks to restore dignity and a sense of personal fulfillment to the dying. The focus is on the patient and the family, rather than on the disease—and the aim is not to extend life, but to improve the quality of the life that remains."

While Randolph's description is general, Section 1811 of the Social Security Act, which was amended by P.L. 97-248, the Tax Equity and Fiscal Responsibility Act of 1982, to provide Medicare reimbursement for covered hospice patients, is fairly specific in what constitutes that care. The act requires that the patient be considered terminally ill with six months to live as diagnosed by a physician licensed in the United States. Care for the patient must center on pain and symptom control provided by an interdisciplinary team of health care professionals including nurses, physicians, social workers, clergy, and specially trained volunteers. The act requires that the majority of a patient's care be rendered in the home, that care be available 24 hours a day, and that the family participate in the care of the patient.

HISTORICAL ANTECEDENTS

Although the appearance of hospice programs in the United States is recent, the concept has existed for centuries. Medical historian David Reisman noted that the concept of hospice antedates A.D. 475 and that there is proof of a hospice founded in the Port of Rome by Fabiola, a disciple of Saint Jerome, to care for pilgrims returning from Africa.[4]

The word "hospice" originally meant a place of shelter for travelers. During the medieval period, hospices were maintained by religious orders as resting places for individuals on pilgrimages to the Holy Land. Hospices were in operation throughout Europe in large, densely populated areas as well as in more rural ones. Some estimates indicate there were as many as 750 in England, 40 in Paris, and 30 in Florence, as well as others in monastic hermitages in wilderness areas, at mountain passes, and near river crossings. Hospices could be found anywhere travelers to the Holy Land might experience the greatest hazards.[5] For centuries, the idea of hospice signified a refuge where people went to be cared for, nourished, and loved in the face of impoverishment, crisis, or impending death. In the fifth century A.D., St. Bridget of Ireland offered hospice care when she provided respite to the lost, the lame, the sick, and the dying. Similarly, the Hospitaler Knights of St. John cared for the Crusaders of the eleventh and twelfth centuries, providing food and open-air rooms for those who would not recover. The Sisters of Charity of Paris, Reverend Fleidner of Kaiserwerth Hospital in Prussia, Elizabeth Fry, the Irish Sisters of Charity in England, and countless others are noteworthy for caring for the sick and dying in a humanitarian way.[6]

As an institution designed primarily for the care of incurably ill persons, however, the modern hospice traces its roots directly to the Irish Sisters of Charity in Dublin. In the mid 1800s, Sister Mary Aikenhead opened a home in Dublin for the dying, calling it "hospice" in consonance with her view of death as part of an eternal journey. A contemporary of Florence Nightingale, Mother Mary, as she was known, was crippled and forced to direct the work of the sisters from her bed. Through her leadership, the Sisters established hospitals for the sick and refuges for the poor and homeless. News of her charitable work spread overseas and in 1900, Mother Mary was invited to come to London by Cardinal Vaughan. Within five years, the Sisters had established St. Joseph's, the first British hospice. Today St. Joseph's is a 100-bed facility located in London's East End, where its four- and six-bed wards provide a place of refuge for terminally ill patients. St. Joseph's also has served as a model for other English hospices, the most notable of which is St. Christopher's Hospice, established in a London suburb by Cicely Saunders, M.D., following seven years of training and study at St. Joseph's.* [7]

It is to St. Christopher's Hospice and its founder, Dr. Cicely Saunders, that the U.S. hospice movement has looked for direction.[8] The Hospice of Connecticut, America's first hospice program, is modeled after St. Christopher's. Although Hospice of Connecticut did not open its doors to patients until 1974, efforts to develop the hospice began in 1963 following a speech given by Dr. Saunders at Yale University. Dr. Saunders' speech paved the way for open discussion of the concept of death and dying. Less than a decade later (spring 1971), the Hospice of Connecticut became incorporated.[9]

---

* The United Kingdom currently has 77 programs: 42 inpatient hospice programs; 12 hospital-based programs; 23 community-based, home-care programs; and 6 day-care units. Fifty percent of the funding for hospice is received from private sources. Other countries with hospice programs include Taiwan, Japan, China, South Africa, Canada, Holland, Israel, and Sweden (see Edwin J. Olsen, "Hospice Care Developing Internationally," *National Hospice Organization Newsletter*, August 1982, 7).

The majority of hospice programs in the United States today are home based; that is, patient care is provided in the home, rather than in an institutional setting. This situation can be traced to the tendency of the original founders to shy away from traditional institutional settings, which exclude family involvement in patient care, as well as to the cost-containment efforts that swept the country.

Many of the early hospice organizers were not medically trained, but rather were clergy, consumers, social workers, funeral directors, etc. They met in living rooms and churches across the country. People gathered and voiced their fears, concerns, and frustrations with the existing practice of caring for the dying. As one early organizer described a local meeting:

> We were all just mad. We sat in my living room . . . like hours. We all had some horror story. We were angry at the doctor, the nurse, someone. After a while we realized that our loved one might have received better care if he was at home. It was the place of care that caused the problem. All of us had had a bad experience with [the] hospital . . . Now we knew what we had to do. . . .[10]

In early stages, hospice advocates discussed the need to be isolated from the traditional medical system. After all, it was the existing system that caused the problems, that failed to provide appropriate care for the terminally ill. Therefore, it followed that change from the status quo meant a break with the medical system and the formation of independent hospice organizations.

Early hospice programs were typically small, voluntary organizations. They had little, if any, program of care of the dying. Some organizers turned to England for guidance; others sought support from leaders such as Elisabeth Kubler-Ross. The dynamics of early program coalescence were described by one woman:

> Let's face it, we didn't know anything. It sounded like a good idea. . . . We thought we knew all the problems . . . we envisioned a cadre of volunteers . . . neighbors, who would help each other during the final stages. The articles we'd read were so appealing. The family, clustered around the dying patient's bed. A small child kneeling, a dog looking in. It was so ethereal. . . . The patient had a smile on his face, he looked so peaceful. The news articles were always the same. They had testimonials from people who described the beauty of death. There wasn't a lot of information back then. We all read Kubler-Ross' book and discussed it. . . . It's funny. Things changed. They became so different once we really got started. We had so many things to think about. We realized we needed to provide more than emotional and social support. We had to do actual physical patient care. This boggled

our minds. We didn't know how or where to begin. . . . I remember, it was one year after we began meeting that we'd heard of this other program in Michigan. It was started by a doctor. We received some information. It looked terribly involved. We decided at that meeting that we had to expand our group.[11]

As collective interest in the experience of dying grew, death itself took on a significant moral and value-laden quality—the inalienable right of everyone to die in a comfortable manner that afforded each individual the most dignity and allowed the dying person to be surrounded by his or her loved ones. The media played an important role in promoting hospices. Elisabeth Kubler-Ross' book *On Death and Dying*, first published in 1969, gained national attention and sold millions of copies. A 1978 article by June Bingham in the *Detroit News* noted, "Hospice is an idea whose time has come—for people whose time has come. . By the time I am dying," she continued, "I hope there will be enough good hospices in the U.S. for one to be near my home."[12] Television and print media began to feature shows about cancer and dying. The NBC "Evening News," "Good Morning America" (ABC), "Donahue" (CBS), "60 Minutes" (CBS), "The MacNeil/Lehrer Report" (PBS), *Time, Newsweek, U.S. News and World Report*, and other television programs and magazines covered the growth and development of hospice programs in cities across the United States. Between 1974 and 1984 hundreds of articles were printed describing the hospice philosophy of care and providing examples of operating programs. An abridged bibliography by Foster and Finn Paradis lists nearly 1,000 journal and book articles dealing with hospice-related topics.[13] Professional publications in pharmacy, nursing, social work, medicine, hospital and nursing home administration, geriatrics, thanatology, and related disciplines devoted considerable space to issues related to death, dying, and hospice care.[14]

Early interest groups pressured legislators to introduce death-with-dignity legislation. In 1972, the Special Committee on Aging of the United States Senate held hearings entitled "Death with Dignity: An Inquiry Into Related Public Issues." Within two years after the opening of Hospice of Connecticut (1974), the National Institutes of Health (NIH) held a symposium on the management of pain and humanitarian care for the dying.

By the late 1970s, hospice organizers stopped calling for programs of care that were separate from the existing medical care system and began to develop strategies for integration. Then Secretary of Health and Human Services, Joseph Califano, called on his staff to devise a number of steps to facilitate the progress of the hospice movement. Through funding from the Hospice of Connecticut, the National Hospice Organization (NHO) was incorporated in 1978. A year later, the NHO received separate funding and became organizationally independent. To speed hospice acceptance, the W.K. Kellogg Foundation provided funding for the development of a model hospice program in Battle Creek, Michigan and in 1981, the Foundation also provided funds to the Joint Commission on Accreditation of Hospitals (JCAH) to develop standards for hospice care. In addition to funding of hospice care by private philanthropy, government also participated in program integration. In 1979, Congress mandated the Health Care Financing Administration (HCFA) to examine the implications of including hospice services in Medicare and Medicaid programs. Contracting with Brown University, the HCFA selected 26 hospices from an applicant pool of 233 to participate in a two-year experimental program to examine hospice services and cost.[15]

By 1981, the National Hospice Organization had become a powerful lobbying force. They shepherded through an amendment to the Tax Equity and Fiscal Responsibility Act of 1982, which provided for hospice benefits to Medicare beneficiaries beginning November, 1983. Later that year, a Senate resolution was passed asking President Reagan to proclaim the week of November 7–14 as National Hospice Week.

Although the number of patients enrolled in hospice programs is small, the hospice movement "has entered the American health care scene with an intensity of a religious revival and a growth rate characteristic of a boom town."[16] The number of hospice programs across the United States has grown from a handful in 1977 to more than 1,500 in 1985, according to the National Hospice Organization.[17] There are planning groups in rural and urban areas throughout the country. The efforts of hospice programs to gain status as legitimate providers of health care for the terminally ill have been successful with the enactment of Medicare entitlements to provide reimbursement for hospice care and with the negotiation of hospice benefits in third-party payment contracts. Under Medicare the hospice reimbursement benefit is an elective benefit, which, when selected, eliminates other patient options. For a more detailed discussion see Chapter 8.[18] Further, 15 states have passed hospice licensing statutes and others are considering passage of regulatory measures. (California, Colorado, Connecticut, Delaware, Florida, Hawaii, Illinois, Kentucky, Maryland, Michigan, Missouri, New Mexico, New York, Virginia, and West Virginia have passed hospice licensing legislation.[19])

SOCIAL FACTORS INFLUENCING HOSPICE DEVELOPMENT

Changing views of death and euthanasia, demographic changes in the population, a growing awareness and fear of cancer, a burgeoning medical technology, issues of health-cost containment, the women's movement, and the home-birth movement have all influenced the development of hospice as a social movement.

The recent U.S. concept of hospice care grew out of a widespread death awareness movement, which, according to Huntington and Metcalf, had its origins in the 1963 publication of Jessica A. Mitford's expose, *The American Way of Death*.[20] The book attacked America's funeral industry, claiming it was excessively commercial and that it capitalized on death. Mitford cited morticians as profiteering through the selling of unnecessarily expensive services and goods to a captive clientele under great temporary stress. Her questioning of the appropriateness of the funeral ritual, especially the elaborate preparation of and display of the corpse, provided a basis for public reassessment of the death ritual. Following Mitford's work, Glaser and Strauss wrote a seminal book entitled *Awareness of Dying*. Just as Mitford attacked the funeral industry, Glaser and Strauss criticized the "moral attitude" of health care professionals, particularly physicians and nurses, who refused to talk openly about death to dying patients. Glaser and Strauss concluded in their opening summary:

> . . . staff members' efforts to cope with terminality often have undesirable effects on both the social and psychological aspects of patient care and their own comfort. Personnel in contact with terminal patients are always somewhat disturbed by their own ineptness in handling the dying. . . .[21]

During the 1960s, as Huntington and Metcalf note, "there began a broader reconsideration of all aspects of the experience of dying and the significance of death in modern society."[22] The movement to understand death was more than challenges to professionals. It addressed the way in which lay persons dealt with the death of family and friends, and criticized existing institutional structures.

By the early 1970s the stage was set for death and dying to become what Blumer called a "general social movement" consisting primarily of "groping and uncoordinated efforts" toward vague goals or objectives.[23] A general social movement lacks organization, leadership, and structure. It grows gradually out of "cultural drifts," which are "gradual and pervasive changes in the values of people." As a general movement begins to form from a cultural drift, it gradually acquires spokespersons who are more like "voices in the wilderness" than real leaders.[24]

In the United States, the leader of the death-with-dignity movement was Swiss-born physician Elisabeth Kubler-Ross. Her book *On Death and Dying* prompted widespread debate on rights of the dying patient and helped foster the concept of "death with dignity." The "classical death of Western nostalgia," presented by Kubler-Ross, provides a memorable example of the genre:

> I remember as a child (in Switzerland) the death of a farmer. He fell from a tree and was not expected to live. He asked simply to die at home, a wish that was granted without questioning. He called his daughters into the bedroom and spoke with each of them alone for a

few minutes. He arranged his affairs quietly, though he was in great pain, and distributed his belongings and his land, none of which was to be split until his wife should follow him in death. He also asked each of his children to share in the work, duties and tasks that he had carried on until the time of the accident. He asked his friends to visit him once more, to bid good-bye to them. Although I was a small child at the time, he did not exclude me or my siblings. We were allowed to share in the preparations of the family just as we were permitted to grieve with them until he died. When he did die, he was left at home, in his own beloved home which he had built, and among his friends and neighbors who went to take a last look at him where he lay in the midst of flowers in the place he had lived in and loved so much.[25]

According to Fox, *On Death and Dying* catapulted Kubler-Ross to the top of a newly emerging specialty, thanatology—the study of death and working with and caring for the dying. "It made her the 'Death-and-Dying Lady,' a national and international celebrity. It launched her on a perpetual round of house calls to dying patients and their families, in the United States and abroad, and a continuous cycle of public lectures and 'Life, Death, and Transition Workshops' attended by thousands of persons."[26]

Fox notes that Kubler-Ross' book contended that the contemplation of death and the acceptance of mortality are not morbid, but life-enhancing, "conducive to respect for life, personal growth, loving relationships, and a happier sense of meaning. She has also consistently affirmed that persons passing through the 'final stages of life' can be our teachers and that those who get close to the terminally ill 'will learn much about the functioning of the human mind, the unique human aspects of our existence and will emerge from the experience enriched . . . perhaps with fewer anxieties about their own finality.' "[27]

Demographic changes in the United States ushered the way for this heightened awareness and pondering of death and dying.[28] Declining fertility and mortality rates have increased both the proportion and number of persons who are living longer. Whereas in 1900 approximately 3 million persons, or 4 percent of the American population, were 65 or older, in 1980, 25 million persons, or close to 12 percent of our population, belonged to this age category.[29]

As sociologist Otto Pollak writes, this "increase in the numbers of persons who live out the full span" has helped to make "the anticipation of dying a national experience" and aging a process of "dying in installments."[30] Pollak states that social and cultural factors are as responsible for these associations between aging and dying as demographic and biological ones:

Old people in the United States live in a society which puts a premium on being young. . . . Youth is hope and hope is life-sustaining. . . .

> Old people symbolize hopelessness, the renunciation of fantasies, the pain and despair of dying. . . .[31]

The growth in our aging population has led to a shift in the cause of death. As Lerner points out, certain chronic illnesses that have not yielded to the progress of medicine are now the primary causes of mortality, among them cancer, heart disease, and stroke. "Diseases of the heart ranked fourth among the leading causes of death in this country during the 1900's; this category caused 137.4 deaths per 100,000 and accounted for 8.0 percent of all deaths. By 1966, however, it had risen so far in importance that it had become the leading cause of death, far outranking all others. Its mortality rate had risen to 375.1 deaths per 100,000 population, and it accounted for nearly 40 percent of all deaths in that year. . . . The pattern of increase for malignant neoplasms (cancer) as a cause of death was quite similar. This disease ranked eighth among the leading causes of death in 1900. It accounted for 64 deaths per 100,000 population and less than 4 percent of all deaths. By 1966, however, its rank among the leading causes had risen to second, its rate per 100,000 to 154.8, and its proportion of the total of all deaths exceeded 16 percent. . . ."[32] In 1983 death from cancer accounted for more than 18 percent or 183 deaths per 100,000 population.

Thus, a considerable portion of the American preoccupation with death and dying is concerned, directly or indirectly, with chronic illness and the care of the chronically ill.* [33] The disease most dreaded and feared in this connection is cancer. It has become the archetypical metaphor of "insidious, malevolent, uncontrollable, ugly, and pain-filled aspects of these chronic-illness-associated problems. . ."[34] Hospice provides a "waystation" for patients suffering from cancer. It is designed to both control pain and attend to the patient's and family's anxieties and fears of death.

The development of hospice programs as social movement organizations (SMOs) is a manifestation of deep cultural changes occurring in our society and in its world view. The upsurge in hospice programs appears at a time when other

---

* Aries (*Western Attitudes Toward Death*, 88) divides changes occurring in the death of populations and attitudes toward death into four stages: "tamed death" (pre-Renaissance); diachrony (Renaissance to Middle Ages); achronic (post Middle Ages); and contemporary. In precontemporary society, death warnings occurred through a "magical premonition"; the dying is prepared for death through steps dictated in traditional ceremony (e.g., lying in bed, in a position, arms crossed over the body, etc.). At the end of the 18th century (beginning of the contemporary period), doctors discovering the first principles of hygiene complained about overcrowding bedrooms of the dying. With the advent of "poor farms" and subsequently hospitals, the isolation of the dying from the family was complete.

Death in the hospital is no longer the occasion of a ritual ceremony, over which the dying person presides amidst his assembled relatives and friends. Death is a technical phenomenon obtained by a cessation determined in a more or less avowed way by a decision of the doctor and the hospital team.

health care and social reforms also are being proposed. For example, in 1968, the *Journal of the American Medical Association* (JAMA) ran numerous articles about legal decisions physicians may face when using biomedical advances to prolong life. Concern surrounding this issue escalated, reaching a peak one decade later when two judicial cases made national headlines: the 1976 Quinlan decision of the New Jersey Supreme Court and the 1977 Saikewicz decision of the Massachusetts Supreme Court.[35] Both courts questioned the patients' physical or legal incompetency to express their own views about continued survival and the morality of using heroic biomedical techniques to prolong life.

The Quinlan case involved the question of withdrawing respirator support from a comatose young woman believed to have suffered irreversible brain damage even though she did not meet the widely accepted Harvard criteria for brain death. The court said the decision properly belongs with the patient's parents and physicians, provided a hospital-appointed ethics committee concurred with their decision. The Quinlan decision was widely acclaimed by the medical profession because it supported long-standing medical tradition. The court's ruling did not appear to call for any major change in medical practice.[36]

In the Saikewicz case, the court emphatically rejected the Quinlan solution, asserting instead that only the courts were qualified to decide life-or-death issues for incompetent patients. Saikewicz, a profoundly mentally retarded man of 67 who developed acute leukemia, had been denied medical treatment at the request of his parents and physicians. As interpreted by some lawyers, the Saikewicz decision established new laws mandating probate judicial hearings before any life-or-death decision could be made for incompetent patients, excepting only emergency cases.[37]

The Quinlan and Saikewicz cases provided a forum for the public to address the issue of euthanasia and the question of whether life-prolonging medical techniques should be applied to forestall the natural death of one who is in an irreversible unconscious state.* [38]

While the medical profession and the courts were debating the utilization of appropriate medical technology and the role of the physician in the care of the terminal patient, other related issues were being publicly addressed. These included the cost of medical technology and of hospital care in general, as well as the consumer's right to choice in health care matters.

---

* Arien Mack in *Death in American Experience* (New York: Schocken Books, 1974, 29) discusses the relation of the physician to the patient as treatment becomes increasingly technical. Using the symbolic interactionist concept of "definition of the situation," Mack writes: "Orientation to the nearly absolute 'commandment' to combat the death of his patient provided a strong definition of the situation for the physician in several respects. It assured the physician that he could act in direct relation to a value of great importance without having to embroil himself in a broad range of difficult problems of meaning. It permitted, indeed required, he pursue the 'saving' of life at almost any cost, that is, by subordinating almost all other value considerations."

Medical costs have been escalating dramatically during the last two decades and have consumed an increasingly larger proportion of our country's Gross National Product (GNP). Figures from the Department of Commerce show that in 1960 health care expenditures were $26.9 billion, or 5.3 percent of the GNP. By 1982 that figure had increased twelvefold to $322.4 billion, or 10.5 percent of the GNP.[39]

Beginning in the early 1970s, the U.S. Congress developed a series of programs designed to contain health care costs. The Social Security Amendments of 1972 (P.L. 92-603) added two relevant sections to the Social Security Act. Section 234 mandated planning by health care institutions as a condition of Medicare participation and Section 1122 specified that health facilities in participating states would receive reimbursement by Medicare, Medicaid, and Maternal and Child Health Programs for claims relating to capital expenditures only if the expenditures were deemed necessary by the state planning agencies. The National Health Planning and Resources Development Act, 1974 (P.L. 93-641), Titles XV and XVI of the Public Health Service Act, passed in 1975, was enacted to create a mechanism for coordination of planning efforts. Title XV established a new program for health planning and resources development. Title XVI revised existing programs for the construction and modernization of health care facilities (the former Hill-Burton Program). The act created a series of state and national planning authorities responsible for reviewing the efficacy of capital expenditure requests by hospitals and nursing homes.[40] In 1982, Congress passed P.L. 97-248, the Tax Equity and Fiscal Responsibility Act (TEFRA), which created ceilings in hospital and physician reimbursement. The use of diagnostically related groups (DRGs) represented a significant change for the existing fee-for-service payment system and forced providers to carefully consider the unit and cost of services rendered. Hospice is considered the first DRG by federal authorities.[41]

The concern over inflation of medical care expenses intrudes into nearly every aspect of health care today. Cost containment is the dominant catchword. The reasons for this phenomenon are varied, but the largest culprit, according to Andrew Hunt, is the expansion of medical technology.

> There seems to be general agreement that much of the excess inflation in medical care is related to expansion of use of technologically complex and costly methods of diagnosis and treatment. While such development is generally welcomed as evidence of scientific medical progress producing higher quality patient care with demonstrably improved results, "over utilization" is becoming the watchword in the struggle to limit costs. That too many patients are hospitalized, that too many hospitals have CAT scanners, that too many laboratory tests and x-rays are done on too many people, and that over use of drugs

and expensive treatment methods are all too common statements being
made with increasing frequency.[42]

Care for terminally ill patients in hospital settings is extremely expensive.
Indeed, people often spend more on medical care during their last two weeks
of life than they spend at any other time. Research by the National Blue Cross/
Blue Shield Association showed that it costs an average of $15,836 (1980 dollars)
for each terminal patient during his or her last six months of life.[43] The majority
of expenses occur in the last month of life when inpatient hospitalization is most
likely; hospital inpatient expenses accounted for 78 percent of the total costs.
The cost savings per patient for hospice care in place of traditional hospital care
range from $800 per patient to over $15,000.[44]

The high cost of care for the terminally ill has lent support to the development
of hospice as an alternative means of care. Stressing the importance of presumably
less expensive, home-based care, hospice programs offer an option to the highly
technological and labor-intensive hospital environment. The hospice care cost
analysis by Case Western Reserve Department of Epidemiology and Community
Health showed that hospice care decreased inpatient hospital use by terminal
patients an average of 4.1 days during the last two weeks of life. This represented
an average cost savings of 39 percent to third-party payers.[45]

The use of the home to care for patients was seen as a potential alternative
to the hospital by another group: those demanding more control for mothers over
the births of their children. Beginning in the early 1970s, a series of books were
published asking why women did not have control over their own bodies.[46] This
question recurred during debates on abortion as well as home birth.

As Fox points out, the death-and-dying movement "intersects with the broad
affirmation of individual rights taking place in American society since the 1960s
and with organized attempts to expand the scope of these rights."[47] Beginning
in 1963 with Betty Friedan's book *The Feminine Mystique* and subsequent formation of the National Organization of Women, the women's movement initiated
discussion of women's rights over control of their bodies and childbirth. The
articulation of the right to die closely paralleled that of the right to choose a
birthing place. In both instances, groups organized to oppose restrictions concerning "constitutionally" guaranteed rights to give birth and to die in the settings
that one wishes without interference from others.

As women met to discuss careers, family life, and the propriety and costs of
gynecological care and childbirth, the doors opened for other types of debates,
including the treatment and care of the terminally ill. The same issues raised in
discussing gynecological care and birth became the focus of a larger societal
phenomenon in which claims for the extension of individual rights, a "self-care
movement," and a patient's rights for choosing the method of birth and death
figure prominently.[48]

While the "death-with-dignity" movement was gaining public support in the early 1970s, a countermovement was beginning to develop that was largely sponsored by "right-to-life" groups. These groups had previously been founded to counter the pro-choice movement sponsored largely by feminist organizations. Robert Veatch of the Hastings Center reported in 1977 that "forty pieces of legislation were introduced into state legislatures during this period in an attempt to legalize one or another aspect of euthanasia."[49] By 1984, 15 states and the District of Columbia had Right to Die bills and similar bills were being introduced in another 28 states.[50] Originally founded in the late 1960s to defeat "pro-choice" (pro-abortion) efforts, the right-to-life movement became concerned with the issue of euthanasia raised by the death-with-dignity movement. One right-to-life organizer wrote in her letter to me,

> Our concern over the abortion issue included the prediction that loss of respect for life at the beginning would lead to a similar loss of respect at the end of life. Our literature, presentations, etc., in the early days of our organizations predicted that this loss of respect would spread to those who were also helpless due to old age, retardation, handicap, etc. In those days, we were told that we were exaggerating, and that it would not happen. The growth of the so-called 'death with dignity' movement confirmed our early predictions.
>
> Euthanasia became an issue with right to life as the various pieces of legislation's court cases began to unfold. It was not unexpected, and as a result, our focus broadened to include not only the unborn, but all human beings whose right to life appeared to be threatened. However, abortion remains the main focus and the reason for the existence of right-to-life organizations.[51]

Michigan Representative Dave Hollister noted, "The meetings my committee held on death-with-dignity legislation were becoming increasingly dominated by members of the Catholic Church and right-to-lifers who worked hard for the defeat of the proposed legislation."[52]

Debate in the 1970s over right-to-death issues led to the development of several factions: those who were unalterably opposed to any legislation that did not support the continued use of life-support mechanisms and heroic surgeries to sustain life; those who were adamantly opposed to continued life-support measures and medical techniques against the wishes of the patient, his or her family, or close companion; and those who were anxious to promote death with dignity, but who focused on the humane aspects of the care for the dying while rejecting any talk of euthanasia. It was this third group that, in most states, became the foundation upon which the current hospice movement is based.

An unofficial alliance between church officials, right-to-life advocates, and death-with-dignity supporters formed and focused on an organized approach to care for the terminally ill. The concept of hospice was promoted as a method of care for the dying that involves traditional health care providers but also gives the patient and the family some choice in the continuation of medical interventions. The hospice movement did not address the issue of families of unconscious patients making any decisions for the patient, but focused instead on care for the conscious and aware terminal patient. This was an important point since early death and dying legislation focused on treatment, or lack of it, for unconscious patients regardless of long-term prognosis.

The hospice concept provided earlier discussions of death and dying with what Blumer terms a "specific" focus.[53] Organizers defined as its goal the development of hospice programs to care for the terminally ill and a revamping of the existing health care structure. As Lyn Lofland points out, death and dying are not salient concepts for many individuals because so many people in our society die in segregated organizational settings. However, once these numbers of "individuals begin to reach a sufficient size, they become aware of themselves as a group and can begin publicly articulating those concerns which its individual members had kept private. The hiatus on death and dying as public discourse ends. The emergence of death and dying as fad, fashion and social movement begins."[54]

The hospice movement highlights the failure of the traditional health care system to provide for the needs of the dying patient. It is a struggle against what Turner and Killian have pointed out is "a wrong which ought to be replaced." That sense of something wrong is sustained by a sense of "righteous indignation. A sense of injustice that is vital enough to have consequences requires not only a situation that appears unfavorable by comparison with some reference group but also an oppressor, so that the situation can be seen as a product of human will."[55]

Some movements—for example, the nuclear power movement, as noted by Useem and Zald—are "fortunate" in facing an opposition that is organized and articulated.[56] The members of these organizations can be identified and personified: the oppressor is real.[57]

Nathanson and Ostling in *Aborting America* describe how the pro-abortion movement focused on the hierarchy of the Catholic Church as an "oppressor of women's rights":

> Historically . . . every revolution has to have its villain. It doesn't really matter whether it's a king, a dictator, or a czar, but it has to be someone, a person, to rebel against. It's easier for the people we want to persuade to perceive it this way . . . now, in our case, it makes little sense to lead a campaign only against unjust laws, even though

that's what we are really doing. We have to narrow the focus, identify those unjust laws with a person or a group of people. A single person isn't quite what we want, since that might excite sympathy for him. Rather, a small group of shadowy, powerful people . . . It's got to be the Catholic hierarchy. That's a small enough group to come down on, and anonymous enough so that no names ever have to be mentioned, but everybody will have a fairly good idea whom we are talking about (pp. 51–52).

However, not all movements have "enemies" that are clearly identifiable. The thing or idea that is found unconscionable is a consequence of the way things are done, the way they have evolved. The practice that is abhorred may be merely a "de facto" creation.

"De facto" enemies are not very useful for creating "righteous indignation." As Lofland writes, "They do not articulate any opposition. They do not seem to be enemies at all. If they are to be useful to a movement, if they are to provide the emotional springboard for a sustained sense of injustice, they must be evoked by the movement itself. If they do not speak for themselves, they must be articulated by the movement."[58]

The hospice movement had no specific enemy (e.g., an individual or group of individuals). However, it was able to sustain an "emotional springboard" by which it set up an ideal and then to point to problems with the existing system. William Goode describes the way in which critics of contemporary family arrangements evoke an ideal that he calls the "classical family of Western nostalgia," by painting a picture of the kinfolk and life on grandma's farm and the harmonious living arrangement.[59]

Philippe Aries provides an example of this view:

For thousands of years man was lord and master of his death, and the circumstances surrounding it. Today this has ceased to be so. . . . Today nothing remains either of the sense that everyone has or should have of his impending death, or of the public solemnity surrounding the moment of death. What used to be appreciated is now hidden; what used to be solemn is now avoided. . . . We have seen how modern society deprives man of his death, and how it allows him this privilege only if he does not use it to upset the living. In a reciprocal way, society forbids the living to appear moved by the death of others; it does not allow them either to weep for the deceased or to seem to miss them.[60]

By creating an image of the ideal or preferable state of affairs, the "ideological crafts-person" then describes the way in which the real world fails to measure up.[61] In doing so, the opposition is "articulated"; a social problem is "created."[62]

Proponents of the hospice movement, in working toward an "ideal way of death," have asserted that the existing system has failed for a number of reasons, that it has viewed secular discussion of death as taboo and prevented public discourse of the subject. The consequences of this denial lead to exorbitant funeral costs and barbaric funeral practices, inhumane handling of dying patients in hospitals, ostracism of the dying from the living, false communication with the terminally ill, rejection of the needs of the dying person's family, a mechanical, nonorganic view of life.

HOSPICE, THE "IDEAL" WAY OF DEATH

St. Christopher's Hospice in England has been viewed as the American hospice prototype.[63] Cicely Saunders wrote in St. Christopher's annual report for 1977–78:

> Our important links with the United States began in 1963 with an invitation to the Yale School of Medicine through an English surgeon, Bernard Lytton, who had carried out a research project at St. Joseph's. Here I met Florence Wald, Dean of the Graduate School of Nursing who, in 1966 when I was again there as a visiting lecturer, invited Elisabeth Kubler-Ross, Colin Murray Parkes and myself to meet in a workshop attended by others already involved in this field. Dr. Kubler-Ross was then carrying out the work on which she later based her best-selling book, *On Death and Dying* (1969) which led to such a surge of interest in this field in the States (p. 16).[64]

Based on these early meetings, a list of essential principles of hospice care developed and these have been adopted in whole or part throughout the country. The National Hospice Organization used these principles when developing its own standards for a hospice care program. The standards include requirements that care be available 7 days a week, 24 hours a day, with integrated inpatient and home care services available. Volunteers are used to serve patient needs and to work with patients and families in their education about death. Hospice care is planned and provided by a medically supervised interdisciplinary team. The standards also require that the patient, family, and others important to the patient are able to work together to assist the patient during the final days of life. Emphasis is placed on cooperation between the family and the medical care team in caring for the patient.

Unlike the medical care personnel studied by Glaser and Strauss[65] who tried to hide impending death from patients, hospice personnel are trained to acknowledge death and to help the patient and family work through its eventuality. Energy is directed toward coping and comforting and not toward denial of the problem. It is a way of providing role models for future dying individuals and for establishing social symbols and language that can be used to describe dying. Words such as "coping with pain," "grief and bereavement," "passive euthanasia," and so on have taken on meaning within American society, and have provided a vocabulary for describing the act of dying. In short, the hospice movement has provided the larger social system with a mechanism for openly communicating feelings, beliefs, and attitudes about death. Thus, it has encouraged specific as well as general social change.

Most important, the hospice movement has provided an option for a patient to leave the sacred confines of a highly praised, technologically intense health care system and retreat to a place of his or her choice. The movement has also alleviated the burden from the shoulders of physicians, nurses, and other personnel who previously were taught to reject death and to view death as a failure rather than a natural part of the life cycle. In achieving these ends the hospice concept has provided more than a program of treatment. It has provided a socially acceptable forum for discussing the meaning of death and the fears associated with dying.[66]

DIVERGENT MODELS FOR TREATING THE DYING

The way in which hospice programs treat terminally ill patients and train staff, patients, and families to cope with dying varies greatly. In the United States, hospice programs of care come in all shapes and sizes. Some programs are located in office buildings or churches and provide home care for the dying and support for bereaved family members. Others are located in hospitals, nursing homes, or home-health agencies and have a variety of agreements with other health providers in the area. Still others involve free-standing hospice facilities, such as Hospice of Connecticut, Hospice of Southeast Michigan, or the Riverside Hospice in Boonton, New Jersey. These facilities have resident staff members, including physicians, nurses, social workers, clergy, physical therapists, and other service personnel.

The General Accounting Office has identified five predominant models, which are described in detail in the next chapter. Briefly, these models are:

1. free-standing hospice
2. hospital-affiliated, free-standing hospice
3. hospital-based hospice
   a. acute-care hospital with centralized palliative care or hospice unit
   b. acute-care hospital hospice team who visit patients
   c. units operated as part of an HMO

4. hospice within an extended-care facility or nursing home
5. home care program only
   a. hospital based
   b. nursing home based
   c. community based

While these models are considered the most common, a variety of others exist, including small, all-volunteer programs and physician-office services. In the former, volunteer staff work cooperatively with existing agencies to provide hospice support services to patients. Some of these programs have volunteer nurses who donate time and resources to serving terminal residents in their communities. Physician-office service programs consist primarily of a patient's attending physician and perhaps some of the office staff who offer "hospice-like" services for patients. Primary care practitioners seem most prone to employ this model.[67]

Exhibit 1-1 Activities in the United States Leading to Hospice Development as a Social Movement Organization

---

1963—Cicely Saunders speaks at Yale University about hospice care in England, sparking development of first U.S. hospice.
—Jessica Mitford publishes critical expose on funeral industry.
1966—National Organization of Women is formed.
1969—Elisabeth Kubler-Ross publishes *On Death and Dying*.
1970—Abortion law is passed in New York State; abortion is legalized.
1972—Right-to-life movement gains strength in the U.S.
—Social Security amendments regarding health planning are passed.
—Senate holds hearings on death-with-dignity legislation.
1973—Supreme Court decision allowing abortion (Doe vs. Bolton and Roe vs. Wade).
1974—Hospice of New Haven, Connecticut, opens doors to patients.
1975—National Health Planning Resource Development Act passed.
1976—Quinlan decision, New Jersey Supreme Court.
1977—Saikewicz decision, Massachusetts Supreme Court.
1978—National Hospice Organization formed.
—Secretary of Health, Education, and Welfare (HEW), Joseph Califano, announces that HEW is requesting proposals for experimental funding.
—Senators Abraham A. Ribicoff, Edward M. Kennedy, and Robert J. Dole ask the General Accounting Office to review the development of hospice across the United States.
—Connecticut becomes the first state to have regulations governing the licensing of hospices.
1981—W. K. Kellogg Foundation funds a Joint Commission for Accreditation of Hospitals, releases a project to draft standards for hospice programs.
1982—Tax Equity's Fiscal Responsibility Act includes a section for Medicare coverage of hospice.
—President Reagan proclaims November 7–14 as National Hospice week.

SUMMARY

Because hospice is a relatively new movement (see Exhibit 1-1), it has not been fully evaluated. Much of the existing literature is characterized by an evangelical flavor extolling the virtues of hospices without objective analysis.[68] Management and planning information is needed about the organization of hospices, their growth over time, their experiences in caring for the dying, their interface with other aspects of the traditional system, and their ability to provide high-quality care at a reasonable cost.

The next chapter provides a foundation for subsequent chapters by examining the divergent models of hospice care and the structural components of each program type. It examines essential principles common to all programs and critically compares the administrative, programmatic, and delivery of care component among all models.

NOTES

1. John R. Flexner, "The Hospice Movement in North America—Is It Coming of Age?" *Southern Medical Journal* 72 (March 1979): 248–250.

2. Basil S. Georgopoulos and Floyd C. Mann, "The Hospital as an Organization," in *The Community General Hospital* (New York: Macmillan, 1962), 5–15.

3. Renee Fox, "The Social Meaning of Death," *The Annals* 447 (January 1980): 32.

———, "The Sting of Death in American Society." *Social Service Review* (University of Chicago: March 1981): 42–59.

4. David Riesman, *The Story of Medicine in the Middle Ages* (New York: Hoeber, 1935).

For the history of the hospice movement, see also Elisabeth Kubler-Ross, *On Death and Dying* (New York: Macmillan, 1969); J. Krom, "Designing a Better Place to Die," *New York Magazine* 1 (March 1976): 43–49; Sandol Stoddard, *The Hospice Movement* (New York: Vintage, 1978); Paul Dubois, *The Hospice Way of Death* (New York: Human Sciences Press, 1980); Marian Osterweis and Daphne Szmuszkovicz Champagne, "The U.S. Hospice Movement: Issues in Development," *American Journal of Public Health* 69 (May 1979): 492–496; Florence S. Wald, Zelda Foster, and Henry Wald, "The Hospice Movement as a Health Care Reform," *Nursing Outlook*, March 1980, 173–178; and Philippe Aries, *Western Attitudes Toward Death: From the Middle Ages to the Present* (Baltimore, Md.: Johns Hopkins University Press, 1974).

5. Sandol Stoddard, *The Hospice Movement*.

6. Greg Owen, *Care for the Dying: A Study of the Need for Hospice in Ramsey County, Minnesota*. A Report to the Northwest Area Foundation from the Amherst H. Wilder Foundation (St. Paul: Wilder Foundation, 1981): 13.

7. Ibid.

8. Sylvia Porter, "Hospices, A Better Way for the Terminally Ill?" *Detroit Free Press* (five-part series) October 14, 1979—October 19, 1979.

9. Robert Fulton and Greg Owen, "Hospice in America: From Principle to Practice" (Paper presented at The International Hospice Conference, St. Christophers Hospice, Sydenham, England, June 4, 1980.)

10. Interview conducted by Lenora Finn Paradis with hospice board chairman who asked to remain unnamed. Michigan. November, 1982.

11. Confidential interview conducted by Lenora Finn Paradis with hospice board member. Michigan. January, 1983.

12. June Bingham, "St. Christopher's in London: Hospice Helps Ease Death's Grip," *The Detroit News,* October 12 1978.

13. Larry Foster and Lenora Finn Paradis. *Hospice and Death Education: A Resource Bibliography.* Allendale, Mich.: Grand Valley State College, 1985.

14. Owen, *Care for the Dying.*

15. David Greer, Vincent Mon, Howard Bunbaum, Sylvia Sherwood, and John Morris. *National Hospice Stud Preliminary Final Report* (Providence Rhode Island: Brown University, November 1983).

16. Kim Cam and Nancy Burns, "Hospice: A Case Study," Working Paper Series 82-11, Arlington, Texas: University of Texas, Arlington, 1982.

17. Phone conversation by author with Ira Bates, staff, National Hospice Organization, November, 1984. The NHO research and evaluation committee had just completed a hospice census. Bates noted that approximately 1,500 programs were surveyed. The census is entitled "The 1984 Guide to the Nation's Hospices," and is by the National Hospice Organization, Arlington, Virginia, 1984.

18. John D. Blum and Dennis A. Robbins, "An Assessment of Hospice Licensure and Accreditation." Paper presented at the National Hospice Organization Convention, Washington, D.C., November 8, 1982.

19. Ibid.

20. Richard Huntington and Peter Metcalf, *Celebrations of Death* (Cambridge: Cambridge University Press, 1979).

Jessica Mitford, *The American Way of Death* (New York: Fawcett Crest, 1963).

21. Barney Glaser and Anselm Strauss, *Awareness of Dying* (Chicago: Aldine, 1965), 5.

22. *Celebrations of Death,* 3.

23. Herbert Blumer, "Social Movements," in *Studies in Social Movements,* ed. Barry McLaughlin (New York: The Free Press, 1969).

24. ———, "Social Problems as Collective Behavior," *Social Problems* 18 (Winter 1971): 298–306.

25. Kubler-Ross, *On Death and Dying,* 5–6.

26. Fox, "The Sting of Death in American Society," 50.

27. Ibid.

28. Fox, "The Social Meaning of Death," vii–xi.

29. U.S. Bureau of the Census, 1980.

30. Otto Pollak, "The Shadow of Death Over Aging," *The Annals* 447 (1980): 1.

31. Ibid.

32. Monroe Lerner, "When, Why and Where People Die," in *Death, Current Perspectives,* 3rd ed. Edwin S. Schneidman, ed. (Palo Alto, Calif.: Mayfield, 1980), 95.

33. Philippe Aries, *Western Attitudes Toward Death: From the Middle Ages to the Present* (Baltimore, Maryland: Johns Hopkins University Press, 1974): 88.

34. Fox, "The Sting of Death in American Society," 44.

35. John Parks, "Court Intervention and the Diminution of Patients' Rights: The Case of Brother Joseph Fox," *New England Journal of Medicine* (October 1980).

36. Arnold S. Relman, "The Saikewicz Decision: A Medical Viewpoint *American Journal of Law and Medicine* 4 (Fall 1978): 233–245.

37. Ibid.

38. Arien Mack, *Death in American Experience* (New York: Schocken Books, 1974): 29.

39. Health Care Financing Administration, *Annual Report of Health Care Expenditures* (Washington, D.C., Department of Health and Human Services, 1983).

40. See Gerald R. Connor, "Summary of Federal Certificate of Need Regulations," *State Health News* (Washington, D.C.: Health Policy Center, March 1977).

41. Lenora Finn Paradis. "The Integration of Hospice Into the Traditional Health Care System: A Sociological Analysis." Unpublished Ph.D. Dissertation, Michigan State University, June 1983.

42. Andrew Hunt, "Medical Education, Cost Containment and Medical Practice Conflicts in Values" (Paper for Medical Humanities Program, Michigan State University, October 1, 1980).

43. J. Gibbs and J. Newman, "Study of Health Services Used and Costs Incurred During the Last Six Months of a Terminal Illness." Prepared under contract with the U.S. Department of Health and Human Services (HEW-100-79-D110) (Washington, D.C.: Research and Development Department, Blue Cross, Blue Shield Association, 1982).

44. See Charles H. Brooks, "The Potential Cost Savings of Hospice Care: A Review of the Literature, *Health Matrix* 1 (Summer 1983): 490–53.

45. Charles H. Brooks and Katherine Smyth-Staruch, *Cost Savings of Hospice Home Care to Third-Party Insurers* (Cleveland, Ohio: Department of Epidemiology and Community Health, Case Western Reserve University, School of Medicine, September 1983).

46. See Barbara Richard, *The Women's Movement* (New York: Harper & Row, 1975); Suzanne Arms, *Immaculate Deception* (Boston: Houghton Mifflin, 1975); Sheila Kitzinger, *The Experience of Childbirth* (London: Victor Gollancz, 1972); Brigette Jordan, *Birth in Four Cultures* (Montreal: Eden Press, 1978).

47. Fox, "The Sting of Death in American Society.

48. Robert M. Veatch and Ernest Tai, "Talking About Death: Patterns of Lay and Professional Change," *The Annals* 447 (January 1980): 29–46.

49. Fulton and Owen, "Hospice in America," 5.

50. Society for the Right to Die. *Handbook of Enacted Laws* (Society for the Right to Die: New York, 1984).

51. Letter from an official of Michigan Right To Life Organization, Lansing, Michigan.

52. Dave Hollister (Democratic Representative from Michigan). Interview in Lansing, Michigan, June 21, 1982.

53. Blumer, *Social Movements*.

54. Lynn Lofland, *The Craft of Dying* (Beverly Hills, Calif.: Sage, 1978).

55. R. H. Turner and L. Killian, *Collective Behavior* (Englewood Cliffs, N.J.: Prentice-Hall, 1972), 259.

56. Bert Useem and Mayer Zald, "From Pressure Group to Social Movement: Organizational Dilemmas of the Effort to Promote Nuclear Power," *Social Problems* 30 (December 1982): 29–46.

57. Bernard N. Nathanson and Richard Ostling, *Aborting America* (Garden City, New York: Doubleday, 1979).

58. Lofland, *The Craft of Dying*, 89.

59. Ibid.

60. Aries, *Western Attitudes Toward Death*, 136–138.

61. Lofland, *The Craft of Dying*, 89.

62. Blumer, "Social Movement."

63. Owen, *Care for the Dying*, 13.

64. Cicely Saunders, Dorothy Summers, and Neville Teller (ed.), *Hospice: The Living Idea* (London: Edward, Arnold, 1981), 9–18.

65. Glaser & Strauss, *Awareness of Dying*.

66. Florence S. Wald, Zelda Foster, and Henry Wald. "The Hospice Movement as a Health Care Reform," *Nursing Outlook* 34 (March 1980): 173–178.

67. Finn Paradis, "The Integration of Hospice into the Traditional Health Care System."

68. Carney and Burns, "Hospice: A Case Study."

Chapter 2

Systematic Planning for Hospice Care

Catherine M. Lamb

At some point, every hospice founder asks whether starting a hospice program is really a good idea. The concept is attractive and symbolizes a departure from the big business of health care and a return to the home as a center for care. But, can a hospice survive in the dollar-conscious health care industry and meet its espoused goals of holistic and dignified care? Is the trend toward hospice care a fad, to be replaced with something more fashionable? Because hospice care is still considered a new phenomenon, there is no real blueprint for success.

As hospice programs develop across the country, varied models for providing hospice care emerge. In some areas, home-based, all-volunteer models of care predominate. In other locations, emphasis is on freestanding or institutionally affiliated hospices. Although the passage of Medicare reimbursement encourages certain organizational patterns of care, a wide range of hospice programs and services exist. These have evolved as a result of the divergent philosophies of program founders, regulatory mandates, and the match between community characteristics and available resources.

This chapter describes an approach for planning hospice services. Planning for hospice care entails consideration of several factors, among the most important community support, marketing strategies, regulatory factors, philosophical considerations, organizational design, and fiscal requirements (Exhibit 2-1). These developmental components interrelate and provide a systematic approach to hospice programming. Within this same framework, five predominant models of hospice care are illustrated (see Appendix 2-A). As planners and administrators utilize a systematic planning process, decisions regarding the appropriate model of hospice care become clear.

COMMUNITY SUPPORT

Each of us can recall instances in which community support was a tangible force contributing to the continuation or demise of a local organization or en-

Exhibit 2-1 Hospice Care: Systematic Planning

Community Support	*Marketing*
• General public	• Target population
• Physicians	• Service needs
• Health and human	• Demand for service
services professionals	• Organizational resources
• Clergy and civic leaders	• Community resources
• Community assessment	
	Regulatory
Fiscal	• Health system agencies
• Reimbursement	• Certificate of need
• Starting costs	• Licensure
• Financial systems	
• Development	
Organizational Design	*Underpinnings*
• Definition of program	• Mission and philosophy
• Management	• Governing body
• Paid and voluntary staff	• Goals and objectives
• Quality assurance	• Evaluation

terprise. The many faces that had patronized one business ignore another. Those supporting one candidate downplay the virtues of the opponent. The commitment to a cause or program by neighborhood leaders and workers often leads to future success. As leaders in a locally based organization, hospice administrators cannot ignore the potential impact of community support. This support not only promotes funding and patronage, but also determines volunteer contributions and staffing patterns. Liaisons with churches, civic organizations, and related groups help promote the concept of hospice care and encourage the contribution of available resources.

For purposes of this discussion, community support for hospice is defined as the widespread belief that hospice is a viable health care option warranting promotion and development. The conviction that hospice care is needed and viable evolves in different ways. The most common involvement with hospice comes through personal experience. Firsthand knowledge of lingering terminal illness frequently brings individuals from many different walks of life into a hospice initiative. For many people, this results from the death of a family member or close associate. Alternately, health care professionals identify the need for hospice care based on the limitations of existing resources to assist dying individuals and their family members.

As groups formally or informally organize to promote hospice care, increased community support is usually targeted as a priority. Public and professional education is a useful vehicle to facilitate understanding and subsequently support of hospice care. Kenneth P. Cohen, who cites ignorance of hospice care as a roadblock to hospice development, suggests that education is needed in the following ways:

- General public: frequent community presentations
- Physicians: education and persuasion rather than criticism; accent on symptom control, team approach, and consultation rather than take over of patients
- Other health care professionals (nurses, psychologists, physical therapists, dieticians, etc.): accent on special needs of the terminally ill
- Other health organizations: determination of who does what; avoidance of duplication of services; maintenance of hospice organization's autonomy
- The media: education to combat their cynicism, biases, and tendency toward sensationalism [1]

The support by health care professionals, public policymakers, and the community at large is an essential component in developing any form of hospice care. Initiation of a broad-based planning group with smaller subcommittees (Exhibit 2-2) is one effective way of soliciting the support of key community

Exhibit 2-2 Committees for a Developing Hospice

Public Relations Committee: To build community relations and handle work in the field of public relations, including the development of a Speakers Bureau.

Fund-Raising Committee: To begin fund raising through plans to solicit individuals, businesses, corporations, and foundations. Someone experienced in writing grant proposals is particularly useful.

Education and Training Committee: To develop training programs for professionals and volunteers who care for patients. Also to develop an immediate orientation program for volunteer organizers.

Home Care/Patient and Family Care: To develop future policies and procedures for patient and family care according to the hospice concept of care.

Certificate of Need and Licensure Committee: To conduct research and lay the groundwork for the writing of the certificate of need and future program licensure. Each state has different regulations.

Reimbursement Committee: An investigative group to study the problems concerning future reimbursement for services through insurance companies and other third-party payers.

Source: Adapted from *How to Start a Hospice Program in Your Community* by Dorothy Garrett with permission of the National Hospice Organization.

leaders.[2] This group should include members of the medical community, as well as health or human services professionals who provide services complementary to hospice care. Interested business leaders who lend their organizational and financial expertise are also invaluable. Local civic leaders and clergy offer a community perspective essential to the multifaceted nature of hospice planning. All of these individuals increase the base of community support and facilitate linkage to professional associations and funding sources.

Community support and decisions related to hospice care require facts about the demographic makeup and economic status of the community; in short, a community-wide assessment. This assessment includes information about available resources such as health and human service organizations, population composition, mortality due to cancer or other diseases, potential program participants, financial resources, media and religious group support. Potential community support is often captured in a market analysis, to be described in detail in the following section. It is important to note, however, that these areas are intricately linked.

An economic profile supplies information about the financial makeup of the community. Statistics about income level and insurance coverage are particularly important. To date, Medicare and some commercial carriers have established hospice benefits. For individuals lacking such coverage, access to hospice care is questionable. An economic profile provides the hospice planner with facts about potential donors and funding sources necessary to support a hospice program. This information is tremendously valuable in planning fund-raising activities and capital development campaigns.

Finally, a community assessment takes into account existing hospices and health care organizations in the area and includes collaborative, reciprocal, and competitive aspects of the potential relationships with these organizations. Collaborative efforts, involving many community agencies, may be the best way to provide hospice care in a rural area. On the other hand, a large city may have the ability to support and utilize many different types of hospice programs.

As community support develops and the decision to start a hospice program takes hold, the evolving hospice involves the combined efforts of individuals and organizations in the community. Keys for success include genuine commitment to the hospice concept, timing, and sufficient involvement on the part of community leaders and special interest groups. Hospice programs may ultimately be delivered through a centralized organizational structure or provided in a decentralized fashion. An example of each follows.

A Centralized Community Effort

The early planning efforts of the Joliet Area Community Hospice Corporation described by Theado and Scarry depict a centralized community-based hospice initiative. The corporation relied heavily on the established health care delivery system.

> In March, 1980, concerned individuals approached nursing admin-
> istration at one of the hospitals in the hope of developing a hospice
> program. Specifically, a staff nurse who saw the need to give more
> attention to the dying, the hospital chaplain, and an instructor from
> the community college, spearheaded this concept. This committee,
> with the help of the continuity care director, developed a hospice
> philosophy and goals and completed a feasibility study. The study
> assessed the community's need for hospice care, the relative propor-
> tions of home and inpatient care needed and an inventory of community
> resources. A review of currently operating hospice models and visits
> to various hospices in Illinois, Wisconsin and Indiana were made.
> Workshops on hospice development were also attended by various
> members of this committee.[3]

Work continued by hospital staff, and although hospital administrators were ready to implement the program, inquiries noted the development of a parallel program.

> That same month, to the surprise of the hospital administration and
> planning committee, it was discovered that a private home health agency
> in the area had also become interested in the hospice concept. They
> announced their interest by scheduling a meeting with community
> hospitals, clergy, and business representatives to discuss the estab-
> lishment of a hospice.[4]

The hospital committee reevaluated its position and commitment to hospice care. The knowledge and expertise gained by hospital staff over the two-year internal planning process needed to be salvaged and utilized in the larger community effort. Competitive programs could result in fragmentation and divisiveness within the community.

The meeting, planned by the home health agency, was held as scheduled and a representative spoke about the hospital's planning efforts. An administrator from another local hospital also indicated an interest in hospice care. After several subsequent meetings, a plan evolved: The hospice would utilize existing community resources, and the administrators at the two hospitals would provide joint direction for development of an autonomous, self-governing hospice.

Representatives of both hospitals, the home health agency, and interested community members became part of a central planning committee that drew on the work of subcommittees and task forces. Committees were composed of members from all areas of the community; a leader from each committee also served on the central planning committee (Executive Steering Committee).

As each of the subcommittees completed its tasks, the planning structure would dissolve, leaving in its stead a permanent hospice organizational structure. The Executive Steering Committee would continue its role as overseer of the project until the subcommittees completed their work and a board of directors was solidly in place. During the final planning phase, the ESC would transfer its working knowledge and authority to the board of directors, who would govern the ongoing hospice.[5]

The rest is history. In September 1982, the hospice was incorporated and plans were made to train staff and admit patients during the first half of 1983.[6]

The preceding illustration involved extensive planning and a willingness to cooperate on the part of several health care organizations. However, it is not uncommon to find that hospices have also developed in a more informal fashion, adopting a decentralized organizational structure.

A Decentralized Approach

Hospice of Warren, Pennsylvania, is located in a small rural community. The hospice relies heavily on existing community resources and volunteer services. The number of patients receiving service is small. Typically two or three individuals receive hospice care at any one time. Volunteers provide the core hospice services. Following a 6-hour training program, each volunteer contributes two or more hours weekly to an assigned patient.

The annual budget of $10,000 is used to pay for nondonated operating costs such as office supplies and mailings. The hospice office space and inpatient beds are donated by an area hospital. Medical and service staff work as volunteers. A nonpaid volunteer patient care coordinator and secretary comprise the administrative staff. They are responsible for volunteer recruitment and training and patient service coordination. Board members contribute a great deal of time to other organizational functions such as fund raising, committee development, and so on.

The hospice emphasizes home care and most patients stay at home until death. The board has determined that a separate hospice facility is unnecessary. Coordination with area agencies is done on an informal basis. This is easily achieved because the patient count is small.

Psychiatric consultations to hospice personnel are provided by another area hospital. Equipment, transportation, and limited funds are provided to patients by the American Cancer Society. Organizations such as Area Agency on Aging, the American Lung Association, Meals on Wheels, and area religious groups make it possible to provide individualized support services to each patient. Hospice of Warren successfully draws on existing community resources and in doing so provides needed hospice care with a small annual budget.[7]

The successful administration realizes that community support is often readily available if pursued. Hospices benefit by leadership from interested individuals, health and human service professionals, physicians, leaders in civic and governmental positions, and clergy. Planning groups, striving to develop community support through public and professional education, are instrumental in gaining widespread community support. Individuals responsible for collecting important demographic and economic data should also analyze the collaborative or competitive nature of existing community resources. Community assessment combined with community support are synergetic in developing a hospice program.

MARKETING

Hospice care is generally a local effort, relying on heavy community support. Hospice programs often achieve 'ocal support through the application of marketing concepts, specifically, the identification and analysis of a potential hospice market. Marketing is concerned with successfully directing goods or services from provider to consumer. Because marketing is historically associated with the profit-making sector, the term often connotes hard-sell techniques and expensive advertising. A good example is the automobile industry, which attempts to create demand for its continuous production of new cars. However, this represents only one end of the marketing spectrum.

At the other end of the spectrum is the approach often taken by health care providers: marketing by word of mouth. This approach is based on the assumption that high-quality service retains clients and attracts new clients by favorable endorsements communicated informally. In reality, all organizations in a community may provide high-quality care and, even if they do not, consumers may not be in a position to judge variations. For example, a hospital may increase utilization and demand for its services by employing more creative marketing techniques than the other hospitals in their community.

In his book entitled *Marketing for Non-Profit Organizations*, Philip Kotler describes a balanced marketing approach, applicable to nonprofit organizations such as hospices.[8] He maintains that both service providers and recipients have a mutually beneficial relationship, which is enhanced through various marketing techniques. Marketing research is an example. Opponents of such research argue that it is intrusive. Proponents respond that well-done marketing research allows the hospice to utilize concrete data in its planning efforts. Furthermore, the information can be garnered from many different sources, avoiding professional bias and facilitating provision of appropriate services.

In the early planning and developmental stages, hospice planners are concerned with determining the target population, identifying their needs, and developing a program that matches the needs of clients with organizational resources. Later on, communication or promotion of services to hospice clients requires more attention. Throughout the planning efforts and all subsequent phases of a successful hospice program, the administrator is concerned with building and maintaining strong community support.

Marketing literature stresses that service providers strive to blend high utilization or demand for a given service and high consumer satisfaction. Service organizations also differ from businesses in that they relate to two main markets: clients and donors. Kotler describes this dual market in the following way:

> The clients comprise the group receiving the services of the organization, in return for which they sometimes pay fees. The fees rarely cover the costs of providing the services and the deficit must be made up by raising money from another public, the donors. It may appear that the donors are not in an exchange relation with the organization, that they make a one-way presentation of gifts to the organization. But their giving does yield a return to them in the form of feelings which have a positive value, which reduce one or more needs they have. A given donor may experience a feeling that some unfortunate people will be better off as a result of his gift, or that the society will be safer, or that he is a worthwhile and unselfish person. These feelings are his return payment. The organization must be capable of returning these feelings to him. If the organization were very weak at stimulating these positive feelings in donors, it would soon lose donors.[9]

Building and maintaining donors requires thoughtful and concerted effort in the early stages of hospice planning and throughout the program's growth and maintenance phases. This is crucial since the hospice will undoubtedly compete with other service organizations for philanthropic support.

The potential market for hospice care is comprised predominately of individuals who must deal with a terminal illness, usually cancer. By virtue of the powerful nature of the situation and their involvement with these individuals, family members and associates are also part of the potential market. Not all of the individuals identified in the potential market will actually use hospice services. Utilization of the hospice program is related to these factors:

- Choice of hospice care by the potential recipient
- Admission criteria established by the hospice program
- The fiscal practices of the organization
- Choice of services provided by the hospice

Choice of Care

In marketing hospice services, planners and managers acknowledge that only a portion of those dying will choose hospice services. The decision to receive hospice care is influenced by various social, cultural, physical, and economic factors. Knowledge of hospice care, feelings about death, preexisting attitudes about health care, reliance upon family versus "others" for assistance, and access to hospice services are all essential elements.

Utilization of a hospice program requires a coherent choice on the part of the dying individual. Acceptance of death may come at a time when death is near and there is little time for the patient to benefit from hospice services. While it is not the purpose of this chapter to explore acceptance of hospice care, planners and administrators should keep these factors in mind when designing a program.

Admission Criteria

The admission criteria established by a hospice program will affect its potential market. The basic criterion for accepting an individual into hospice care is that death is imminent. Many hospices establish a three- to six-month prognosis of life expectancy, based on a physician's statement. In addition, acknowledgment by the client and family members that curative means have been exhausted and the disease process is no longer in remission is an important admission criterion.

Because our national experience with hospice care is limited and predicated on service to individuals with cancer, the disease is often cited in the admission criteria for hospice care. Conditions such as multiple sclerosis or chronic obstructive pulmonary diseases, which ultimately cause their victims to deal with approaching death, may also be considered in determining the potential market for a hospice.

The 1983 death rate from cancer is estimated at 187 deaths per 100,000 population in the United States. This rate varies considerably by state, as well as type of cancer and age, sex, and race.[10] Nationally, the death rates per 100,000 population in 1979 for malignant neoplasms (cancer) and chronic obstructive pulmonary diseases were 183.3 and 22.4, respectively.[11] The incidence of such chronic diseases fluctuates from one locale to another and may increase the number of people who might appropriately utilize hospice care. While it is more difficult to determine when treatment for a chronic condition changes from curative to palliative, hospice services provided to the dying individual and family members would theoretically be needed and valued.

Additional criteria for admission may include residence within a specified geographical area, the presence or availability of a caregiver in the home, the individual's and/or family's desire to receive hospice care, and the age of the terminally ill person. Hospice care for children presents planners or administrators with additional considerations and it may be expedient to begin with service to adults and later expand to include dying children. Chapter 6 describes elements for consideration in pediatric hospice programming.

Fiscal Practices

Historically, hospices have not used ability to pay or insurance coverage as admission criteria. This is due largely to the voluntary, subsidized nature of many programs, particularly those cooperating with community service agencies where another provider of care receives third-party reimbursement. However, this trend is quickly changing. The advent of the Medicare benefit for hospice care and increased programmatic integration into the existing health care system has mandated charges for hospice care. This is discussed further in the fiscal section of this chapter.

Service Options

The choice of services to be provided by a hospice is based on many considerations. Because the hospice philosophy embraces family members and associates of a terminally ill person, respite care and bereavement counseling for those individuals are viewed as part of hospice care. The Medicare benefit specifically defines the services that must be provided by a Medicare-certified hospice—for example, medical support, skilled nursing, counseling, and bereavement programming. (These are outlined in detail in Chapter 8.) Other third-party and commercial carriers are following this example and beginning to require that specific services be included in reimbursed hospice care.

Services provided by a hospice may include group counseling or a children's support group for surviving family members, educational programs concerning hospice care, cancer treatment, and pain control for the community at large, or continuing education for professional staff. These additional services provide hospices with indirect benefits such as community recognition, positive image building, volunteer or staff recruitment, and financial support.

Market Analysis

Market analysis is an essential part of the systematic planning process. It requires utilization of operational "givens" and is necessarily based on certain assumptions such as demand for service and the organization's ability to provide a certain percentage of that service. While hindsight may reveal that some factors were overlooked, it provides substantive information to infer a level of demand for hospice care and to envision the type and scope of hospice care needed in a given locale.

Jack Zimmerman, author of *Complete Care for the Terminally Ill*, delineates the method used by Church Hospital, Baltimore, Maryland, to estimate the market for hospice care. This method is particularly useful for hospital-based programs and could be modified for divergent models.

Step 1. Determine areawide hospital utilization rate: 132.4 admissions per 1,000.

Step 2. Determine the year's medical/surgical admission projection: 9,288

Step 3. The hospital's use-rate per population base therefore is:
$$\frac{9,288}{132.4} = 70.15 \times 1,000 = 70,150$$

Step 4. Approximately 50% of the hospital's admissions are from Baltimore City and about 50% are from Baltimore County and the four adjacent counties. City use-rate population base: 35,000; county use-rate population base: 35,000.

Step 5. Cancer death rates for the Baltimore area are city, 288/100,000; county, 196/100,000.

Step 6. To determine the annual number of cancer deaths from Church Hospital's use-rate population base the following computations were made: 35,000/100,000 × 288 = 100.8 patients from Baltimore City; 35,000/100,000 × 196 = 68.6 patients from the four counties.

Step 7. The hospital estimates, therefore, that the hospital's present market share from its service area will provide approximately 170 admissions per year to the hospice program.[12]

The publication entitled *Hospice: Time for Decision*, from the Maryland Hospital Education Institute delineates another system for establishing the potential market for hospices (Table 2-1).[13] This methodology was utilized by the Metropolitan Health Planning Corporation (MHPC), which is the Health Systems Agency for the Cleveland area, and entailed the following steps:

• Projection of cancer-related deaths for the region for a five-year period.
• An estimate that one of four individuals (25 percent) with a terminal illness would be candidates for hospice care.

Table 2-1 Projected Number of Cancer Deaths and Potential Hospice Patients in MHPC's Area, 1980–1984

Year	1980	1981	1982	1983	1984
Projected cancer deaths	4,460	4,517	4,568	4,613	4,652
Potential hospice patients with cancer	1,115	1,129	1,142	1,153	1,163
Total potential hospice patients	1,239	1,255	1,269	1,281	1,292

Note: Computed by applying hospice patient formula as developed by MHPC to the Ohio Department of Health and Vital Statistics.

Source: Reprinted from Hospice: A Time for Decision with permission of Maryland Hospital Education Institute, © 1980.

- An increase of ten (10) percent in the preceding estimation to reflect individuals with non-cancer illness who might be admitted to hospice.[14]

The MHPC study also estimated that 60 percent of the hospice patients would die at home and 40 percent would die in a hospice setting and/or inpatient units in the region. While certain assumptions used in this methodology vary from community to community, its application in planning and developing hospice programs is valuable. In light of these projections, MHPC goals called for a hospice system with seven hospice care teams and 40–50 inpatient hospice beds in no more than five facilities throughout the region.[15]

In their article "Analyzing the Hospice Market," Breindel and O'Hare detail a three-step process through which a hospital analyzed its potential market for a hospice program. First, the authors investigated the type of service envisioned by the organization: a program designed for individuals with an incurable disease and life expectancy of three months or less. Second, they identified the number of patients within the organization's service area: those individuals served by the hospital who had died from cancer or a chronic disease within the past year. Finally, they prepared a summary and recommendations that were presented to the hospital's board as part of their planning efforts. Their conclusion: Without the market analysis, the board's ability to assess hospice as a viable program would be subjective and limited.[16]

REGULATORY

In the early phases of the hospice movement, almost anyone could begin a program of care for the terminally ill and call it hospice. Today this is no longer the case and new, as well as established hospice planning groups, must be sensitive to a number of regulatory concerns. Who can start a hospice program? Is there a limit to the number of hospices in a community? Can a hospice be part of an existing facility such as a nursing home or a hospital? What about licensure? To what extent do hospice planners need to be concerned about regulations? To understand the potential impact of state and federal regulatory mandates, a brief review of national regulatory endeavors will be useful.

Health care planning has received mandated guidelines through federal and state legislation. Title XV of the Public Health Service Act requires the designation of a Health System Agency (HSA) in each of the health service areas in the United States. An HSA may be a nonprofit, private corporation, a public regional planning body, or a single unit of local government. It has responsibility for a designated health services area and is charged with:

- developing a health systems plan (HSP) and an annual implementation plan for meeting health needs of the community
- reviewing and recommending new or expanded programs or capital expenditures proposed by health care facilities as stipulated in state certificate of need laws.[17]

To guide the development of health services in a consistent and systematic manner, the act stipulates that each HSA develop a five-year health systems plan in accordance with federal and state guidelines and in cooperation with state planning agencies. The plan is to include short- and long-range goals and identify changes required in the amount, type, organization, and distribution of health services. It is to be modified annually to reflect new information, program changes, and priorities for action not previously addressed.

Through plan development, plan implementation, and regulatory activities, HSAs respond to health planning issues. Furthermore, the congressional act mandates that decisions and recommendations of the HSA be based on its health systems plan. In this way, the HSA can review proposed changes or additions to health systems as they relate to the stated goals for the region, thus restraining increased costs and duplication of services or facilities in the region. Through a "project review" process, an HSA has authority to make initial determinations regarding the need for hospice services. This authority is then modified by individual state certificate of need laws.[18]

The individual state certificate of need (CON) laws or regulations delineate the type of health care services and projects subject to HSA review. A certificate of need is issued by a governmental body to an individual or organization for provision of a new or different health service, for acquisition of major new equipment, or for construction or modification of a health facility. The CON recognizes that the service or facility will be needed by those for whom it was intended. Many states presently require a CON before a hospice program can be established.[19]

Licensure, another form of regulatory authority, is the process through which a state-established authority grants permission to an individual or organization to lawfully engage in certain activities or services. The process requires the licensing organization to identify standards in order to protect the health, safety, and welfare of individuals receiving care or services. Licensing of hospice programs varies from state to state, and a majority of states still require no licensure.[20] State licensure and its relationship to reimbursement for services will be discussed further in Chapters 8 and 9.

It becomes obvious that, depending upon the state, regulations pertaining to CON and/or licensure need early consideration in the planning process. It is also helpful to be alert to the following situations:

- In many states, home health agencies are not subject to review by the HSA. As a result, a developing hospice program sponsored by a home health agency would not have to be reviewed.
- When a hospital or an inpatient facility increases or redistributes some of its beds from one category to another, a CON may be necessary. For example, if a hospital wishes to change its bed capacity by converting 5 of those beds into "hospice beds," most states require a CON.
- In most states, CON laws mandate review of only those facility changes or projects that cost more than $150,000. Outside of a new building, start-up costs of a hospice would seldom exceed $150,000.
- Hospice services may be considered new or innovative and as such may require review by the HSA.
- A CON may be a requirement of licensure of the facility or service. For example, state licensing requirements for establishing a hospice might include a CON.[21]

It is incumbent upon hospice planners and administrators to identify regulatory mandates affecting the development of a hospice program early in the planning process. Licensure and/or certificate of need conditions may facilitate, impede, or cause modification in plans. Licensure and/or a CON may be required only for hospice programs seeking Medicare certification or for developing a freestanding, inpatient unit; however, the requirements and processes vary from state to state. Furthermore, either process can be lengthy and drastically delay the actual implementation of a hospice program.

UNDERPINNINGS

Governing Body

The governing body of an organization is responsible for establishing overall policies and overseeing implementation of those policies by the officers and/or directors and employees of the organization. Presently, the most typical legal arrangement for a hospice is a nonprofit corporation that qualifies for tax-exempt status under the Internal Revenue Code, Section 501(c)(3). It is established by filing Articles of Incorporation with the Secretary of State and governed by a board of directors.

The Articles establish the corporate purpose and name the first board of directors. These directors adopt corporate bylaws that govern the operation of the corporation. The bylaws specify composition and operating procedures for the board of directors, duties of the officers, and rights of the shareholders or members. One of the most important responsibilities of the governing body is to appoint the organization's chief executive officer or executive director.[22]

The extent to which a board is involved with hospice services depends upon the nature of the organization. In other words, is the organization devoted solely to hospice care or is it organized to deliver many different types of care including hospice? The latter relationship is usually found in conjunction with a hospital or home health agency. Either arrangement is directly related to the impetus for hospice development and availability of resources.

Factors such as reimbursement of hospice care by Medicare may ultimately alter the legal structuring and governing bodies of hospices. If it is possible to realize a profit, individuals and organizations with either private, nonprofit, or proprietary status will begin offering hospice care.

In short, the governing body is a function of the legally organized structure supporting a hospice program. Such legalities are complex and laws governing legal aspects vary from state to state. (General legal issues involving hospice caregivers are discussed in Chapter 9.) Because the legal structure serves as a vehicle to accomplish an organization's mission, hospice planners benefit from competent, professional legal assistance.

Mission and Philosophy

Mission and philosophy statements serve to conceptualize the intent of a hospice program. The mission statement explains why the organization exists and the philosophy statement delineates the overriding beliefs of the organization.

The mission and philosophy may be developed by the planning group, members of the organization sponsoring a hospice program, or key hospice staff. The following questions would facilitate formulation of mission and philosophy:

1. Why do we exist?
2. What "business" are we in?
3. What is our most important product/service?
4. Who are our clients? Volunteers? Donors?
5. Why do they come to us?
6. How have we changed in the past five years?
7. What are our organization's unique strengths and major weaknesses?
8. What philosophical issues are most important to us?
9. What would be lost if we ceased to exist?[23]

Although these questions were prepared by the Public Management Institute for an organization involved in long-range planning, they are very applicable for an evolving hospice program. They will raise controversy and discord. People working side by side in a hospice initiative may find themselves in disagreement regarding fundamental aspects of the program.

Statements of mission and philosophy are far too important to be made by acclamation. Exploration of divergent views allows a choice between alternatives and movement toward logical compromises. It facilitates development of a common ideology regarding definition of the program, the reality of the organization and, in the long run, enhances organizational effectiveness.

After the governing body formally adopts the mission and philosophy statements, the hospice has a basis for establishing the goals, objectives, and action plans that follow. As time goes on, an organization finds that well-defined mission and philosophy serve as primary guideposts in planning, implementing, and evaluating decisions.

Goals and Objectives

Goals, objectives, and action plans are a natural outcome of a clearly stated mission and philosophy. Goals broadly define the intent or expected outcome, while objectives are specific, concrete, and measurable. In addition, objectives specify results in terms of what and when, thus providing the framework for action plans.[24]

Examples of hospice-related goals and objectives follow:

> Goal: To facilitate opportunities for individuals who are terminally ill to live as fully as possible through provision of a comprehensive, multidisciplinary hospice program.

Objective: To complete education and training of health professionals
serving in the hospice program by July 1, 1985.
Objective: To establish admission criteria for the hospice program by
June 1, 1985.

It is clear that goals and related objectives provide direction necessary to mobilize the energies and resources of the organization. Sharing written goals and objectives with all those responsible for implementation of the hospice program promotes efficient teamwork. Well-developed objectives provide a framework for evaluation of specific programs and attainment of goals.

Evaluation

A major responsibility for hospice program administrators is attainment of desired goals and objectives in a cost-effective manner. Program evaluation, as discussed in Chapter 3, provides the mechanism to make judgments regarding success in meeting objectives. It focuses on five distinct areas:

1. *Appropriateness:* the extent to which programs are directed toward concerns that have the greatest importance; e.g., hospice care matches the needs of the community.
2. *Adequacy:* the extent that a problem or situation is eliminated/rectified by a particular program; e.g., hospice care is provided to 50 percent of the projected number of individuals who are terminally ill.
3. *Effectiveness:* the extent to which established program objectives are attained as a result of program activities; e.g., all personnel have completed the hospice training program.
4. *Efficiency:* the cost in resources of attaining established objectives; e.g., bereavement counseling was provided at $X per recipient; this usually entails comparison with past experience or the experiences of other hospices.
5. *Side effects:* desirable or undesirable effects of program operation other than attainment of objectives; e.g., a contribution of a van or loss of good will from one hospital due to location in a competing hospital.[25]

Because evaluation utilizes comparison with a standard, the standard for comparison in a new program is often the attainment of goals planned prior to program implementation. As a result, the administrator will find varying degrees of disparity between the expected and actual accomplishments or outcomes.

If the expected and actual outcomes are close, the administrator may be very satisfied with the program. If there is disparity, intervention may manifest itself in revised objectives, additional objectives, increased activities, higher quality activities, or even abandonment of a certain aspect of the program. In addition, the conceptual meaning of many activities, for example, the unit of service, requires clarity from the service level through the governing body.[26]

Hospice planners and administrators are charged with the responsibility of building a solid foundation for the hospice program. Definition of the role and responsibilities of the governing body, attention to the mission and philosophy of the organization, establishment of meaningful goals and objectives, and responsive evaluation are the cornerstones. With these underpinnings in place, the envisioned hospice can successfully materialize.

ORGANIZATIONAL DESIGN

Definition of Program

The first task of organizational design is to define the hospice program. Realistically, definition evolves throughout all aspects of systematic planning and, in particular, as the underpinnings of the hospice are formalized.

In Chapter 1, "hospice" was defined as a program providing home and inpatient care for the terminally ill patient and family. What is the most effective model to deliver this care? Institutionally initiated programs usually start with inpatient care and expand to include home care. Conversely, community-based services establish home care first and seek linkage with institutions for inpatient coverage. In each case, the key variables are the provision of hospice or hospice-like care and reimbursement of the services provided by the organization.

In terms of reimbursement, when patient care is delineated as hospice care, an organization is eligible for Medicare and limited third-party revenue. Because hospice care entails a certain philosophical approach or attitude in providing care in addition to a defined set of activities (e.g., bereavement counseling, volunteer utilization, and palliative care practices), hospice or hospice-like care provided in the hospital or via a home health agency is reimbursed primarily through acute or home health benefits.[27] With the passage of Medicare this will change. A program must be certified by the government before it is eligible for Medicare hospice reimbursement.

Are your hospice services defined by reimbursement? While the question raises a circuitous debate, it also marks an important aspect of program definition. Fiscal considerations and models for hospice care receive further discussion in the following sections; however, hospice planners should realistically weigh the program for hospice care in terms of both stated service and reimbursement.

Management

Susan T. McLaughlin identifies the need for proper management of a hospice program.

> Organizationally, hospices often begin in a highly collegial mode. Decisions are made by consensus; opportunities and philosophical positions are discussed daily as a team. As the hospice becomes more complex, the reporting lines drawn in accordance with early loyalties may be unclear or unwise. Decisions requiring consensus may be delayed or pushed through precipitously.[28]

The hospice manager may be short on the educational preparation or intuitive skills needed for effective management. As happens in every facet of the health care system, the successful clinician promoted to a management position may not be a successful manager. Management requires a unique set of skills and special knowledge to meet the needs and expectations of the organization. The manager may be working in a loosely defined and evolving organizational structure that calls for flexibility and adaptation.

The first task is to develop a job description that clearly identifies the manager's position. Second, interviewing procedures that include board or committee members with expertise in management must be instituted. Utilization of hypothetical situations requiring management skills in the interviewing process provides a picture of the applicant's skills. Third, following employment, the manager must be involved in decision making, receive administrative support, and facilitate professional development to increase his or her ability to meet the demands of the position.

As a hospice program becomes a Medicare-certified provider or simply grows as an organization, even the successful manager may find the additional responsibilities and activities too demanding. Effective systems, designed to handle routine matters and to flag exceptions for the manager's attention, are important. A well-run hospice program requires effective management practices by the hospice planner or administrator.[29]

Paid and Voluntary Staff

Hospice personnel requirements include individuals with clerical, financial, management/administrative, and clinical skills. In the area of clinical services, the multidisciplinary team consists of home health aides, physical, speech, and/ or occupational therapists, social workers, nutritionists, pharmacists, nurses, physicians, volunteers, and clergy.

Unique to the hospice concept is the practice of utilizing extensive volunteer services to provide both support services and direct patient services. Direct patient services include professional services, which may be provided in the institutional or home setting. The amount and type of care required is established with the patient and family and evaluated via multidisciplinary team conferences.[30]

Utilization of volunteers demands recruitment, retention, and coordination of volunteers by a volunteer supervisor or coordinator. Since voluntary staff are organizationally and legally required to follow the policies and procedures of the hospice, their need for orientation, inservice education, and supervision matches that of salaried staff. Furthermore, as John Blum notes in Chapter 9, considerations regarding liability insurance and legal sanctions appropriate for salaried and voluntary staff should be addressed prior to implementation of the hospice program.

Medical direction in a hospice setting presents special areas for administrative attention. Physicians are typically asked to determine, by virtue of admission criteria, the patient's right to hospice care. As discussed in Chapters 12 and 14, these are large expectations. Philosophical issues arise. For example, a physician may not feel that hospice care is in the patient's best interest or simply dislike a given hospice program. Administrative and board involvement in resolving such issues and building physician support is crucial for an effective hospice program.

Quality Assurance

Quality of Care: That care which implements the most up-to-date knowledge and techniques available to the health sciences. Its aim is to achieve the most desired effect for the patient which those techniques make possible.[31]

Quality assurance has one main purpose: to improve patient care. It involves evaluating what is actually happening with patients and based on that information, improving care or maintaining good care. To assess patient service, an organization evaluates its care against established standards of care such as those generated by the National Hospice Organization or developed internally by the organization. These monitoring activities, including record audits or patient interviews, provide cumulative information to bring about indicated changes.

Because hospice care extends across many different service settings, continuity of patient care presents a unique challenge. As a result of an accreditation study conducted by the Joint Commission on Accreditation of Hospitals, researchers identified the following:

During the pilot test surveys conducted in 1982, continuity of care was the single most influential factor on the quality of care. While care may be comprehensive and adequate in one setting, usually the one controlled by the hospice program, once the patient was admitted to the inpatient setting or to the home from the responsible hospice program, care appeared to breakdown. . . . Orders and intervention initiated by the non-hospice program were often in conflict with those initiated by the hospice staff, leaving the patient's and family's needs unmet and attending physicians confused.[32]

A quality assurance program designed to achieve the most desired effect for the patient considers philosophical, policy, and procedural factors. To accomplish this, administrators should implement a planned and systematic process for monitoring and evaluating the quality of hospice services. Such input is garnered from clients and staff in all service settings. The results are then used to adjust the organizational design of the program and shape the attitudes and practices of all of the staff associated with the hospice program.

Program definition establishes a framework from which management devises systems for maintenance, monitoring, and problem solving related to the hospice program. Utilization of volunteers and unique personnel required by a hospice is taken into account. A quality assurance system is established to ensure delivery of services that are professionally sound and make sense to the recipients. Furthermore, organizational design is clearly influenced by all the components represented in the systematic planning process.

FINANCIAL

Information pertaining to hospice financing and revenue is crucial to planners and administrators. In 1979, Congress mandated a study to examine the implications of including hospice services in the Medicare and Medicaid programs. The Health Care Financing Administration (HCFA) selected 26 hospices to participate in a two-year experimental program. These demonstration sites received reimbursement otherwise unavailable under existing Medicare. Routine Medicare reimbursement coinsurance and deductible provisions were also waived.[33]

In addition to the 26 demonstration sites, the National Hospice Study included 14 non-demonstration hospices and 14 conventional care settings. The latter two groups were chosen by Brown University (the evaluation center for the project). The research questions and analysis of the results of the National Hospice Study are thoroughly covered in Chapters 7 and 8. However, a brief overview is useful.[34]

The HCFA study produced considerable financial data, some of which is still under debate among hospice care providers. Information most pertinent to the discussion of financial considerations follows:

- Some 3,900 patients were admitted to the demonstration hospices. Of these, 1,143 were admitted to hospital-based programs and 2,746 were admitted to home-care hospices.
- The average length of stay in hospice was 72 and 62 days among home-care and hospital-based patients, respectively. The median number of days spent in hospice was 37 and 33 days for the two groups.
- Over 65 percent of patients stayed less than 60 days. Over 5 percent stayed for over 210 days. Ninety percent of the hospice patients were dead when discharged from hospice.
- Hospital-based patients averaged 18.2 days in an inpatient setting, compared with 5.2 days for home-care patients. Of all patient days, 7.2 percent and 29.2 percent were spent in an inpatient setting for home-care and hospital-based patients, respectively.
- Total costs of home and inpatient services per patient were $5,890 for hospital-based and $4,758 for home-care hospices.
- The total cost per patient excludes physician and outpatient services; also, the extent of included overhead costs is not clear.[35]

This summary is taken from the preliminary report; the cost analyses are based upon the first year of demonstration admissions. However, the study does indicate that the hospice approach to terminal care is different and patients are less likely to receive aggressive treatment modalities. Cost savings appear to be associated with reduced use of inpatient facilities and costly ancillary services. The Medicare benefit, implemented in November of 1983, is based on the results of this study.

The Blue Cross and Blue Shield Association (BCBSA) places the conventional health care costs for terminally ill patients during the last 6 months of life at nearly $16,000. This study, based on claims histories for 1,504 cancer patients, was funded by the U.S. Department of Health and Human Services and revealed that:

- Hospital expenditures account for 78 percent of the total costs of conventional terminal cancer care.
- Expenditures for physician services make up 16 percent of the total costs.
- Home care and care in skilled nursing facilities constitute less than 1 percent of the total costs of conventional terminal cancer care.
- Cancer patients in the study averaged 37.7 days of hospital care and spent 15 days of their final month in the hospital.
- The last month alone accounts for 35 percent of all hospital inpatient care during the terminal year.[36]

A major consequence of the BCBSA study is the establishment of a benchmark for comparing conventional costs of terminal illness with the costs of hospice programs. It also provides information about patterns and utilization of health services by the terminally ill. While figures should be adjusted upward for inflation, this information provides baseline data for the hospice planner or administrator.

In another study sponsored by Blue Cross of Northeast Ohio and the Hospice Council for Northern Ohio, the cost of hospice care is shown to be lower than the expense of traditional hospital care. Chapter 7 details the results of the study. However, a few facts are useful here. Based on records for 1,031 Cleveland area residents (1981), results of the study indicated that:

- In the last 2 weeks of life, non-hospice patients spent an average of 6.7 days in the hospital while hospice patients were hospitalized for only 1.6 days.
- The average total third-party payment in the last four weeks of life was $1,290 for the hospice patient compared with $3,557 for other patients.
- In the last eight weeks of life, Medicare and/or private insurance coverage provided payments averaging $1,669 for a hospice patient, $5,509 for patients receiving traditional care.[37]

Hospice planners recognize that determination of costs and projections about the financial viability of any hospice program cannot be separated from standards of care. This was illustrated in the New York State Hospice Demonstration Project, which included extensive evaluation of 12 hospital or community-based hospices. Major conclusions of the study included the following:

- According to results of interviews with primary care providers, the level of satisfaction with hospice care was very high.
- Based upon estimates of the cost of conventional care for terminally ill patients, hospice care was less expensive than conventional care for enrollment lengths of up to 120 days, and the overall savings generally increase with longer enrollments.
- The average charge per patient day varies from $76.35 among community-based programs to $89.36 and $115.67 for hospital-based, autonomous unit programs and hospital-based, scattered-bed programs, respectively. The overall average is $95.10 per patient day.
- The average charge per inpatient day tends to be highest for hospital-based, scattered-bed programs.
- The average charge per hospice patient in New York State was $5,385.

- The average length of enrollment varies among the three models: community-based (38.7 days), hospital-based, autonomous unit (59.4 days), and hospital-based, scattered-bed (76.2 days).
- As expected, the average charge per patient day in New York State hospice programs decreases substantially as the length of enrollment increases.
- The use of volunteers varies among programs. In community-based programs, 36.1 percent of the hours in all program activities were attributed to volunteers. This percentage is 16.0 percent in hospital-based, scattered-bed programs and 38.9 percent in hospital-based, autonomous unit programs.[38]

Carol C. Oviatt, in *Development of Hospice Programs*, reviews and analyzes approximately 20 public and private hospice studies (1977–1983). These data depict home care costs ranging from $40 to $91 per patient day and inpatient costs ranging from $143 to $307 per patient day. The cost per episode of hospice care is shown to extend from $668 to $5,918; the lower cost is primarily associated with home care programs.[39]

Interpretation of cost findings is difficult because of substantive variations in study design. Certain factors, such as the care provided by family members or volunteers and variance in the quality of service, affect the costs of a program. Utilization of charge information rather than actual program costs is also significant. Additional cost comparisons between hospice and traditional care and among various hospice models are still necessary to determine the actual costs and cost effectiveness of hospice care.

Reimbursement

Today, when the vast majority of Americans are covered by some form of health insurance, third-party reimbursement is critical to hospice development. In his book entitled *Hospice: Prescription for Terminal Care*, Kenneth P. Cohen reports on the results of a survey of insurance companies in the United States. Requests for information about hospice coverage yielded responses from over 200 insurance companies. Of these companies, 17 percent reported hospice benefits under hospital or medical plans; only a few policies covered hospice care as a defined benefit.[40]

What is covered by a defined hospice benefit? Generally this refers to coverage for services furnished by a hospice under basic, major medical or comprehensive plans; however, most companies exclude custodial care for terminally ill patients. Blue Cross and commercial carriers usually reimburse direct nursing services for the terminally ill. Generally, benefits do not cover counseling or spiritual and bereavement services. Traditional Medicare benefits are directed toward skilled nursing and rehabilitative services typically emphasized in home health or inpatient services. For an organization, the net effect is reimbursement of portions of hospice care by existing insurance plans, or piecemeal coverage.[41]

Patricia J. Berger-Friedman reports that there are increasing options for hospice coverage.*

> In October 1981, the Health Benefits Consulting Group of the Frank B. Hall Consulting Company surveyed 11 major carriers and found only nominal support among third-party payers for comprehensive hospice services. But by October 1982, the situation had changed dramatically. Many carriers that were not making a hospice option available to their policy holders in 1981 invested significant amounts of time and money to the development of a hospice product in 1982. Some carriers now have products that are being marketed or are planned for release.
>
> In 1981, the carriers indicated that the lack of uniform standards for hospice care, as well as the lack of conclusive evidence on cost savings, presented formidable obstacles to their offering hospice coverage. By 1982, carriers had begun reimbursing hospices, even though standards and data still were lacking. Though respondents in the 1982 survey generally indicated a moral and social responsibility to provide appropriate care to dying patients and their families, this commitment alone cannot account for the dramatic shift in private carrier reimbursement. Apparently, competitive pressure exists among carriers to evaluate and consider cost-effective alternatives to acute care for terminally ill patients.[42]

Medicare Hospice Reimbursement

A discussion of reimbursement is incomplete without detailing the Medicare hospice benefit mandated as part of the Tax Equity and Fiscal Responsibility Act (TEFRA) of 1982. The statute allows reimbursement of hospice services to organizations that meet the hospice conditions of participation. State survey agencies, such as the Department of Public Health, are used to determine a hospice's compliance with the conditions and subsequent approval as a provider of certified hospice services.[43] (See Chapter 8 for a detailed discussion of TEFRA requirements for a hospice.)

TEFRA requires that the hospice employ an interdisciplinary team to plan and deliver care to the client and family. The team must include at least one of the

---

*Reprinted by permission from *Hospitals*, vol. 57, no. 16, August 16, 1983. Copyright 1983, American Hospital Publishing, Inc.

following professionals: a licensed physician, registered nurse, social worker, and counselor. These professionals provide "core" services and must be employed directly by the hospice. Volunteer services are mandated for the hospice program. Other required services can be provided either directly by the hospice or under arrangements with other providers. These services include physical therapy, occupational therapy, speech/language pathology, homemaker/home health aide services, medical supplies (drugs, biologics, and appliances), counseling (including dietary), and short-term inpatient care including respite care and acute inpatient care.[44]

The regulations also mandate a form of prospective reimbursement establishing four per diem rates:

1. *Routine Home Care.* A flat, per diem rate (about $52, weighted geographically) for intermittent services furnished at home. This is all-inclusive, and must cover all wages, drugs, equipment, overhead, and other services.
2. *Continuous Home Care.* A flat, hourly rate (up to $358 per diem) for intensive nursing care delivered by licensed personnel, when the need for such care exceeds 8 hours per day.
3. *Inpatient Respite Care.* A flat per diem rate (about $55, weighted geographically) for inpatient respite care.
4. *Inpatient Acute Care.* A flat per diem rate (about $271, weighted geographically) for inpatient acute care.[45]

All payment for hospice services comes to the hospice; in turn, the hospice is responsible for paying others with whom it has arrangements. A provider (the hospice) submits bills to the designated fiscal intermediary (FI) indicating the services rendered and the name of the recipient. Reimbursement is at the aforementioned rates. A cap on reimbursement of $6,500 per client and a ratio of 80 percent home care and 20 percent inpatient care is also mandated. Basically, an end of the year fiscal reckoning occurs.

The $6,500 is an aggregate cap; calculations entail the total number of patients served during the fiscal year. For example, if 100 patients were served, the FI will multiply this by $6,500 (the amount set as the cap in regulations) and derive the total of $650,000. Following determination of the 80-20 requirement for home care and inpatient days (again, aggregate), the FI reviews the hospice's cost report. Even if the hospice incurred more than $650,000 in "allowed" expenses, Medicare would reimburse no more than $650,000.

Certification as a Medicare hospice provider carries an inherent financial risk for the hospice. TEFRA includes a provision stating that once a hospice accepts a patient, it cannot discontinue care due to inability to pay. For example, if a hospice patient requires hospitalization for acute hospice care and accrues a bill of $15,000, the hospice must pay for the hospitalization even though reimbursement of $6,500 or less is received from Medicare. Furthermore, there is no bad debt allowance within the regulations; consequently a hospice may find itself subsidizing patient care costs.[46]

Starting Costs

The fiscal management of health care organizations is a complex process. Budgeting and fiscal practices are well documented in current literature and the hospice planner or administrator is wise to use resources that allow application to a hospice program. To set the stage, certain fundamental aspects of the financial planning and budgeting process are highlighted.

A budget is the organization's plan expressed in monetary terms; it is based on anticipated outcomes and predetermined goals. Table 2-2 illustrates the expense and revenue budget for a Medicare-certified hospice serving 20 patients annually. For the organization, the budget becomes a definitive statement of mission and goals. Internally, it serves as a control mechanism and management tool.

The annual operating budget for the hospice program entails four separate but mutually dependent components: the expense budget, the revenue budget, the capital budget, and the cash budget. These four components provide a framework to assess intended actions in terms of anticipated expenses, revenue-generating potential, capital needs, and cash flow requirements. Capital and cash budgets are of particular import to new hospice programs.[47]

Working capital is needed in the following areas:

- Capital required to open the doors of the organization (legal or application fees, salaried personnel, or organizational promotion).
- Capital for fixed assets (equipment, furniture, or tenant finish).
- Capital for short-term operating reserves plus needed cash.
- Capital for a temporary period to cover operating expenses during a delay in funding or third-party reimbursement (expected to be paid back within first year).

The quantity of working capital held is directly related to the amount of incoming dollars and it is advantageous to keep working capital costs to a minimum. This requires thoughtful forecasting and planning for financial needs, as well as timely financing strategies. It makes good sense to elicit the assistance of financial consultants or accountants for this aspect of the planning process.[48]

To determine starting costs for a hospice program, it is helpful to seek advice from a similar, already existing program. Formal data on the funds necessary to start a hospice program are limited. A 1979 General Accounting Office (GAO)

Table 2-2 Hospice: Sample Annual Budget for a Medicare-Certified Hospice (Average Daily Census: 20 Patients/Families)

	Expenses		Assumptions
Full-time Equivalents (FTEs)	Staff Salaries		
1.0	Administrator	$ 20,000	● A considerable amount of office
1.0	RN Coordinator	19,000	work is performed by volunteers
.5	Volunteer Coordinator	8,000	● Chaplain will volunteer services
.5	Bereavement Coordinator	9,000	● One nurse can serve 10 patients/
.5	Chaplain	—	families
.25	Physician	15,000	
1.0	Administrative Assistant	14,000	● Bookkeeper, with outside accounting consultation and assis-
1.0	Bookkeeper	16,000	tance, can perform all accounting,
2.0	Registered Nurse	37,000	billing, and reporting functions
2.0	Home Health Aide	18,000	
1.0	Homemaker	8,500	● Professional management of in-
1.0	Social Worker	17,500	patient care can be handled by the described staff
	Subtotal	$182,000	
	Fringe benefits @ 20%	36,400	● Continuous care can be provided by R.N.s and home health aides (equally divided at $12/hour and $7/hour, respectively)
	Total Salaries and Fringes	$218,400	

Overhead Expenses		
Office rent	—	● Donated office space
Utilities	$ 4,000	
Telephone	3,000	● Reduced fees for legal and ac-
Accounting/audit	2,500	counting help
Legal	1,000	
Office equipment	8,000	
Supplies	4,000	
Travel	8,000	
Insurance	15,000	
Printing, etc.	5,000	
Miscellaneous	10,000	
Total Overhead	$ 60,500	

Table 2-2 (Continued)

Expenses		Assumptions
Home Care Ancillaries		
Drugs ($3.00/day × 6,570 days)	$ 19,710	● Ancillaries obtainable at noted costs
Supplies and oxygen ($4/day × 6,570 days)	26,280	● That in a hospice with 20 patients/families on a given day, 18 will be in home care—either routine or continuous (18 patients/
Equipment ($1/day × 6,570 days)	6,570	families × 36 days = 6,570 home care days per year)
Therapies ($2/day × 6,570 days)	13,140	
Total Home Care Ancillaries	$65,700	
Patient Care Contracts		
Inpatient general (686 days × $271)	$185,906	● Inpatient care can be purchased at $271 per day (including ancillaries)
Inpatient "outliers" (22 days × $450/ day)	9,900	● "Outliers" (abnormally difficult or costly cases) can be addressed
Inpatient respite (22 days × $60/day)	1,320	for $450 per day and that these cases will be limited to 3% of all
On call ($2/hour; $15/visit)	15,000	inpatient days
Continuous care (2,364 R.N. hours × $12/hour)	28,368	● Respite care can be purchased for $60 per day
(2,364 home health aide hours × $7/hour)	16,548	● That in a hospice with 20 patients/families on a given day, 2 will be in hospice inpatient care
Total Patient Care Contracts	$257,042	(respite, general, or "outlier")
TOTAL EXPENSES	$601,642	2 patients/families × 365 days/ year = 730 days

Respite: 3% of 730 = 22 days
Outlier: 3% of 730 = 22 days
General: 94% of 730 = 686 days

Table 2-2 (Continued)

Revenues*		Assumptions
Routine Home Care (6,373 days × 85% × $46.25/day)	$250,539	● That in a hospice with 20 patients/families on a given day, 18 will be in home care and 2 will be in-patient care
Continuous Home Care (197 days × 85% × $358.67/day)	60,059	● 70% of all patient days will be covered by Medicare
Inpatient General Care (708 days × 90% × $271/day)	172,681	● 15% of patient days at home and 20% of inpatient days will be covered to same degree as Medicare through other third-party payments and self pay
Inpatient Respite Care (22 days × 85% × $55.33)	1,035	
Physicians' Services (104 visits × $50/visit)	5,200	
TOTAL REVENUES	$489,514	● 15% of patient days at home will be a combination of free care and bad debt
NET INCOME (LOSS)	($112,128)	● 10% of inpatient days will be a combination of free care and bad debt
		● That of all home care, 97% is routine; 3% is continuous. That of inpatient care, 94% is general; 3% is respite; and 3% is "outlier"

*Note: Revenue assumptions based on national unadjusted daily rates.
Source: Reprinted from "Financial Planning and Budgeting for Hospice Survival" with permission of the National Hospice Organization.

report surveyed 42 hospices to determine the sources and amounts of funds needed to begin a hospice program. Initial funding ranged from $100 to $3 million; the latter represents costs associated with inpatient facilities. Hospice programs associated with home care programs reported the lowest start-up costs.[49]

Financial Systems

It is incumbent upon any health care organization to monitor both delivery of service and fiscal operations. Historically, evolving hospices adopted goals with a primary emphasis on service delivery not financial systems. For hospices receiving third-party reimbursement or operating within a larger organization, financial systems are imposed by the fiscal intermediary or the larger organization.

The hospice planner or administrator has the opportunity to define a financial system that blends the delivery of service and practical skills needed to keep the organization alive. The proactive decision making framework advocated by J. B. Silvers (Figure 2-1) places the essential fiscal services of accounting, budgeting, and analysis in the larger organizational context. It suggests there are no purely financial or organizational actions, but rather administrative or governance decisions that, in reality, are expressed in financial or organizational terms.[50]

In order to actualize proactive decision making, it is necessary to collect information and maintain internal fiscal mechanisms. These include:

1. An accrual-based accounting system.
2. A system for identifying and comparing on a monthly, quarterly, and yearly basis, revenues, expenses, and cost flow by line item and by program.
3. A clear audit path.
4. An annual outside audit.
5. Written procedures for day-to-day accountability in receiving income and paying bills.
6. A procedure for reviewing bad debts in a timely manner.
7. A system for collecting client data.
8. An on-going internal cost analysis of each service.
9. Review of capital expenditures.
10. A procedure for annual review of the investment portfolio
11. A procedure for annual financial review of and reapplication for all grants and contracts.[51]

The fiduciary relationship between the governing body of the hospice and the organization demands knowledge of expenses, revenues, and cash flow as well as investments and solicitation of grants, foundations, or private sources (see following section). Members of the governing body or financial consultants provide the hospice planner or administrator with expertise to ensure the financial planning and well-being for the present and future security of the hospice.[52]

Financial security gained through wise investments is an important aspect of the financial management process. Agency investments may include real estate, savings accounts, certificates of deposit, stocks and bonds, or money market funds. Endowments may be designated for a specific purpose or left to the discretion of the hospice. The governing body has primary responsibility for the investment portfolio and will expect to review it at least annually.

As part of its review, the governing body should establish policies regarding the management of investments. What percentages will be short- and long-range

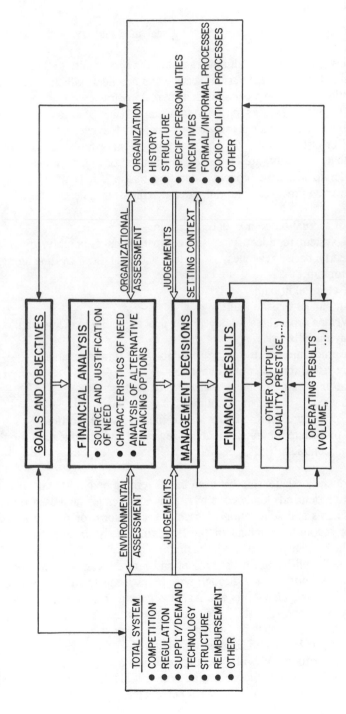

Figure 2-1 Proactive Decision Making Framework

Source: Reprinted from "'Identity Crisis: Financial Management in Health" by J. B. Silvers, *Health Care Management Review*, vol. 1, no. 4, Fall 1976, Aspen Systems Corporation, © 1976.

investments? How will the investment income be used? What is the future plan for the investment portfolio? Financial advice may be provided by bank trust departments, brokerage houses, or private investment counselors. It makes sense for the hospice to seek the best possible return on its investments.

Development

Crucial to successful financial management are investments, grants, and philanthropic contributions supporting the nonreimbursed aspects of the hospice program and providing seed money for special projects. As in the provision of service, the characteristics of the community and the underpinnings of the organization influence the goals and activities related to financial development.

As an illustration, certification for third-party reimbursement requires an established fee-for-service. Do the mission and philosophy state that hospice care is provided regardless of the clients' ability to pay? If so, can the hospice subsidize this unreimbursed service through grants or philanthropy? If not, is there a limit to the amount of subsidized service that will be provided? Are appropriate members of the governing body and service staff involved in determining the criteria for subsidized service? How is subsidized service interpreted in the community, by patients and family members, by the service staff?

Grants designed to initiate or support hospice services are awarded by many private foundations or corporations. Such grants may be available from the state or federal government, e.g., the HCFA hospice demonstration project. The latest foundation directory from The Foundation Center (79 5th Avenue, New York, New York) and related resources are found in designated Foundation Center collections. Local universities and colleges are excellent sources for obtaining information about state and federal grants or contracts.[53] Members of the governing body are also useful conduits regarding opportunities to increase program resources.

Grants and contracts should be related to the local community, its health needs, and the hospice program's ability to meet those needs. The grant or contract will probably mandate an evaluation system and require additional data or procedures beyond what presently exists within the organization. It is important to evaluate the expense of applying for and administering the funded program. In addition, the hospice needs to consider the desirability of funding the project after the grant or contract elapses.

Donations from individuals are an important aspect of philanthropy. Donations result from the donor's interest in hospice care, satisfaction with hospice services received, or direct solicitation by a person or a committee associated with the hospice program. As discussed in the marketing section, donors receive an intangible return from their contribution to a hospice program. An internal system, which provides acknowledgment and concrete appreciation for an individual's investment in the hospice program, is important.

All of the expected revenue from grants, contracts, and individuals are forecast as part of the budget process and the overall financial management process. Expectations for community or foundation grants and individual contributions are translated into goals and objectives for appropriate staff or committees. Continuing the example of providing subsidized service to financially needy patients, the hospice administrator can project the extent of service and related cost. Based on this estimate, a development council or similar group related to the governing body could be challenged to raise money earmarked for charity care.

The goals, results, and activities related to financial development are part of agency evaluation. The governing body should review and approve an annual plan. In addition, they should receive periodic progress reports regarding fundraising and development. Recognition of volunteers lending their expertise and direction to fundraising, particularly by the governing body, is crucial to long-term development efforts. Finally, proposed changes or additions to the hospice program are included in the plan for financial development.[54]

The financial system of a hospice encompasses potential reimbursement for services, starting costs, internal control mechanisms, a budgeting process, and development of outside funding and philanthropic sources. Communication among the members of the governing body, program, personnel, and finance committees, administration, supervisors, and clinical service staff is inherent in the process. Financial decisions are weighed and balanced in terms of delivering hospice services.

SUMMARY

The planning and management of hospice programs are challenging processes. The concept is new and still experimental. This chapter has presented suggestions for basic program development. Hospice administrators, like other health care executives, must assess their base of community support, understand funding sources, have an extensive organizational committee structure in place, and have a clear idea of organizational goals and objectives. Individuals typically became involved in hospice care because of their philosophical beliefs and are committed to promoting the idea. Many early founders never envisaged a system of Medicare funding and other types of third-party reimbursement. As hospice programs develop over time and become more involved with the traditional health care system, success will be largely determined by program management. For administrators, this means a thorough understanding of the hospice market, a clear idea of the costs involved, and a ready supply of resources and the flexibility to initiate programs capable of meeting community needs.

NOTES

1. "The 'How-To' of Hospice Care," Third National Hospice Symposium, Dominican College Campus, San Rafael, Calif., May 26-28, 1977, in *Hospice: Prescription for Terminal Care*, Kenneth P. Cohen (Rockville, Md.: Aspen Systems, 1979), 175.

2. Dorothy Garrett, *How to Start a Hospice Program in Your Community* (Arlington, Va.: National Hospice Organization, no date), 7-8.

3. Grace C. Theado and Kathleen D. Scarry, "Networking Community Services; Politics of Hospice Development," *Nursing and Health Care* 4 (1983): 568.

4. Ibid.

5. Ibid., 671.

6. Ibid., 568-572. This discussion summarizes the material presented in the article by Theado and Scarry.

7. Roger Mesmer and Judith Cerra, "Tapping Area Resources Helps a Hospice Thrive," *Hospitals* 57, no. 4 (1983): 37.

8. Philip Kotler, *Marketing for Non-Profit Organizations* (Englewood Cliffs, NJ.: Prentice-Hall 1975).

9. Ibid., 32.

10. *Cancer Facts and Figures: 1983* (New York: American Cancer Society, 1982), 9.

11. U.S. Bureau of the Census, *Statistical Abstract of the United States: 1982-83*, 103rd ed. (Washington, D.C.: U.S. Government Printing Office, 1982), 77.

12. Jack M. Zimmerman, *Complete Care for the Terminally Ill* (Baltimore: Urban and Schwarzenberg, 1981), 145-146.

13. *Hospice: Time for Decision* (Lutherville, Md.: Maryland Hospital Education Institute, September 1980).

14. Ibid.

15. Ibid.

16. Charles L. Breindel and Timothy O'Hare, "Analyzing the Hospice Market," *Hospital Progress* 60 (October 1979): 10.

17. Susan S. Addiss, "Area Health Planning," *Monday Comments* (Comprehensive Health Planning Council-Southeastern Michigan), no. 10, April 2, 1984.

18. *A Glossary of Health Care Delivery and Planning Terms* (Madison, Wisc.: Institute for Health Planning, August 1981).

19. Section 1122 of the Social Security Act provides that payments will not be made under Medicare or Medicaid with respect to certain disapproved capital expenditures. These expenditures would be determined inconsistent with state or local health plans. P.L. 93-641 requires states participating in the section 1122 program to have the State Health Planning and Development Agency serve as the section 1122 agency for purposes of the required review. U.S. Congress, House of Representatives, Committee on Interstate and Foreign Commerce, *A Discursive Dictionary of Health Care* (Washington, D.C.: U.S. Government Printing Office, 1976).

20. *A Glossary of Health Care Delivery and Planning Terms*; "Certificate of Need Issue Heats Up; State Hospice Laws Moving In: Survey of the 50 States' CON and Licensure Laws," *Home Health Line* 8 (May 30 and June 6 (combined issue), 1983): 14.

21. David Tannenbau, "Planning Amendments Highlight of Year," *Hospitals, JAHA* 54, no. 7 (April 1,1980): 156; Authur Vining Davis Foundation, *Delivery and Payment of Hospice Services: Investigative Study, Final Report* (Vienna, Va.: National Hospice Organization, September 1979).

22. *Legal and Ethical Responsibilities for Board Members of Not-For-Profit Organizations* (Chicago: The National Easter Seal Society, 1984).

23. Paul Hennessey and Research and Development Staff, *Managing Nonprofit Agencies for Results: A Systems Approach to Long Range Planning* (San Francisco: Public Management Institute, 1978).

24. Ibid.

25. Committee on Evaluation and Standards, *Glossary of Evaluative Terms in Public Health* (New York: American Public Health Association, 1970): 1546–1547.

26. C. Lynn Deniston and Irwin M. Rosenstock, "Evaluating Health Programs," *Public Health Reports* 85, no. 9 (September 1970): 835–840.

27. Richard P. Ames, "Starting a Hospice Requires Tenacity, High Standards," *Hospital Progress* 61, no. 2 (February 1980); George David "Hospice Reimbursement Issues," *Caring* (National Association for Home Care) 2, no. 6 (June 1983): 56–59.

28. Susan T. McLaughlin, "Avoiding Common Hospice Pitfalls," *Caring* 2:6 (June 1983): 18.

29. Ibid.

30. *Standards of a Hospice Care Program* (Arlington, Va.: National Hospice Organization, 1982).

31. *Criteria and Standards for Home Health Care* (Comprehensive Health Planning Council of Southeastern Michigan, November 21, 1979).

32. Barbara McCann, "JCAH Hospice Project: Proposed Standards," *Caring* (National Association for Home Care) 2 (June 1983): 17.

33. *National Hospice Study, Preliminary Final Report, Extended Executive Summary* (Providence, R.I.: Brown University, November 1983).

34. Ibid., 8–14.

35. Ibid., 20.

36. Health Services Foundation, *Research and Development Terminal Illness Study* (Chicago: Blue Cross and Blue Shield Association, 1983).

37. *Cost Savings of Hospice Home Care to Third Party Insurers* (Cleveland: Hospice Council for North Ohio Blue Cross of Northeast Ohio, Case Western Reserve University, 1983).

38. *An Analysis and Evaluation of the New York State Hospice Demonstration Project* (Albany, N.Y.: New York Department of Health, December 1982).

39. Carol C. Oviatt, *Development of Hospice Programs* (Madison, Wisc.: Institute for Health Planning, February 1984).

40. Kenneth P. Cohen, *Hospice: Prescription for Terminal Care*, 103–118.

41. Ibid.

42. Patricia J. Berger-Friedman, "Paying for Hospice Care," *Hospitals*, August 16, 1983, 106.

43. "Medicare Program; Hospice Care," *Federal Register* (Washington, D.C.: Health Care Financing Administration, Department of Health and Human Services, December 16, 1983), 56008–56036.

44. Ibid.

45. NAHC Report (No. 21) (Washington, D.C.: National Association for Home Care, April 15, 1983).

46. Ibid.

47. Howard J. Berman and Lewis W. Weeks, *The Financial Management of Hospitals*, 4th ed. (Ann Arbor, Mich.: Health Administration Press, 1980).

48. "Sample Annual Budget," National Hospice Organization, in "Hospice 84" (Regional Training Conferences in Hospice), *Financial Planning and Budgeting for Hospice Survival* (Dearborn, Mich.: June 1, 1984).

49. U.S. General Accounting Office, *Hospice Care—A Growing Concept in the United States* (Washington, D.C.: (HRD 79-50), March 6, 1979).

50. J. B. Silvers, "Identity Crisis: Financial Management in Health," *Health Care Management Review* 1, no. 4 (Fall 1976): 31–40.

51. *Administrator's Handbook for Community Health and Home Care Services* (New York: National League for Nursing, 1984), 26.

52. Ibid., 21–32; Berman and Weeks, *The Financial Management of Hospitals*, 63–99.

53. Boris Frank, Proposal Writing Workshop, Dearborn, Mich.: Boris Frank Associates, March 17, 1983.

54. *Administrator's Handbook*, 26.

BIBLIOGRAPHY

Addiss, Susan S. "Area Health Planning." *Monday Comments* (Comprehensive Health Planning Council-Southeastern Michigan) no. 10, April 2, 1984.

Administrator's Handbook for Community Health and Home Care Services. New York: National League for Nursing, 1984).

Aitken-Swan, Jen. "Nursing the Late Cancer Patient at Home." *The Practitioner* 183 (July 1959): 64-69.

Alderson, M. R. "Terminal Care in Malignant Disease." *British Journal of Preventive and Social Medicine* 24 (May 1970): 120–123.

Ames, Richard P. "Starting a Hospice Requires Tenacity, High Standards." *Hospital Progress* 61 (February 1980): 56–59.

An Analysis and Evaluation of the New York State Hospice Demonstration Project. Albany: New York Department of Health, December 1982.

Berger-Friedman, Patricia J. "Paying for Hospice Care." *Hospitals*, August 16, 1983, 106–108.

Berman, Howard J., and Weeks, Lewis W. *The Financial Management of Hospitals*, 4th ed. Ann Arbor, Mich.: Health Administration Press, 1980.

Bloom, Bernard S., and Kissick, Priscilla D. "Home and Cost of Terminal Illness." *Medical Care* 18 (May 1980): 560–564.

Blumstein, James F., and Zubkoff, Michael. "Public Choice in Health: Problems, Politics and Perspectives on Formulating National Health Policy." *Journal of Health Politics, Policy and Law* 4 (Fall 1979): 382–413.

Breindel, Charles L. "Management Issues Regarding Hospice Programs and Nursing Homes." *Long Term Care and Health Services Administration* 4 (Spring 1980): 43–47.

Breindel, Charles L., and Boyle, Russell M. "Implementing a Multiphased Hospice Program." *Hospital Progress* 60 (March 1979) 42–45, 76.

Breindel, Charles L., and O'Hare, Timothy. "Analyzing the Hospice Market." *Hospital Progress* 60 (October 1979): 52–55.

Butler, Robert N. "The Need for Quality Hospice Care." *Quality Review Bulletin* 5 (May 1979): 24.

Cancer Facts and Figures: 1983. New York: American Cancer Society, 1982.

Coale, Jack. "The Hospice in the Health Care Continuum." *Quality Review Bulletin* 5 (May 1979): 22–23.

Coburn, Karen. "Oncology Nursing in the Local Community." *Cancer Nursing* 4 (August 1979): 287–295.

Committee on Evaluation and Standards. *Glossary of Evaluative Terms in Public Health*. New York: American Public Health Association, 1970.

Cost Savings of Hospice Home Care to Third Party Insurers. Cleveland, Ohio: Hospice Council for North Ohio Blue Cross of Northeast Ohio, Case Western Reserve University, 1983.

Council of Home Health Agencies and Community Health Services, National League for Nursing. "Statement on Hospice." New York: National League for Nursing, January 1979.

Criteria and Standards for Home Health Care. Comprehensive Health Planning Council of Southeastern Michigan, November 21, 1979.

David, George. "Hospice Reimbursement Issues." *Caring* (National Association for Home Care) 2 (June 1983): 10–11.

Davidson, Glen W. "Five Models for Hospice Care." *Quality Review Bulletin* 5 (May 1979): 8–9.

Davidson, Glen W. *The Hospice: Development and Administration*. Washington, D.C.: Hemisphere, 1978.

Dellabough, Robin. "Four Models of Hospice Care." *Hospital Form* 23 (January/February): 6–10.

Deniston, C. Lynn, and Irwin M. Rosenstock. "Evaluating Health Programs," *Public Health Reports* 85, no. 9 (September 1970): 835–840.

Dennis, Jeanne. "Implementing the Hospice Concept in a Small Hospital." *Journal of Nursing Administration* 10 (June 1980): 42.

Dorang, Edith S. "A VNA-Organized Hospice Volunteer Program." *Nursing Outlook* 29 (March 1981): 170–173.

"Experts Probe Issues Around Hospice Care." *Hospitals, JAHA* 54 (June 1, 1980): 63–67.

Fath, Gerald. "Pastoral Care and Hospice." *Hospital Progress* 60 (March 1979): 73–75.

Frelik, Robert W. "Hospice: What Is It? What Is Its Future?" *Forum On Medicine* 3 (June 1980): 390–394.

Garrett, Dorothy. *How To Start a Hospice Program in Your Community*. Arlington, Va.: National Hospice Organization (no date), 7–8.

"Certificate of Need Issue Heats Up; State Hospice Laws Moving In: Survey of the 50 States' CON and Licensure Laws." *Home Health Line* 8 (May 30 and June 6 (combined issue), 1983): 14–18.

A Glossary of Health Care Delivery and Planning Terms. Madison, Wisc.: Institute for Health Planning, August 1981.

Greenberg, Bernard G. Dean, UNC-CH, School of Public Health, Chapel Hill, North Carolina. Interview, 28 February 1980.

Greene, H. Rex. "Getting Hospicized." *Hospital Physician* 15 (October 1979): 54–55.

Grobe, Mary Ellen. Director of Hospice Project, Mayo Clinic, Rochester, Minnesota. Telephone Interview, 2 June 1980.

Hadlock, Daniel C. "Hospice Care: Its Implications and Influence on Current Health Care Concepts." *Long Term Care and Health Services Administration* 4 (Summer 1980): 132-154.

Halper, Thomas. "On Death, Dying and Terminality: Today, Yesterday, and Tomorrow." *Journal of Health Politics, Policy and Law* 4 (Spring 1979): 11–29.

Health Services Foundation. *Research and Development Terminal Illness Study*. Chicago: Blue Cross and Blue Shield Association, 1983.

Hennessey, Paul, and Research Development Staff. *Managing Nonprofit Agencies for Results: A Systems Approach to Long Range Planning*. San Francisco: Public Management Institute, 1978.

Hinton, John M. "The Physical and Mental Distress of the Dying," *Quarterly Journal of Medicine* 32 (January 1963): 1–21.

Hinton, John. "Comparison of Places and Policies for Terminal Care." *Lancet* 1 (January 6,1979): 29–32.

Hospice, Inc. *Frequently Asked Questions About Hospice.* New Haven, Conn.: Hospice Inc., 1978.

Hospice: Time for Decision. Lutherville, Md.: Maryland Hospital Education Institute, September 1980.

Hospice: Prescription for Terminal Care, Kenneth P. Cohen. Germantown, Md.: Aspen Systems, 1979.

Johnson, Richard L. "Hospital Buildings Have Few Alternative Uses." *Hospital Progress* 60 (October 1979): 42–70.

Kaluzny, Arnold D., et al. *Management of Health Services.* Englewood Cliffs, N.J.: Prentice-Hall, 1982.

Kolbe, Richard. "Inside the English Hospice." *Hospitals, JAHA* 51 (July 1, 1977): 65–67.

Kotler, Philip. *Marketing for Non-Profit Organizations.* Englewood Cliffs, N.J., Prentice-Hall, 1975.

Krant, Melvin J. "Expectations of Patient and Family." *The Hospital Medical Staff* 7 (February 1978): 1–6.

Lawrence, Susan V. "New Hospice Opens in Nursing Home." *Forum on Medicine* 1 (September 1979): 18–20.

Legal and Ethical Responsibilities for Board Members of Not-For-Profit Organizations. Chicago: The National Easter Seal Society, 1984.

Levey, Samuel, and Loomba, N. Paul. *Health Care Administration*, Philadelphia: J. B. Lippincott, 1973.

Lyons, Marge. "Hospital Provides Special Care for Dying Patients and Their Families." *Health Care and Social Policy* 52 (November 6, 1978): 123–126.

Markel, William M., and Sinon, Virginia B. "The Hospice Concept." *Ca—A Cancer Journal for Clinicians* 28 (July/August 1978): 225–237.

Martin, M. Caroline. "Cooperation Marks Development of Hospice." *Hospitals, JAHA* 53 (July 16, 1979): 32, 41, 44.

Martin, M. Caroline, and Brink, Gerald R. "Setting Up an In-Hospital Hospice." *Journal of the Association of Western Hospitals* 23 (January/February 1980): 12–17.

McCann, Barbara. "JCAH Hospice Project: Proposed Standards." *Caring* (National Association for Home Care) 2, no. 6 (June 1983): 15–17.

McLaughlin, Susan T. "Avoiding Common Hospice Pitfalls." *Caring* 2, no. 6 (June 1983): 18–19.

"Medicare Program; Hospice Care." *Federal Register.* Washington, D.C.: Health Care Financing Administration, Department of Health and Human Services, December 16, 1983, 56008–56036.

Mesmer, Roger, and Cerra, Judith. "Tapping Area Resources Helps a Hospice Thrive." *Hospitals* 57, no. 4 (1983): 37.

Meyer, Katherine A. "The Hospice Concept Integrated with Existing Home Health Care." *Nursing Administration Quarterly* 4 (Spring 1980): 49–54.

Millett, Nina. "Hospice: Challenging Society's Approach to Death." *Health and Social Work* 4 (February 1979): 130–150.

Montefusco, Ann. Staff, National Hospice Organization, Vienna, Va. Telephone interview, 9 June 1980.

Mount, Balfour M. "Palliative Care for the Terminally Ill." *Royal College Lecture*. Presented at the annual meeting of the Royal College of Physicians and Surgeons of Canada, Vancouver, British Columbia (January 27, 1978).

NAHC Report (no. 21). Washington, D.C.: National Association for Home Care, April 15, 1983.

National Hospice Study Preliminary Final Report, Extended Executive Summary. Providence, R.I.: Brown University, November, 1983.

Naylor, David B. and Machul, Audrey E. "Adding a Hospice: Issues To Consider." *Michigan Hospitals* no. 19 (June 1983): 38–41.

Osterweis, Marian, and Champagne, Daphne Szmuszkovicz. "The Hospice Movement: Issues in Development." *American Journal of Public Health* 69 (May 1979): 492–496.

Oviatt, Carol C. *Development of Hospice Programs*. Madison, Wisc.: Institute for Health Planning, February 1984.

Parkes, C. Murray, "Home or Hospital? Terminal Care As Seen by Surviving Spouses." *Journal of the Royal College of General Practitioners* 28 (January 1978): 19–30.

Parks, Patricia. "Evaluation of Hospice Care Is Needed." *Hospitals, JAHA* 53 (November 6, 1979): 68–70.

———. "Hospice Care for Dying Patients: A Look at the Issues." *Trustee* 32 (October 1979): 29–32.

———. Staff, Division of Medical Services, American Hospital Association, Chicago. Telephone interview, 9 June 1980.

Boris Frank. Proposal Writing Workshop. Dearborn, Mich.: Boris Frank Associates, March 17, 1983.

"Proposed Hospice Regulations Reviewed." *Caring* (National Association for Home Care) 2 (June 1983): 6–8.

"Questions Remain Unanswered in Hospice Care Movement." *The Hospital Medical Staff* 8 (October 1979): 24—28.

Rakove, Roberta. "Hospice Care: A Planning Perspective." *Quality Review Bulletin* 5 (May 1979): 10–12.

"Hospice 84" (Regional Training Conferences in Hospice), "Financial Planning and Budgeting for Hospice Survival," Dearborn, Mich., June 1, 1984.

Saunders, Cicely. "Hospice Care." *The American Journal of Medicine* 65 (November 1978): 726–728.

Schneidman, Edwin S., ed. *Death: Current Perspectives*. Palo Alto, Calif.: Mayfield, 1979.

Silvers, J. B. "Identity Crisis: Financial Management in Health." *Health Care Management Review* 1, no. 4 (Fall 1976): 31–40.

Simione, William, Jr. and DeVita, Richard. "Hospice Fiscal Planning and Reimbursement." *Caring* (National Association for Home Care) 2 (June 1983): 8–9.

Spiegel, Allen D. *Home Health Care*. Owings Mills, Md.: National Health Publishing, 1983.

Standards of a Hospice Care Program. Arlington, Va.: National Hospice Organization, 1982.

Storck, Mick. "Getting Death and Dying into the Curriculum." *The New Physician* 27 (May 1978): 29.

Sweetser, Carleton J. "Integrated Care; The Hospital-Based Hospice." *Quality Review Bulletin* 5 (May 1979): 10–13.

Tannebau, David. "Planning Amendments Highlight of Year." *Hospitals, JAHA* 54, no. 7 (April 1, 1980): 156; *Delivery and Payment of Hospice Services: Investigative Study, Final Report*. Authur Vining Davis Foundation. Vienna, Va.: National Hospice Organization, September 1979.

Theado, Grace C., and Kathleen D. Scarry. "Networking Community Services; Politics of Hospice Development." *Nursing and Health Care* 4 (1983): 568-572.

U.S. Bureau of the Census, *Statistical Abstract of the United States: 1982-83* (103rd edition) U.S. Government Printing Office, Washington, D.C., 1982.

U.S. Congress, House of Representatives, Committee on Interstate and Foreign Commerce. *A Discursive Dictionary of Health Care.* Washington, D.C.: U.S. Government Printing Office, 1976.

U.S. General Accounting Office. *Hospice Care—A Growing Concept in the United States.* Washington, D.C.: (HRD 79-50), March 6, 1979.

Walker, Norman T. *Hospice Pilot Project Report.* Hayword, Calif.: Kaiser Permanente Medical Center, 1979.

Ward, Audrey W. M. "Terminal Care in Malignant Disease." *Social Science and Medicine* 8 (July 1974): 413-420.

Ward, Barbara J. "Hospice Home Care Program." *Nursing Outlook* 26 (October 1978): 646-649.

Wegmann, JoAnn, Miller, Nancy, and Perlia, Mildred. "An Oncology Unit Model." *Nursing Management* 15 (January 1984): 46-48.

Widmer, Geraldine, Briu, Roberta, and Schlosser, Adela. "Home Health Care: Services and Costs." *Nursing Outlook* 26 (August 1978): 488-493.

Wilkes, Eric. "Terminal Cancer at Home." *Lancet* 1 (April 10, 1965): 799-801.

Woodward, Kenneth, et al. "Living with Dying." *Newsweek* 91 (18) (May 1, 1978): 52-63.

Zimmerman, Jack M. *Complete Care for the Terminally Ill.* Baltimore: Urban and Schwarzenberg, 1981.

Models of Hospice Care: Anticipating the Planning Process

Chapter 1 cited five predominant models of hospice care identified by the Government Accounting Office. They included variations of home-based, institutionally based, and freestanding programs. Using the management approach described in this chapter, we can assess the advantages and disadvantages of each of the models outlined below. Each type of hospice program is examined according to the planning and administrative elements described earlier. While all hospice programs must ultimately address the planning issues raised in this chapter, no one model is ideally suited to the needs and aspirations of a specific community. Planners and organizers must eventually relate the best-suited hospice program to the community being served.

FREESTANDING OR HOSPITAL AFFILIATED HOSPICE

Structure

- A *distinct facility* providing both inpatient and home hospice care.
- May be a renovated facility or one built expressly for hospice care.
- Includes patient lounge(s), special kitchens where family members may cook, meditation room or chapel, a children's nursery, community or activity room, or outpatient facility.

Community Support

- Easily recognized; promotes involvement of community members and volunteerism.
- Limits access by health professionals and mainstream health care system.
- Allows creative adaptations for the terminally ill and their extended families.

Marketing

- Easily identified as a hospice; facilitates referrals.
- Provides a central location for additional services such as counseling or education.
- Negative connotations may arise due to emphasis on terminal illness and death.

Regulatory

- Designation of a hospital unit or a separate facility usually requires CON.
- Probably requires state licensure.

Underpinnings

- May have own governing body or function as semiautonomous unit of parent organization.
- Mission and philosophy developed by governing body if free-standing; for semiautonomous unit, mission and philosophy complements the parent organization.
- Goals, objectives, and program evaluation are substantively developed and directed by the hospice.

Organizational Design

- Promotes continuity of care between hospice and home health care.
- Limits opportunities to share health care resources; contractual arrangements are always possible.
- Facilitates recruitment and retention of staff committed to caring for terminally ill.
- Lends itself to an effective quality assurance system.
- Facilitates full, interdisciplinary hospice care.

Fiscal

- Certified hospice providers receive reimbursement via Medicare hospice benefit.
- Limits reimbursement by traditional Medicare and Blue Cross/commercial carriers.

- Requires higher starting costs and long-term financial development.
- Discrete service setting facilitates financial planning and development.

HOSPITAL-BASED HOSPICE; DESIGNATED UNIT

Structure

- A *distinct unit* of the hospital providing inpatient hospice care; may be called a palliative care unit.
- Requires home care arrangements through a hospital-based or community-based home care agency.
- May necessitate remodeling to physically implement the hospice concept.

Community Support

- Less autonomy than freestanding; impacts identification, volunteer involvement, and financial development.
- Access to medical and health professionals.
- Allows utilization of the hospital resources, including volunteer services.
- Allows creative adaptations for the terminally ill and their extended families.
- If serving the entire community, identification with a particular institution may be strength or weakness.

Marketing

- Increases marketing opportunities; identification of hospice separately or as part of the hospital.
- Hospital facilities available for patients and families as well as additional services such as counseling or education.
- Consider hospital atmosphere or restrictions.

Regulatory

- Designation of beds may require CON.
- Separate licensure is probably unnecessary.

Underpinnings

- Governing body and organizational structure designated by hospital.
- Mission and philosophy complements that of the hospital.

- Goals, objectives, and program complement overall hospital operations.
- Program may be under auspices of designated hospice committee, specific supervisor, and/or department.

Organizational Design

- Promotes continuity of care, if home care component is arranged.
- Facilitates recruitment and retention of staff committed to caring for terminally ill.
- Cost-efficient use of facility and staff; unit may have "swing" beds to accommodate hospice or nonhospice patients (depends on size of unit).
- Facilitates full interdisciplinary hospice care.
- Lends itself to an effective quality assurance system.

Fiscal

- Certified hospice providers receive reimbursement via Medicare hospice benefit.
- Reimbursement possible through traditional insurance plans.
- Cost-efficient use of existing facility.
- Budgeting and financial reporting part of larger hospital system; less control of hospice costs

HOSPITAL-BASED HOSPICE; HOSPICE TEAM

Structure

- A *distinct team* within the *hospital* providing interdisciplinary hospice care or consultation to other staff.
- Frequently called the "scattered bed" approach.
- Requires home care arrangements through a hospital-based or community-based agency.

Community Support

- Less autonomy than separately identified unit; limits identification, volunteer involvement, and financial support.
- Ready access to medical and health professionals.
- Allows utilization of hospital resources, including volunteer services.

- If serving the entire community, identification with a particular institution may be strength or weakness.

Marketing

- Affects marketing opportunities; more difficult to identify hospice care within the context of the whole hospital.
- Hospital facilities available for patients and families as well as for additional services such as counseling or education.

Regulatory

- Depending upon emphasis, designated beds may or may not require CON.
- No separate licensure.

Underpinnings

- Governing body and organizational "slot" within hospital structure.
- Program may be under auspices of designated hospice committee, specific supervisor, and/or department.
- Goals, objectives, and program complement the overall hospital operations.

Organizational Design

- Promotes continuity of care, if home care component arranged.
- Direct supervision of hospice team may be responsibility of many different supervisors.
- Direction of the hospice program may be under a designated supervisor and/or department; separate from supervision of individual team members.
- Cost-efficient use of staff.
- Depending on organizational support of team, facilitates full interdisciplinary hospice care.
- Quality difficult to monitor.

Fiscal

- Prohibits certification as a Medicare hospice provider.
- Reimbursement possible through traditional insurance; both inpatient and home health.
- Cost-efficient use of existing facility.

- Budgeting and financial reporting part of larger hospital system; reduced control of hospice costs.

HOSPITAL-BASED HOSPICE; HMO ARRANGEMENTS

HMO arrangements could take on any of the previously described hospital-based characteristics.

While the Government Accounting Office identified HMO units as hospital-based, it is likely that HMOs will offer hospice care to members through a free-standing, hospital-based, or home-care hospice.

HOSPICE AFFILIATED WITH AN EXTENDED CARE FACILITY OR NURSING HOME

Structure

- A *distinct unit* or an extended or skilled nursing care facility (SNF) or nursing home providing inpatient hospice care.
- Requires home care arrangements through a facility-based or community-based home health agency.
- May necessitate remodeling to physically implement the hospice concept.

Community Support

- Less autonomy than freestanding hospice.
- The smaller size of many SNFs and nursing homes impacts identification and promotion of the hospice program; recruitment of volunteers.
- Limits access by health care professionals and mainstream health care system.
- If serving the entire community, identification with a particular facility may be strength or weakness.
- Allows creative adaptations for the terminally ill and their extended families.

Marketing

- Complements the services provided by the SNF or nursing home and increases marketing opportunities.
- Facility may have limited space for visiting or familylike activities.
- Depending on type of facility and location of beds, atmosphere may lend itself to hospice care.

- Many patients in a nursing home have a terminal illness; allows utilization of hospice care by those individuals and/or families.

Regulatory

- Designation of beds may require CON.
- Separate licensure is probably unnecessary.

Underpinnings

- Governing body and organizational structure designated by facility.
- Mission and philosophy complements that of the SNF or nursing home.
- Program under auspices of designated hospice committee, supervisor, or specific department.
- Goals, objectives, and program complement the overall SNF or nursing home operation.

Organizational Design

- Promotes continuity of care; home care component arranged.
- Staff involved in different types of care; impedes recruitment and retention of hospice staff.
- Promotes cost-efficient use of existing staff.
- Full interdisciplinary hospice care requires additional direct or contracted staff.
- Since most facilities do not provide home health, the home care component is arranged or not provided.
- Allows effective monitoring and evaluation of quality.

Fiscal

- Certified hospice providers receive reimbursement via Medicare hospice benefit.
- For an SNF, reimbursement available through traditional benefits.
- Limited reimbursement by traditional Medicare, Blue Cross, or commercial carriers.
- Budgeting and financial reporting part of larger system; reduces control of hospice costs.

HOSPICE HOME CARE; HOSPITAL-BASED

Structure

- A *hospital-based home health agency* providing home hospice care.
- Requires inpatient hospice care arrangements with the hospitals, SNFs, and nursing homes.

Community Support

- Less autonomy than freestanding hospice; impacts identification, volunteer involvement, and financial development.
- Access to health care professionals.
- Allows utilization of the hospital's resources including volunteer services.
- If serving the entire community, identification with a particular hospital may be a strength or weakness.

Marketing

- Increases marketing opportunities; identification of hospice separately or as part of the home care program.
- Hospital facilities available for patients and families as well as additional services such as counseling or education.

Regulatory

- Designation of hospice program may require CON.
- Licensure varies among states.

Underpinnings

- Mission and philosophy complements the home care program of the hospital.
- May function as semiautonomous program of home health agency.
- Program under auspices of designated hospice committee, supervisor, or specific department.

Organizational Design

- Facilitates continuity of care, particularly if inpatient arrangements are with the same hospital.

- Facilitates shared resources; maximizes services of both home health and hospice programs.
- Staff involved in home care or dedicated to hospice care only; impacts recruitment and retention of interested staff.
- Ready access to medical and health care professionals.
- Full interdisciplinary hospice care requires additional direct or contracted staff; also volunteer services.
- Lends itself to effective quality assurance system.

Fiscal

- Certified hospice providers receive reimbursement via Medicare hospice benefit.
- Requires low starting costs; maximizes reimbursement.
- Allows reimbursement through traditional home health benefits; provision of hospicelike care.
- Budgeting and financial reporting part of larger system.

HOSPICE HOME CARE; NURSING-HOME BASED

Hospice home care that is nursing-home based presents essentially the same picture as a hospice program located in a nursing home. Inpatient care would be arranged with the nursing home; arrangements for acute care would also be necessary.

HOSPICE HOME CARE; COMMUNITY-BASED

Structure

- A *community-based home health agency* providing home hospice care.
- Requires inpatient hospice care arrangements with hospitals or other inpatient facilities.

Community Support

- Less autonomy than a freestanding hospice, impacts identification, volunteer involvement, and financial development.
- Many voluntary or nonprofit home health agencies have cultivated community support; benefits both hospice and home health programs.
- Limits access to health care professionals.

- Draws on existing expertise of agency in providing services in the home setting.

Marketing

- Increases marketing opportunities; identification of hospice care separately or as part of the entire agency.
- Agency facilities available for additional services such as counseling or education.

Regulatory

- Designation of hospice program may require CON.
- Licensure varies from state to state.

Underpinnings

- Mission and philosophy complements that of the home health agency.
- Hospice could function as semiautonomous program.
- Goals, objectives, and program under auspices of designated hospice committee, supervisor, or specific department.

Organizational Design

- Impacts continuity of care; inpatient arrangements.
- Facilitates shared resources; maximizes services of both home health and hospice programs.
- Staff involved in different types of home care or dedicated to hospice care only; impacts recruitment and retention of interested staff.
- Full interdisciplinary hospice care requires additional direct or contracted staff; also volunteer services.
- Lends itself to an effective quality assurance system.

Fiscal

- Certified hospice providers receive reimbursement via Medicare hospice benefit.
- Requires low starting costs; maximizes reimbursement.
- Allows reimbursement through traditional home health benefits; provision of hospicelike care.
- Budgeting and financial reporting part of larger system.

Chapter 3

Evaluating Hospice Care*

T. Neal Garland and David M. Bass

The healing professions and occupations in the United States are strongly identified with the scientific approach to problem solving. This approach demands empirical evidence in support of any claim before it is granted any significant degree of credibility. Yet, as Mumford points out,[1] very few of even the most widely used treatment modalities in Western medicine have been scientifically evaluated to assess their effectiveness.

The idea that methods of treatment used in health care *should* be evaluated is not new. Christoffel and Lowenthal note that nearly a century and a half ago Dr. Pierre C. A. Louis, a French physician and statistician, urged his colleagues to rigorously demonstrate the effectiveness of their treatment procedures in order to be sure these procedures were accomplishing their intended goals.[2] Florence Nightingale, in the middle of the nineteenth century, proposed a method of recording surgical procedures that included information about the patient's age, sex, and occupation as well as information about the disease or other cause of the operation, the date of the patient's recovery from the operation, and a description of complications.[3] Such data would provide the beginnings of a systematic evaluation of the dangerousness and effectiveness of a particular surgical procedure for male and female patients of varying ages and occupational backgrounds.

In spite of the requests by these and other early pioneers in health care, as Schulberg and Baker note,[4] in the 1970s, systematic evaluation of health care was only beginning to qualify as a scientific endeavor. At the same time, the necessity for evaluation of health care was growing as a result of several sources

* The study reported in this chapter was supported in part by faculty research grants 681, 725, and 789 provided by the Graduate School of The University of Akron and in part by a grant from The Ritchie Foundation, provided through the Visiting Nurse Service, Akron, Ohio.

of pressure. Health care professionals were searching for the most effective and the most efficient means for treating patients, and thus were becoming ever more interested in systematic evaluation of both new and traditional methods of treatment. As the cost of health care escalated, third-party payers—including the federal government—began demanding empirical evidence that specific approaches to treatment did, in fact, accomplish intended goals with maximum efficacy.

The trend toward increased pressure for systematic evaluation of health care treatment methods and of health care programs has continued to grow during the 1980s. Now, more than ever before, health care providers, program administrators, federal and state legislators, funding agencies, third-party payers, and patients desire—and increasingly *demand*—hard, factual evidence upon which to base their decisions. In this type of atmosphere, hospice planners and managers need objective evaluations of programs if the concept of hospice care is to gain and maintain a significant position within the American health care system. In order to understand the benefits that evaluation studies can offer to hospice programs, it will be helpful to first examine the general nature of evaluation research.

WHAT IS EVALUATION RESEARCH?

In the social sciences, as in the other sciences, a distinction is made between *basic* research and *applied* research. Basic research is research carried out for the purpose of advancing knowledge, without any attempt to demonstrate how that knowledge can be used. Applied research, on the other hand, is conducted in order to find an answer to a very practical problem: the results are intended to be useful in the "real" world of everyday activities. Evaluation research belongs to the larger category of applied research. Louise Kidder notes,

> Applied research, as its name suggests, is carried on for practical reasons—to produce findings that are applicable, practical, immediately useful. Evaluation research is a special form of applied research, designed to evaluate programs, usually ameliorative social programs such as remedial education, welfare reforms, innovative teaching methods, health care delivery systems, job training programs and the like. The results of evaluation research are not meant merely to add to our store of knowledge or develop theories. They are used, often immediately, to decide whether programs should stop or go, whether budgets should expand or contract, whether personnel should be hired or fired—all based on whether the program accomplished what was intended.[5]

The conclusions reached by evaluation researchers potentially have direct effects on programs, program personnel, and clients. It is necessary to emphasize the word *potentially* here, for the results of even the best-designed evaluation study may be ignored by managers and policymakers. For example, President Richard Nixon commissioned a massive study of the effects of pornography on sex crimes. The study, which was conducted by highly qualified social scientists and followed rigorous standards of evaluation research, concluded that there was no evidence to support the claim that use of pornography induces people to commit sex crimes.[6] President Nixon chose to ignore the results of this study, either because he did not believe the research findings or because it was politically expedient to do so. Such has been the fate of many evaluation research projects.

On the other hand, in many cases the decisions affecting the fate of programs often must be made by people who are far removed from the day-to-day activities of those programs—legislators, boards of directors, members of funding bodies—and such people increasingly demand facts rather than opinions to guide their decisions. Programs that can produce the results of well-designed and carefully carried out evaluation studies are in a much stronger position when they are arguing in favor of continued funding or favorable legislation.

EVALUATING HOSPICE PROGRAMS: MAJOR ISSUES TO CONSIDER

In order to ensure that state and national credentialing and regulatory agencies and funding agencies accept the results of an evaluation study as legitimate evidence of a program's performance, the hospice program manager or administrator should take certain issues into consideration. These include choosing evaluators, working effectively with evaluators, setting program goals, interpreting results of the evaluation, and applying the results to program planning and improvement.

Choosing Evaluators

The hospice program manager or administrator who wishes to have an evaluation study conducted has two basic choices regarding who should conduct the study: "internal" or "external" evaluators.[7] "Internal" evaluators are members of the program's own staff. "External" evaluators are brought in from a university, research firm, or other research-oriented organization.

There are benefits and costs associated with each type of evaluator. Internal evaluators tend to be more familiar with the goals, personnel, and actual operation of the program, and thus may be able to develop an adequate evaluation research design more quickly than outsiders. On the other hand, insiders may be so involved in the program that they are unable to be objective in their research. There is a danger that the evaluation study produced by insiders may simply support existing biases without providing information that could lead to important improvements in the program.[8]

It must be kept in mind that those to whom the results of the study are to be presented (legislators, funding sources, etc.) are likely to question the credibility of evaluation conducted by insiders. Often it will be assumed that the insider has a vested interest in making the program look good and that he or she will consciously or unconsciously stack the cards to produce a favorable outcome. Also, except in the case of very large and/or well-funded agencies, it is unusual for a health agency to have a professionally trained evaluation researcher on the staff. The insider who is chosen to conduct an evaluation study necessarily will have to divert time and energy from his or her normal duties (which must be covered by someone else) in order to learn or to brush up on research techniques. This may constitute an unacceptable drain on the agency's resources.

Outside evaluators most often will be professional researchers who are thoroughly familiar with the intricacies of research design, statistical techniques, and computer capabilities. They are less likely to have a vested interest in the outcome of the study. Further, the outcome is more likely to have a high level of credibility in the eyes of funding and regulatory bodies. However, the outsider may fail to adequately understand the goals of the program or the unique historical background of the agency.

Weiss suggests several factors that the program administrator should consider regarding the choice of insider or outsider evaluations[9]:

1. *Administrative confidence.* How much confidence does the administrator have in the professional skills of those who propose to conduct the evaluation? In some cases the administrator may feel that members of the agency's staff are inadequately prepared to conduct good research and will prefer the professional researcher from the outside. In other situations, the administrator may feel that researchers based in academic settings are too oriented toward the ivory tower and that they fail to understand everyday agency operations.

2. *Objectivity.* Who is more likely to produce a highly credible study? Can the shadow of vested interest be effectively dispelled if the evaluation is conducted by insiders? How? On the other hand, what is the reputation of the outside evaluator? Are studies conducted by this evaluator generally held in high regard by the people to whom this evaluation will be submitted? What evidence can the outside evaluator present to demonstrate his or her level of credibility?

3. *Understanding of the program.* An effective evaluation must be based on accurate perceptions of what the program is trying to accomplish and of how the agency actually functions on a day-to-day basis. Generally speaking, insiders will have an advantage here, although perceptive outsiders may also be highly accurate in their understandings if given the cooperation of the staff.

4. *Potential for utilization.* When the results of the evaluation are in, the administrator must decide how to use them. Insiders may be especially helpful here, for they may more easily see how these results can be applied to the needs of the program and they can more easily argue in favor of a course of action in staff meetings. However, outsiders may offer a different kind of advantage in that their prestige as professional researchers and the greater objectivity they are presumed to possess may lend greater weight to their suggestions.

5. *Autonomy.* Because outsiders generally have less vested interest in the program, they can more freely suggest large and dramatic changes in the agency's structure and functioning. Such changes may be extremely helpful in extricating an agency or a program from a disagreeable situation. Insiders are more likely to take the basic structure, values, and functioning of the agency for granted and to suggest changes that leave these basic features intact. Insiders' suggestions may be more helpful if the program administrator has little leeway in the kinds of changes the agency's rules allow.

Working With the Evaluator

Gerald Barkdoll points out that once an evaluator has been hired, there are three different "evaluator styles" that he or she can exhibit.[10] The first is the "Lone Ranger" style, where the evaluator is the "good guy" and the members of the program staff are the suspected "bad guys." The task of the Lone Ranger evaluator is to get the goods on the bad guys so they can be forced to become law-abiding citizens. The second style is that of the "value-free scientist." The value-free scientist single-mindedly seeks to discover TRUTH regardless of its cost, consequences, or utility for the program being evaluated. The third style Barkdoll identifies is the "consultative" evaluator. The consultative evaluator attempts to work with members of the agency or program in a cooperative manner. The evaluator's goal in this style is to reach a consensus with members of the program regarding the goals, methods, and applications of the evaluation study.

Each of the styles of evaluation can be of benefit in the appropriate circumstances. However, it is likely that the consultative style will be the most useful to the agency in a majority of cases.[11] The hospice administrator should discuss these evaluation styles with potential evaluators to make sure all parties understand the evaluator's role. The consultative or cooperative style usually maximizes input from program administrators and staff regarding the evaluation design. It also maximizes the probability that the study will produce relevant and useful results.

The administrator who considers hiring an evaluator who utilizes the consultative style should expect the evaluator to ask the administrator and staff to become involved in developing aspects of the study such as the specification of program goals, definition of program success, and a methodological focus.

Specifying Goals of the Program

It is often assumed that program goals can easily be identified. However, Nay and associates note that it has been impossible to evaluate the success of many federally funded programs because the program goals have been so abstract or so unclear that there is no way to measure progress toward them.[12]

Before contacting an evaluation researcher, the program administrator should reach some tentative conclusions regarding what his or her program is attempting to accomplish. Official documents of the agency often include specification of the agency's intended purpose. Frequently, however, these specifications will be limited to extremely broad statements (e.g., "to improve the quality of life among the poor in this community"). Such statements serve as useful starting points in discussions with evaluators, who can help the administrator develop more sharply focused goals that can be measured in an objective manner.

Seldom does an agency have only a single goal toward which it is working. The more common situation is for the agency to have several goals that may or may not be closely related to each other. Some of the agency's goals are likely to be more important than others, so the program administrator must develop a hierarchical ranking of goals. It would be inefficient for an agency to expend funds for a highly sophisticated evaluation of the degree to which it is achieving a minor goal while at the same time leaving its movement toward a major goal unevaluated.

Agencies often have both short-term and long-term goals. The usual plan is to have accomplishment of short-term goals contribute toward the achievement of long-term goals. The hospice program administrator should decide whether to have the evaluation focus on long-term or short-term goals, or both. If short-term goals are chosen as the target for the evaluation, the evaluator may be able to clarify the coordination between short-term and long-term goals.

The administrator may also want to consider the extent to which the agency has both overt and covert goals. For example, the overt goal of the agency may be to provide hospice services for the terminally ill. At the same time, the agency's covert goal may be to increase the amount of its power relative to other health care agencies in the local community. It is possible that the agency may be succeeding at one of these goals but failing at the other. Which of these goals does the administrator want evaluated? Can both be evaluated at the same time? Is it desirable to evaluate both?

Another factor to consider is that different people may have different goals for the same program.[13] Agency administrators, primary service personnel, clients, and funding bodies may all have somewhat different views as to what it is the program is attempting to accomplish. One positive function served by a program evaluation study is that it can reveal the extent to which various relevant parties concur with the agency's intentions. The administrator must decide, if viewpoints differ, how the various views can be integrated so that the evaluator knows what to evaluate. Another approach is to clearly state the program's goals as they are understood by each of the relevant parties. Either way, the evaluator must know what it is that he or she is expected to evaluate.

Defining "Success" for the Program

The basic idea behind evaluation research is quite simple: determine the goals of the program, measure the extent to which those goals are being met, and decide on the extent to which the program is succeeding.[14]

However, few things are as simple as they first appear. Evaluation research is no exception. For example, program A may be accomplishing its goal, but not as well as program B. Is program A "successful"? Program A may have several goals. If it is accomplishing three of these goals very well and failing miserably on four others, is it successful? Or, program A may have a single stated goal, with several departments in the agency working toward that goal. If almost all of the success in movement toward that goal is due to the efforts of one department (or even one person) while the other departments either contribute nothing or actually detract from movement toward the goal, is the program successful?

Just as administrators and staff may have different views as to a program's goals, so they may differ in their views as to what constitutes program success. For example, a funding body may see the program as successful if it provides services for a specified number of clients each year. The service providers themselves may not be satisfied with the quality of service they were able to offer and may therefore see the same program as unsuccessful regardless of the number of clients "processed." Managers and staff should specify as clearly as possible the criteria used to decide the degree to which the program has been successful. This is best done in cooperation with the evaluator to ensure that relevant measurements are collected.

In addition to the general problems of defining success for purposes of evaluation, the hospice program administrator is faced with a unique problem. "Success'' in health care traditionally has been defined as curing the patient. In hospice care, this definition does not apply because it has been agreed that the patient will not be cured. Patients are not admitted to hospice programs unless their physicians have decided that death is highly likely within six months or less. Therefore, a new definition of success is necessary.

The hospice philosophy provides guidelines for developing this new definition: hospice care can be regarded as successful if it helps the patient live out his or her remaining time in as enjoyable and constructive a manner as possible, free from the distractions of pain and other debilitating symptoms. Likewise, it can be seen as successful if it helps surviving family members cope with bereavement in a constructive and satisfying manner. But this definition leads to certain measurement problems. During the final stages of illness the patient may be unable to answer questions, and after death occurs one cannot ask the deceased about the quality of his or her life during the last days. Likewise, determining whether or not survivors are coping in a constructive and satisfying manner may be difficult. How long after the patient's death should such a determination be made? Which family members should hospice care be most concerned about? Conceptualizing or defining success is easier than objectively measuring it.

Methodological Matters

Even though the evaluator is the technical expert when it comes to research methodology, it is likely that he or she will request input from hospice program administrators and personnel on several important methodological issues. Dialogue among evaluator, staff, and administrators regarding these issues ensures that everyone understands the purpose of various research procedures. It also will help the evaluator stay in touch with the realities the program faces. Foremost among the methodological matters are such things as the study design, specification of the unit of analysis, selection of a sample, and the development of valid and reliable data collection instruments.

Research Techniques and Designs in Evaluation Studies

Evaluation researchers utilize all of the same research techniques and study designs as investigators involved in basic social science research. These include systematic sampling of the population being studied, the development of questionnaires or interview instruments, the use of statistical tests to analyze the data, and an objective point of view.

For many investigators, the classical experiment is the ideal research design.[15] In this design, the researcher begins with a group of research subjects and randomly assigns each subject to either an experimental or a control group. Random assignment ensures that the subjects in the two groups will be as nearly equal as possible on all relevant factors (age, sex, race, education, health status, etc.). Both groups first are measured on whatever it is that the experiment is attempting to affect (e.g., attitudes toward physicians, dietary practices). The experimental group then receives a stimulus or treatment designed to modify members' attitudes, behavior, or condition in some way deemed desirable (e.g., they are shown a movie about physicians, receive a lecture about dietary practices), while the control group does not receive this stimulus. Then the initial measurement is repeated. While both groups should be approximately equal on this measure the first time it is administered, if the stimulus is effective there will be a difference between the two groups on the second administration of the measurement. Statistical tests enable the researcher to estimate the likelihood that any differences appearing between the groups at the time of the second measurement are due to random or chance fluctuations in measurement. If the differences are larger than can reasonably be expected by chance alone, it is logical to conclude that the experimental stimulus did, in fact, make a difference.

Of course, evaluation research does not usually take place in a laboratory where all relevant variables can be controlled by the investigator. Instead, evaluators must conduct their studies within the context of ongoing programs. In the health care field it seldom is possible or even desirable to randomly assign some patients to receive a given treatment while others receive no treatment. Certainly, this is the case with hospice care. Evaluation studies most often must make skillful use of quasi-experimental research designs.

In a quasi-experiment, one or more of the elements of the true experiment is missing.[16] There is no control group, for example, or it is impossible or impractical to obtain before-and-after measures. Some social scientists argue that because of these missing elements, the conclusions reached through the use of quasi-experiments are less valid than those based on the classical or "true" experiment.[17] Others[18] feel that use of the experimental design produces misleading results in many situations.

Whichever side of this debate one chooses to support, in most situations evaluators are called upon to investigate, it is impossible to utilize a true experimental design. Constraints of ethics, time, funds, personnel, and other resources must be considered. In the final analysis, the researcher can do only what the administrators of the program being evaluated allow. Because the administrators' jobs, or the expansion or continuation of the program, may depend on the outcome of the evaluation, the research design must be negotiated with those in charge of the program. The major factors guiding such negotiations must, in the end, be common sense and consideration of the rights of all parties involved.

Choosing the Unit of Analysis

The term "unit of analysis" refers to the person or persons from whom data are to be collected. The concept is similar to that of "unit of care" in health care delivery. The hospice philosophy identifies the patient and his or her family as the basic unit of care. That is, hospice providers are concerned with meeting the needs of both the terminally ill individual and his or her family. In addition, the interdisciplinary hospice team is composed of numerous health care and service providers trained in different fields. These individuals may approach their tasks with somewhat varied assumptions as to what constitutes good care. The evaluators, program administrators, and staff must specify whose point of view is to be utilized in the evaluation. In the ideal situation, the evaluator considers the views of persons receiving or delivering hospice care as well as the interrelationships among these views. This method ensures that the evaluator gains a comprehensive perspective of program goals. If the unit of analysis includes more than one category of respondents, data must be collected from all categories.

Selection of a Sample

In social science research, a sample is a subset of items chosen from a larger population. The sample is selected so that the characteristics of the sample accurately represent those of the population. Social scientists most often utilize samples in their research rather than entire populations because of time and money considerations. Information collected from a carefully chosen sample accurately reflects the information that would have been obtained had the entire population been studied. Because of the relatively small size of most hospice programs, this issue of sampling usually is not a problem. However, administrators of programs serving several hundred patients should discuss sample selection with the evaluator. This will ensure that findings can be generalized to the entire patient population with a high degree of confidence.

Before selecting the sample, the administrator and the researcher should decide what characteristics a patient/family unit must possess to be eligible for inclusion. This will help make it clear to what types of patient/family units the results can be generalized once the study has been completed.

If the unit of analysis for the evaluation is the patient and his or her family, then the sample should include both groups. This can be accomplished in one of two ways. Patients and their families can be selected from the program's records and become part of the sample. Or patients and family members can be regarded as distinct populations from which samples are drawn independently. The method chosen depends on the purposes of the evaluation.

Regardless of the approach taken, it is important that samples are chosen randomly—that is, every member of the population should have an equal chance of being included in the sample. This will ensure that findings from the sample can be generalized to the population. Because individuals selected for the study may decide they do not wish to participate, it is not possible to obtain a truly random sample. The researcher's goal, however, is to have the sample be as nearly representative of the population as possible.

Measurement of Program Effects

The authors of a highly respected research methods textbook point out that "The quality of research depends not only on the adequacy of the research design but also on the quality of the measurement procedures employed."[19] If the measurement instruments utilized by the evaluator do not accurately measure the concepts being studied, the results of the evaluation will be useless or, worse yet, misleading. Therefore, it is essential that questionnaires or interview guides used in an evaluation study be both valid and reliable. The administrator and program staff should discuss these issues with the evaluator.

Determining whether responses to questionnaire items are due to exposure to the program or to other factors is difficult.[20] In fact, it is impossible to construct a completely valid questionnaire. However, there are techniques that can maximize the validity of an instrument. The evaluator should be familiar with these techniques and explain them to the hospice staff.

A concept closely related to the concept of validity is reliability. The term has come to have several meanings for social science researchers, including

> The aspects of reliability that have received most attention are the *stability* of individuals' positions from one administration of the measure to another; the *equivalence* of individuals' positions on different instruments intended to measure the same characteristic or on a given instrument as administered by different people at essentially the same time or as scored by different judges; and *homogeneity*, the extent to which individuals' responses to the various items or other components of a measure are consistent.[21]

If researchers could be certain that their measurement instruments were completely valid, the issue of reliability would not present a problem. However, since the researcher seldom can be sure of the validity of the measurement instrument, he or she pays attention to the instrument's reliability. A highly reliable instrument is more likely to be valid. While this assumption can be questioned, it sometimes is necessary to accept this less than optimal situation. Hospice administrators and staff members should ask the evaluator to explain the reliability level of the evaluation data collection instrument(s) employed.

Interpreting Results

Though research findings typically are reported in neutral terms, they may mean quite different things to different people. The interpretation a person assigns to a set of findings generally depends largely on that person's position in the program. The bureaucratic division of labor that typifies most organizations ensures that certain aspects of the evaluation will be relevant to some and ir-relevant to others. The concerns of direct service providers, such as nurses or caseworkers, are different from the broader concerns of agency administrators, whose concerns are, in turn, different from those of regulatory or funding bodies.

The administrator, members of the staff, and the evaluator should carefully review findings and determine how persons in various positions might interpret them. It is surprising how findings that appear self-evident from one point of view can be anything but self-evident when seen from another perspective.

Applying the Results

Many evaluation studies result in little more than a research report occupying a spot on a dusty shelf. Numerous reasons have been offered for this state of affairs. Schulberg and Baker, for example, suggest that perhaps the evaluator was laboring under a false assumption.[22] The evaluator may have assumed that it was possible to determine whether or not the program was accomplishing a particular goal and to suggest techniques for improvement. However, the ad-ministrator may find these suggestions impossible to implement. A hospice may have many goals. It is possible that the evaluator's suggestions can be followed only at the cost of endangering the hospice's ability to meet other, more important goals. The evaluator should understand, from the outset, how the program or service activity under evaluation fits into larger institutional missions.

Historically, there has been a large communication gap between researchers and service providers. The hospice program administrator should make sure that negotiations with the evaluator include provisions for the researcher to com-municate findings to relevant agency personnel in clear, nontechnical language. Halpert suggests several ways to maximize the chances that evaluation research results will be communicated in understandable, useful ways.[23] These include:

1. Ask researchers to prepare abstracts of reports for distribution to staff members.
2. Clearly identify which research findings are relevant to which practitioners by preparing specialized (as well as general) reports. *Don't ignore lower-level employees.* Research clearly indicates that the success or failure of many programs is decided by the individuals who actually deliver hands-on care to clients.[24]
3. Consider having the evaluators assist in preparing manuals to help staff members become familiar with results of the study.
4. Consider having evaluators assist in presenting inservice training sessions and/or interdisciplinary conferences for members of the staff.
5. Consider asking the evaluators to serve as ''shirt-sleeve consultants'' who participate in service delivery to show members of the agency how to apply findings.

6. Locate "opinion leaders" in the agency or on the board and be sure that they understand the implications of the research findings. They can play a leading role in implementing changes in the program if their support is obtained.
7. Consider the possibility of making structural changes in the agency that make it easier to follow through on the implications of the research.

Evaluation research consumes time and other valuable resources. The prudent hospice manager must seek out ways to use the findings to strengthen his or her agency.

THE EVALUATION OF A HOSPICE PROGRAM: AN EXAMPLE

The remaining sections of this chapter describe an actual evaluation study of a hospice program. This study illustrates points made earlier. It also provides insights into ways an evaluation study can be helpful to the administrator and staff beyond merely meeting requirements of funding and/or regulatory bodies.

The Setting

The hospice program serving as the research site for this investigation is staffed by nurses from a home health care agency. Serving patients since 1978, the program emphasizes home care. A majority of the actual care is provided by two hospice teams, each of which is composed of three registered nurses. In addition, home health aides, social workers, therapists, dieticians, volunteers, and other care professionals provide services as necessary. The program has no inpatient beds of its own, although arrangements have been worked out with local hospitals so that hospice patients can receive inpatient care.

Demographic characteristics of patients who use the services of this hospice are similar to those of hospice patients nationwide.[25,26] The predominant prognosis is cancer and most patients are over 55 years of age. Findings from this evaluation therefore may be relevant for hospice programs across the country.

Choice of Evaluators

Program administrators chose researchers from the sociology department of a local university to conduct the evaluation study. This choice was made because the health care agency did not have trained social science researchers on its staff and because the prestige of the university in the community would add to the study's credibility. An additional advantage was that the researchers, as "outsiders" to the agency, would have no vested interest in the outcome. This would further add to the credibility of the findings.

Specification of Program Goals and Definition of Success

The written guidelines of this agency specify a number of goals for the hospice program.[27] The goal chosen to serve as the focus of this evaluation was: "To assist the patient in maintaining maximum independence and to live each day of life to its fullest." This is a very abstract goal. The problem facing the evaluators was to translate it into specific components that could be measured.

This goal has two parts: (1) helping the patient to maintain maximum independence and (2) helping him or her to live each day of life to the fullest. It was decided to measure the first part by recording whether the patient died at home or in a hospital or other health care facility. It was assumed that being at home gives the patient the maximum opportunity for independence, while being in a hospital or other facility minimizes this opportunity.

The second part of the goal, "leading life to the fullest," is even more abstract than the first. A reasonable approach to measuring goal attainment for this part is to identify whether the needs of patients are met while they are enrolled in the program. To create this measurement, a list of major needs of terminally ill patients was constructed.

To develop an empirically measurable list of patients' needs, evaluators sought advice of the hospice administrators and care team members. Based on this input, researchers conducted a survey of the literature on death and dying in order to develop a list of needs for terminally ill patients and their families. This list was compiled and shared with the hospice nurses. The nurses examined it and indicated their feelings about the appropriateness of each item. The nurses suggested the addition or deletion of certain needs. Several meetings between the evaluators and the nursing teams were held and a list of patient/family needs was agreed upon. The list of patient needs appears as Appendix 3-A at the end of this chapter.[28] Success of the program was measured by the extent to which these needs were met while the patient was enrolled in the hospice program. The list includes items such as the need to control pain, the need to know that medical care will be available at any time of the day or night, and the need to have one's wishes respected by the hospice nurses.

Methodological Matters

The following discussion presents a brief overview of some of the major methodological issues discussed in meetings with staff. In attendance were evaluators, program administrators, and the hospice nursing teams. Consensus was reached on each issue before the study was initiated.

The Research Design

The research design is best described as a before-and-after quasi-experimental design with no control group.[29] While this design is less rigorous than might be desired, it was deemed adequate for the purpose of this evaluation: to measure the program's success in meeting the needs of patients and families while patients were enrolled in the hospice program. In this discussion we will deal only with measurement of the degree to which needs were met for patients. Need fulfillment for the patients' primary caregivers also was measured, but is not reported here. If the purpose of the evaluation had been to compare the impact of the hospice program with the impact of nonhospice care of terminal patients, a control group would have been necessary.

A questionnaire was constructed based on the list of needs of terminal patients and their families mentioned above. The patient's primary caregiver was chosen as the appropriate person to answer the questions. Most often this is the patient's spouse or other close family member. It was decided not to ask patients to respond to the questionnaire because, even at the time of entry into the program, many of them were too ill to answer questions.

For each need item, the respondent was asked to estimate the extent to which he or she felt the patient's need had been met. The respondent was contacted and asked to fill out the questionnaire approximately five months after the patient's death. Preliminary research showed that this timing resulted in a better response rate than either a shorter or a longer time after the death.

The questionnaire also asked for various types of demographic and other information about both the patient and the caregiver. This was done so researchers could see if these characteristics were related to whether the patient's needs were met.

The hospice team assigned to the patient was also asked to fill out a questionnaire after the patient's death. This questionnaire was identical to the one given to the primary caregiver and required nursing team members to indicate the extent to which each need was met for the patient.

The Unit of Analysis

The patient and the members of his or her family were defined as the unit of analysis. Under ideal conditions, information should have been collected from the patient and all members of his or her family. Due to constraints of time, funds, and the realities of terminal illnesses, one family member—the primary caregiver—was asked to serve as a "proxy" for the patient. In other words, the primary caregiver was asked to estimate how the patient would have answered the questions had he or she been able to do so. The primary caregiver also was asked to indicate the extent to which his or her own needs had been met during the time the patient was enrolled in the hospice program.[30]

Selection of the Sample

The criteria for including the patient and family caregiver in the study sample were as follows:

1. The patient has a specific individual serving as the primary caregiver.
2. The caregiver is perceived by the hospice providers as emotionally stable.
3. The patient received at least three home visits from the hospice care team.

Of the 385 patients who enrolled in the hospice program during the two-year study period, 264 met the above criteria. Because researchers could not randomly select sample participants, given the nature and sensitivity of hospice work, the survey was sent to all eligible individuals. Following the hospice team's third visit to these patients, a hospice nurse presented the caregivers with a letter explaining the purposes of this study, a consent form, and a stamped, addressed envelope to be used to mail the consent form to the university research team. The nurse also verbally explained the nature of the study to the caregiver and answered any questions.

The nurses emphasized that the hospice care teams would not know the identity of the study participants. Nurses also emphasized that the caregivers' decisions in this regard would not, in any way, affect the services they or their family received from the hospice program. One hundred thirty-five of the caregivers consented to participate in the study. One hundred six caregivers completed the study.

Measurement of Program Effects

This evaluation measured the extent to which certain needs were met for various types of patients. It did not measure whether hospice care did a better job of meeting those needs than other forms of nonhospice care.

The evaluators utilized three different measures of program success. Two of these measures were attitudinal and the third was behavioral. First, the patient's caregiver was asked to estimate the extent to which the needs of the patient were met. Second, the hospice nursing team assigned to the patient was asked to estimate the extent to which his or her needs were met. Finally, the site of the patient's death (at home or in a hospital or other health care facility) was noted. It was assumed that the patient's dying at home indicated a higher level of need satisfaction than if he or she died elsewhere. It must be emphasized that the validity of this behavioral measure of patient satisfaction is open to question, although at least one study[31] has found a higher level of satisfaction reported for patients who died in a hospice program than for those who died during hospital terminal care.

Utilization of three different surveys enabled the researchers to compare scores on each to assess validity and reliability. Consistent scores on all three measures would increase the reliability of the surveys and the utility of their results in further hospice programming.

Each primary caregiver's responses to the need items were summed and the result divided by the number of need items. This produced a mean "success" score for each patient. A mean score of 1.0 indicates that none of the patient's needs were met at all, while a score of 7.0 indicates all of the needs were met. For the total sample, the mean score for primary caregivers' estimates of the degree to which patients' needs were met was 5.9.

A similar procedure was used to compute a mean "success" score based on the responses of the hospice nursing teams. The mean score for nurses' estimates of the success in meeting patients' needs was 5.1.

The behavioral measure (place of death) showed that 64.2 percent of all patients died at home. Evaluating the meaning of this finding is difficult because there is no standard for comparison. This figure simply indicates that nearly two-thirds of patients had the type of hospice experiences they wanted as measured by the absence of a facility admission. On the other hand, a large segment of patients, more than one-third, had at least one facility admission and thus a potentially less successful hospice experience.

Results of the Study

Results of any statistical analysis can be presented in a number of ways, not all of which are valuable to the hospice manager. In this study, the overall success ratings showed that both caregivers and nurses felt patients' needs were met quite well. However, nurses perceived patients as having somewhat less successful experiences than did caregivers. While the difference between the nurses' estimates and the caregivers' estimates was not large in absolute terms (5.1 versus 5.9), the evaluators showed program administrators that this difference was larger than would be expected by chance (i.e., the difference was statistically significant). Thus, nursing staff was less confident of their patients' satisfaction than were the primary caregivers.

The behavioral measure (place of death) showed that most patients (64.2 percent) maintained their in-home status for the duration of their hospice stays and also died at home. Therefore, this measure also indicates that a majority of the hospice patients had a successful hospice experience.

These results represent group averages. They present an overall picture of the program outcome, but they do not provide many important details. The evaluators utilized other techniques to provide program administrators with a more useful analysis of the data.

Several factors were tested to see if they had a statistically significant relationship to the three measures of success. These factors were (1) the age of the patient, (2) the patient's social class, (3) the patient's state of physical deterioration at the time of entry to the hospice program, (4) the degree to which the patient was aware of his or her terminal condition, and (5) the extent to which the primary caregiver had difficulty with care procedures. The results of this step in the analysis are shown in Table 3-1.

Table 3-1 Relationship between Selected Factors and the Three Measures of Success

Factor	Measure of Success		
	Caregivers' Scores	Nurses' Scores	Facility Admissions
Age of Patient	N.R.*	N.R.	N.R.
Social Class of Patient	N.R	N.R.	N.R.
Patient's State of Physical Deterioration	More deteriorated patients received higher success scores.	More deteriorated patients received lower success scores.	More deteriorated patients were less likely to be admitted (greater success).
Patient's Awareness of His or Her Terminal Condition	N.R.	The more aware patients were of their terminal status, the higher the success scores assigned to them by nurses.	N.R.
Caregiver's Difficulty With Care Procedures	N.R.	The fewer the difficulties experienced by the caregiver, the higher the success rating assigned to the patient by the nurses.	The fewer the difficulties experienced by the caregiver, the less likely the patient was to return to a health care facility (greater success).

*N.R. = No Relationship

Age of the Patient

Butterfield-Picardo and Magno suggest that hospice developed to respond to the needs of the elderly population.[32] This may have resulted because of the increasing size of the aged population and their high rates of affliction with chronic diseases.[33] The sensitivity of hospice care to the needs of the aged may also relate to societal values that define the death of an elderly person, compared with that of a younger person, as more acceptable.[34] It was hypothesized that the close link between the status of the aged population and hospice care would result in elderly patients having more successful hospice experiences. However, as Table 3-1 indicates, the age of the patient was not significantly related to any measures of success. Therefore, hospice program managers have no reason to expect that their programs will be more or less successful for patients in particular age categories.

Physical Deterioration

Patients who have severe physical deterioration when they enter hospice care generally are considered less likely to have a successful hospice experience.[35] Very deteriorated patients are unlikely to benefit from the holistic style of care mandated by the hospice philosophy[36] because care for these patients deals primarily with physical concerns, to the exclusion of social, emotional, and daily functioning needs. Therefore, it was hypothesized that patients with very deteriorated conditions would have less successful hospice experiences.

This expectation was supported in terms of nurses' perceptions of success. Nurses tended to rate more deteriorated patients as having less successful hospice experiences. Caregivers, on the other hand, tended to rate their patients as having more successful outcomes when the patients entered the program in a more deteriorated state. To some degree, program success as measured by the facility admissions coincided with caregivers' ratings. The more deteriorated patients were when they entered the program, the less likely they were to have a facility admission.

The findings imply that nurses were the only parties who believed that deterioration in the patient's condition impeded success. One explanation may be that the caregiver felt the patient was not ready for hospice care until the patient's condition was severe. When the patient reached this stage, hospice care became undeniably appropriate. Hospitalizations were also not considered as a necessary course of action for patients in worse condition. By the time patients had become severely deteriorated, the hospital clearly offered little benefit. In addition, the decision to keep the patient at home was made in light of his or her severe deterioration. Continued decline did not motivate a return to a facility. Home hospice care was selected by the client despite the patient's condition.

This finding has practical value for the program administrator. Administrators often protest that the hospice program is seen by many physicians simply as a "dumping ground" for patients whom they no longer can help and for whom death is very near. Such patients may not be welcomed by hospice care providers, because these patients are unable to experience hospice benefits. Data from this study, however, suggest that the state of the patient's deterioration upon admission is not unrelated to the caregiver's perception of the program's success. One explanation for this finding is that caregivers indicated satisfaction based on their assessment of the extent to which the program helped *them* in the arduous task of caring for a seriously ill patient. Since the patient *and the members of the patient's family* are seen as the unit of care in hospice programs, this finding suggests that severely deteriorated patients should not be regarded as unsuitable for hospice care. The members of their families may, in fact, be more in need than anyone else of the assistance a hospice program can offer.

Awareness Context

Hospice patients are expected to be aware of their terminal status.[37] Patients who openly accept their terminal status are portraying an attitude more consistent with the hospice philosophy of care. It was therefore hypothesized that the greater the patient's awareness the more successful the hospice experience. Results showed that the degree to which patients were aware of their terminal status had no relationship to the level of success as perceived by caregivers, or to the likelihood of facility admissions. However, results differed for nursing staff. Nurses tended to rate patients who were more openly aware of their terminal status as more likely to have their needs met than those who were less aware of their status.

This implies that hospice nurses were more concerned with the patient's awareness of his or her terminal status than were the caregivers. Nurses' perceptions of success were related to the patient's awareness, whereas caregivers' perceptions of success were unaffected by this factor. One explanation for this finding is that nurses are highly committed to the hospice philosophy of care. A mandate of this philosophy is that patients should be openly aware of their terminal status. Patients who do not comply with this mandate may be considered less successful since they are not showing an acceptance of the hospice philosophy. Caregivers, on the other hand, may be unconcerned with the hospice philosophy. Their interest may simply be to manage their patient at home, keeping him or her as comfortable as possible. Similarly, the awareness context of the patient is not of central importance in affecting whether or not the patient returns to a facility or remains at home for the entire hospice stay.

This finding raises questions for program managers. In what ways do the philosophical views of staff members affect the quality of care? Can providers become so devoted to a point of view that this dedication impedes the quality of care?

Caregiver's Difficulty with Procedures

Patients who enroll in home-based hospice care are expected to have a family member or friend to provide the vast majority of patient care.[38] Participation by the primary caregiver is perceived as being beneficial to the emotional status of the patient and caregiver.

A question has been raised as to whether it can be realistically assumed that caregivers can adjust to the intense responsibilities of caring for a terminally ill patient.[39] There are many aspects of caregiving that may cause problems. Consideration in this investigation focused on the amount of difficulty caregivers had performing procedural aspects of care. It was hypothesized that the more difficulties caregivers experienced with procedures, the less successful hospice care would be for the patients.

Findings for this factor varied depending on which of the three measures of success one considers. Success, as measured by caregivers ratings, was unaffected by the amount of difficulties they encountered. However, nurses' assessments of success showed that patients whose caregivers had less difficulty were rated as having higher levels of success. In contrast, in terms of facility admissions, the fewer the difficulties caregivers experienced, the higher the probability of the patients being admitted to a facility and thus the lower the rate of success.

Nurses' ratings of success for patients were affected by the amount of difficulties the caregiver experienced with procedural aspects of care, while caregivers' ratings of success, on the other hand, were unaffected by difficulties with procedures. The probability of the patient having a facility admission actually *decreased* with an increase in the amount of difficulties caregivers had in performing procedural aspects of care.

One explanation for this finding may be that nurses and caregivers use different criteria in evaluating factors affecting success. Nurses feel that problems with procedures lead to negative outcomes. Caregivers may experience difficulties, but these difficulties do not result in a lowering of the caregivers' perceptions of success.

This finding also has a practical implication for the program administrator. It is possible—and perhaps even probable—that nurses (and administrators) and clients assign different meanings to the same act. Such differences can easily lead to misunderstandings and to communication problems. The hospice administrator may find it beneficial to develop an information-sharing system that will allow all parties involved in the care process to share viewpoints and develop an assessment of specific care procedures.

Interpretation and Applications

A patient who was rated as having a successful hospice experience by his or her primary caregiver did not necessarily receive a successful rating by the nursing team or die at home. In other words, the three different measures of success were not strongly related to each other. Lack of congruence between the measures of success suggests that (1) one or more of the measures may not have been valid, (2) the three different measures may have been measuring different types or aspects of success, or (3) the members of the different respondent categories may have used different criteria in evaluating program success.

Methodological and practical implications can be derived from comparing the indicators of success. Methodologically, administrators interested in evaluating program success should understand problems in defining the concept. Since success connotes different things to different people, evaluation of hospice programs can be effective only if success is considered to have many dimensions. A program may be very successful in one respect, but not in others. In fact, the achievement of one form of success may impede the attainment of alternative forms.

From a programmatic viewpoint, findings from this study show that different parties involved in hospice care use different criteria in evaluating the hospice's success. Logically, primary caregivers who felt that hospice care successfully met their patients' needs should be less likely to have cared for a patient who returned to a facility. Statistical analysis indicated that this was not the case. Similarly, it was expected that nurses would evaluate a patient's outcome as successful if the patient maintained his or her home care status for the duration of the stay in hospice. This, however, was not supported by the data. Caregivers and nurses did not agree on the extent to which hospice care was successful for a given patient. Nor were their success ratings strongly related to program success as measured by the facility admissions. Therefore, program managers interested in improving their program may find that not all persons involved in a hospice program can be pleased at the same time. Improvement or the achievement of success becomes a relative phenomenon.

The problematic task of evaluating such elusive concepts as quality and success is best accomplished by utilizing the input of divergent professionals and consumers of care. It is through the influence and motivations of these individuals that program outcomes can be measured and shaped.

Characteristics of patients who used the hospice in the past can be used to predict the probability of patients' success. By knowing this, hospice administrators can give special attention to patients who have a high probability of having less successful outcomes. This would increase the likelihood that these patients would have more successful outcomes in the future.

An example of the utility of this evaluation is found in the analysis of facility admissions. One characteristic related to a patient's facility admission is the amount of difficulty the hospice nurses feel the patient's caregiver has providing care. On the basis of this finding, an administrator interested in reducing hospital utilization might request that nurses estimate their perceptions of the amount of difficulty caregivers experience. Any caregiver assessed as having a greater than average amount of difficulty could be given special assistance with care procedures. Hopefully, this would reduce the likelihood of the patient being returned to a facility from the home hospice program. Success, as defined by the number of facility admissions, would then be increased.

Summary

Evaluation is an important aspect of hospice programming. A well conducted evaluation study can identify program strengths and weaknesses and provide administrators with important information for future service delivery. There are varied approaches and types of program evaluation. The hospice manager and planner should carefully consider his or her information needs and the requirements of external funding agencies and third-party payers when designing an evaluation.

The hospice evaluation described provides administrators and service providers with an illustration of the divergent uses of evaluation research. The results of the study emphasize the importance of looking at any issue from more than one point of view. The extent to which patients in this program had a "successful" hospice experience varies according to the measure of success employed. This awareness will help administrators predict how similar types of patients and caregivers may react to the hospice program.

Furthermore, the results show that a majority of the hospice patients sampled had their needs met successfully. The empirical evidence supporting this statement will be helpful to program administrators in their negotiations with funding and regulatory agencies.

NOTES

1. Emily Mumford, *Medical Sociology: Patients, Providers, and Policies* (New York: Random House, 1983), 86.

2. J.D. Christoffel and M. Lowenthal, "Evaluating the Quality of Ambulatory Health Care: A Review of Emerging Methods," *Medical Care* 5 (November, 1977).

3. Florence Nightingale, *Proposal for Improved Statistics of Surgical Operations* (London: Savil & Edwards, 1863). Cited in Frank Baker and Carol B. McPhee, "Approaches to Evaluating Quality of Health Care" in *Program Evaluation in the Health Fields*, Vol. II, ed. Herbert C. Schulberg and Frank Baker (New York: Human Sciences Press, 1979).

4. Herbert C. Schulberg and Frank Baker, "Evaluating Health Programs: Art and/or Science?" in *Program Evaluation in the Health Fields*, Vol. II, ed. Herbert C. Schulberg and Frank Baker (New York: Human Sciences Press, 1979), 3–33.

5. Louise H. Kidder, *Sellitz, Wrightsman, and Cook's Research Methods in Social Relations*, 4th ed. (New York: Holt, Rinehart and Winston, 1981), 83.

6. Maurice Yaffe and Edward Nelson, eds., *The Influence of Pornography on Behavior* (New York: Academic Press, 1982).

7. Carol H. Weiss, *Evaluation Research: Methods for Assessing Effectiveness* (Englewood Cliffs, N.J.: Prentice-Hall, 1972).

8. Aaron Wildavsky, "The Self-Evaluating Organization," *Program Evaluation in the Health Fields*, Vol. II, ed. Herbert C. Schulberg and Frank Baker (New York: Human Sciences Press, 1979).

9. Weiss, *Evaluation Research*, 20–21.

10. Gerald L. Barkdoll, "Type III Evaluations. Consultation Consensus," *Public Administration Review* (March/April 1980): 174–179.

11. Michael Quinn Patton, *Practical Evaluation* (Beverly Hills, Calif.: Sage, 1982).

12. J. N. Nay et al., "If You Don't Care Where You Get To, Then It Doesn't Matter Which Way You Go," in *The Evaluation of Social Programs*, ed. C.C. Abt (Beverly Hills, Calif.: Sage, 1979).

13. Weiss, *Evaluation Research*, 26–30.

14. Ibid., 24–25.

15. D.T. Campbell and J.C. Stanley, *Experimental and Quasi-Experimental Designs for Research* (Chicago: Rand McNally, 1966).

16. Thomas D. Cook and Donald T. Campbell, *Quasi-Experimentation: Design and Analysis Issues for Field Settings* (Chicago: Rand McNally, 1979).

17. Campbell and Stanley, *Experimental and Quasi-Experimental Designs*, 34–37.

18. Weiss, *Evaluation Research*; Irwin Deutscher, "Toward Avoiding the Goal Trap in Evaluation Research," in *Readings in Evaluation Research*, ed. F.G. Caro (New York: Russell Sage, 1977); Mumford, *Medical Sociology*.

19. Claire Sellitz, Laurence S. Wrightsman, and Stuart W. Cook, *Research Methods in Social Relations*, 3rd ed. (New York: Holt, Rinehart and Winston, 1976).

20. Ibid., 169.

21. Ibid., 183.

22. Herbert C. Schulberg and Frank Baker, "Program Evaluation Models and the Implementation of Research Findings," in *Program Evaluation in the Health Fields*, ed. Herbert C. Schulberg, Alan Sheldon, and Frank Baker (New York: Behavioral Publications, 1969), 562–572.

23. Harold P. Halpert, "Communication as a Basic Tool in Promoting Utilization of Research Findings," in *Program Evaluation in the Health Fields*, ed. Herbert C. Schulberg, Alan Sheldon, and Frank Baker (New York: Behavioral Publications, 1969), 497–505.

24. Robert Bogdan et al., "Let Them Eat Programs: Attendants' Perspectives and Programming on Wards in State Schools," *Journal of Health and Social Behavior* 15 (June 1974): 142–151.

25. Robert W. Buckingham and Dale Lupu, "A Comparative Study of Hospice Services in the United States," *American Journal of Public Health* 72 (May 1982): 455–461.

26. David S. Greer et al., *National Hospice Study Preliminary Final Report, Extended Executive Summary* (Providence, R.I.: Brown University, 1983).

27. Visiting Nurse Service, *Visiting Nurse Service Demonstration Project: Objectives* (Unpublished document, Akron, Ohio: The Visiting Nurse Service, July 20, 1979).

28. For a complete list of patient and family needs, see David M. Bass, "An Evaluation of the 'Success' of a Home Based Hospice Program" (Ph.D. diss., The University of Akron, 1985).

29. Campbell and Stanley, *Experimental and Quasi-Experimental Designs*.

30. Bass, "An Evaluation of the 'Success' of a Home Based Hospice Program."

31. David Naylor, "Quality of Life as an Outcome of Hospice Care" (Ph.D. diss., The University of Akron, 1984).

32. Helen Butterfield-Picardo and Josefina Magno, "Hospice the Adjective, Not the Noun," *American Psychologist* 37 (1982): 1254–1259.

33. Lenora Finn Paradis, "The Integration of Hospice Programs into the Traditional Health Care Systems: A Sociological Study" (Ph.D. diss., Michigan State University, 1983).

34. R. A. Kalish, "The Aged and the Dying: The Inevitable Questions," *Journal of Social Issues* 21 (1965): 87–96; Robert J. Kastenbaum, "Death, Dying, and Bereavement in Old Age," *Aged Care and Services Review* 1 (1978): 200–207; John F. Potter, "A Challenge for the Hospice Movement," *New England Journal of Medicine* 302 (1) (1980): 53–55.

35. Fred P. Pestello and David M. Bass, "Goal Impediments in Two Hospice Programs." *Nursing and Health Care* 4 (September 1983): 397–399; Nannabell Cook et al., "Sources of Stress and Stress Reducers in Hospice Nursing" (Paper presented at the North Central Sociological Association Annual Meetings, Cleveland, Ohio, 1981).

36. National Hospice Organization, *Standards of a Hospice Program of Care*, 6th rev. ed. (McLean, Va.: National Hospice Organization, 1979).

37. Roberta Lyder Paige and Jane Finkbiner Looney, "Hospice Care for the Adult," *American Journal of Nursing* (November 1977): 1812–1815; Sylvia Lack, "Philosophy and Organization of a Hospice Program," *Proceedings of the First National Training Conference for Physicians on Psychological Care of the Dying Patient*, University of California School of Medicine, San Francisco, Calif., April 19–May 1, 1976.

38. Butterfield-Picardo and Magno, "Hospice the Adjective."

39. Robert Fulton, "The Sociology of Death," *Death Education* 1 (1977): 15–25.

Appendix 3-A

List of Needs of Terminally Ill Patients

	Not important at all					Extremely important		Don't know or not sure/ No response
	1	2	3	4	5	6	7	9
1. The need to know that medical care will be available at any time, day or night	1	2	3	4	5	6	7	9
2. The need for help with financial worries resulting from the illness	1	2	3	4	5	6	7	9
3. The need to finish up any "unfinished business," such as seeing friends or places again	1	2	3	4	5	6	7	9
4. The need to maintain as close to normal relationships with the family as possible	1	2	3	4	5	6	7	9
5. The need for close contact with family members	1	2	3	4	5	6	7	9
6. The need to feel that he/she will not be a burden to the family	1	2	3	4	5	6	7	9
7. The need to control pain	1	2	3	4	5	6	7	9

	Not important at all					Extremely important		Don't know or not sure/ No response
	1	2	3	4	5	6	7	9
8. The need to discuss appropriate plans for the future	1	2	3	4	5	6	7	9
9. The need for assistance in caring for pets	1	2	3	4	5	6	7	9
10. The need for help with any legal matters related to his/her illness	1	2	3	4	5	6	7	9
11. The need to understand the reasons for any medical procedures	1	2	3	4	5	6	7	9
12. The need to know that family members will have help with financial problems other than expenses resulting from his/her illness	1	2	3	4	5	6	7	9
13. The need to know that family members will have open and honest communication with his/her doctors	1	2	3	4	5	6	7	9
14. The need to have his/her wishes respected by the hospice nurses	1	2	3	4	5	6	7	9
15. The need to choose the place where he/she will receive medical care (home or in the hospital)	1	2	3	4	5	6	7	9
16. The need for help with grocery shopping or running errands	1	2	3	4	5	6	7	9
17. The need to know the course his/her illness is going to take	1	2	3	4	5	6	7	9

	Not important at all					Extremely important		Don't know or not sure/ No response
	1	2	3	4	5	6	7	9
18. The need to know that the doctors and nurses will consider his/her individual needs rather than treating him/her as just another patient	1	2	3	4	5	6	7	9
19. The need for help with emotional difficulties	1	2	3	4	5	6	7	9
20. The need to know that the family will have a clear understanding of the illness and the course it is going to take	1	2	3	4	5	6	7	9
21. The need to discuss his/her feelings about the illness	1	2	3	4	5	6	7	9
22. The need for a friendly person who is not a member of the family to talk with	1	2	3	4	5	6	7	9
23. The need for help with housework or household tasks	1	2	3	4	5	6	7	9
24. The need to have transportation assistance to and from the hospital or other medical facility	1	2	3	4	5	6	7	9
25. The need to know that family members will have help with any emotional difficulties they may experience as a result of his/her illness	1	2	3	4	5	6	7	9
26. The need for medical supplies (other than medication)	1	2	3	4	5	6	7	9

	Not important at all					Extremely important		Don't know or not sure/ No response
	1	2	3	4	5	6	7	9

27. The need for some-one to talk to about religious or spiritual concerns	1	2	3	4	5	6	7	9
28. The need for honest and open communica-tion with the doctors and nurses	1	2	3	4	5	6	7	9
29. The need to have doctors and nurses ask his/her permission to perform any medi-cal procedures	1	2	3	4	5	6	7	9
30. The need for help in caring for his/her chil-dren	1	2	3	4	5	6	7	9
31. The need to have his/her wishes respected by physicians	1	2	3	4	5	6	7	9
32. The need for help in preparing meals	1	2	3	4	5	6	7	9
33. The need to know that family members will be able to obtain help with any trans-portation difficulties	1	2	3	4	5	6	7	9
34. The need to know that family members will have open and honest communication with his/her hospice nurses	1	2	3	4	5	6	7	9

Please add any additional needs not listed that you feel will be very important for the patient.

_____

_____

_____

Part II

Hospice Programming:
Applying Divergent Models

Chapter 4

The Application of Hospice Principles in Long-Term Care

Greg Owen

During the past ten years in the United States, hospice programs for the dying have experienced unprecedented growth. As noted in Chapter 1, nearly 1,500 hospice programs can be identified throughout the United States today. Most metropolitan areas have one or more hospice programs in operation and many smaller communities, if they do not have programs, are examining the prospects for developing hospice services. The concept of delivering appropriate and compassionate care to the terminally ill has found widespread support and acceptance among many health care professionals as well as the lay public.

It may appear that hospice programs have found their niche in the American health care scene as evidenced not only by their phenomenal growth, but also by the availability of their services under a new Medicare option. In form, however, hospice programs continue to show enormous variation and resist rigid classification. Despite the efforts of many hospice advocates to codify standards and promote accreditation, the hospice concept remains fluid in American society and can be found as a component in many types of institutional arrangements.

Program variations notwithstanding, the hospice philosophy has focused on the following aspects of care:

- The relief of social, emotional, and physical distress, particularly pain in all of its forms
- The value of home care or a homelike environment in which care can be provided
- The potential role of family members, friends, and volunteers in performing various caregiving functions
- The need to carefully monitor the symptoms and progress of an illness while keeping patients and families informed
- The need to support, assist, and respect the wishes of families as well as patients

- The importance of having health professionals available to help patients and families when needed
- The usefulness of a medically directed team approach in meeting the needs of patients and families
- The value of bereavement follow-up with families after a patient's death
- The importance of providing hospice services to all dying persons regardless of their ability to pay

To the extent that hospice represents a set of ideal values associated with care for the dying, health care administrators and planners from various settings are asking, "What relevance does hospice have for my organization? Do we need a full-fledged hospice program or should we simply borrow and use what seems to apply here?"

The questions are not academic. J. Albin Yokie, Executive Vice President of the American College of Nursing Home Administrators, believes that while

> there are not many hospice programs serving nursing home patients in the United States today . . . the nursing home administrator can identify the needs of the dying patient, recognize that the nursing home staff is already oriented toward death and dying patients and build upon this experience to develop a strategy to provide hospice care.[1]

He argues that "the perceived need to provide hospice care in the nursing home and the increasing public interest in the provision of this care should encourage nursing home administrators to explore ways to provide such care."[2]

It appears that others in the nursing home industry agree. With planning that began in 1977, the Evangelical Lutheran Good Samaritan Society implemented a hospice program in 1981 in one of its long-term care facilities located in Moscow, Idaho. A short time later, another Good Samaritan facility in Windom, Minnesota, developed a similar program. Both were founded on the belief that dying patients and their families need the comfort, support, and relief that hospice care provides. Both emphasize an interdisciplinary team approach, control of pain and other symptoms, social and emotional support of patients and families, and bereavement care for the family. Home care, although not available through the facility, can be arranged for through other community providers. Most care costs are covered by Medicare, Medicaid, or an insurance provider, with the balance of cost to be "paid privately according to a patient's means."[3]

The idea of putting the hospice concept to work in nursing homes is not a new one. In fact, many nursing home administrators and staff contend they have been "doing hospice for years" without the hospice designation. There is, to be sure, some justification for this claim considering the substantial numbers of persons who spend the last months of their lives in nursing homes and who are cared for until death by long-term care personnel. Nonetheless, the hospice concept offers a specific focus, as well as a set of clearly defined standards, toward which to strive.

Nursing homes contain mixed populations. Some residents will live a long time and participate in a variety of therapeutic experiences during their stay. Others die shortly after admission. Some are clear-headed and communicate their concerns easily. Others are frequently or always confused or disoriented. Many have families and many do not. Some will die miserable, painful deaths and some will enjoy the support and relief provided by well-trained and compassionate caregivers. Individual nursing homes vary considerably in the quality of care and expertise they are able to bring to the dying patient's bedside.

Nursing homes of all shapes and sizes, of all levels of quality, have begun to recognize the contribution hospice principles and protocols can make in the long-term care environment. This chapter explores the relationship between hospice care and long-term care through an examination of the incidence of deaths in nursing homes, the history and public perceptions of nursing home care, the way the hospice concept works in some nursing homes, and the promise and problems to be expected by the integration of hospice and long-term care.

DEATHS IN NURSING HOMES

One of the by-products of twentieth-century science, with the control of disease and the extension of the average life span, has been the clustering of deaths at the end of the age spectrum. At the turn of the century, more than half of all deaths occurred among children under age 15. Today, children under 15 account for only 3.3 percent of all deaths. Persons over 65, however, now account for 67 percent of all deaths.[4] While nursing homes may, at any one time, house only 4 to 5 percent of those over 65, statistics on place of death show that between 20 and 25 percent of deaths of persons age 65 and over occur in nursing homes.[5,6] For 1980, that means approximately 312,650 deaths of persons 65 and over occurred in America's 23,000 nursing homes.[7] This figure does not include residents transferred to a hospital to die during the last days of life.

The numbers are compelling and indicate a need to address issues of terminal care in the long-term care facility. However, there is another problem that cannot be as easily represented, that is, the image and public perceptions of nursing homes.

HISTORY

Hospice programs and nursing homes do not share a common history. Chapter 1 describes the emergence of the hospice concept during the Middle Ages as a refuge for the sick and homeless, a place for weary travelers who needed rest.

The service was almost always dispensed by members of a religious order as part of their commitment to serve others.

During the nineteenth century, the Irish Sisters of Charity offered care to those suffering from typhus and cholera in Dublin and established their hospice as a service to the dying and destitute. When the Irish Sisters were invited to London at the beginning of the twentieth century, they established St. Joseph's Hospice in London. St. Joseph's later became the training ground for Dr. Cicely Saunders, the woman who became the leader of the modern British hospice movement. The needs she recognized among dying patients led her to establish St. Christopher's Hospice in 1967, which later became the prototype for the first American hospice programs.

Work at St. Christopher's Hospice is based on the ethic that "no dying patient anywhere should suffer unrelieved relievable distress."[8] This focus, along with an emphasis on spiritual values, has had an important impact on American hospices. In particular, it has meant that American hospice providers, for the most part, see their work as a moral commitment to the dying.

In contrast, nursing homes have their roots in almshouses and poorhouses of the late nineteenth and early twentieth century.[9] These were not desirable places, but a growing elderly population (three million over 65 by 1900) made such facilities necessary. Early nursing homes typically were managed by a matron and organized to be self-supporting through the operation of a farm. People who lived in such settings were called inmates. Services consisted of food and shelter and not much more. A report prepared by the Department of Labor in 1925 found the conditions in the typical almshouse "deplorable."[10]

One of the problems with the almshouse system was that it housed the infirm elderly alongside the insane, the retarded, and the depraved. The only common attribute was poverty. When the Social Security Act was passed in 1935, it established a system of cash benefits for old age assistance (OAA) allowing eligible recipients to spend their benefits as they chose. However, the act prohibited anyone living in a public institution from receiving benefits.[11] When it became clear that many OAA recipients could not be maintained in their own homes, the services of proprietary homes (including rest homes and convalescent centers) looked attractive, particularly since they could be paid for with OAA benefits. Conditions in these facilities, however, were less than desirable and the government exhorted owners to upgrade them.

By the early 1940s, some changes were visible in the nursing home industry. "Private entrepreneurs were offering nursing and personal care services over and above what boarding homes had traditionally provided. Private homes for the aged began to provide health services for their residents."[12]

With the end of World War II, the federal government began substantial investment in hospital construction with funds made available through the Hill-Burton Act. In 1954 this act was amended to also provide funds for nursing home construction. During the same time period, the Social Security Act was amended to provide payments to persons in public institutions and to allow the federal government to match payments by state and local welfare providers to the suppliers of nursing home services. In addition, the legislation required states to license nursing homes.

With the advent of the Kerr-Mills law in 1960, medical assistance for the aged was made available and vendor payments for nursing home care increased. The passage of Medicare[13] and Medicaid[14] legislation in 1965 opened up additional funding sources for nursing homes. However, there was still a pervasive view that "most nursing homes were inadequate, incapable not only of meeting the objectives of the 'extended care' philosophy but even more modest goals of decent custodial service."[15]

Medicare was important in shaping the reimbursement system for nursing homes and in providing payments based on reasonable costs. Medicare law required round-the-clock nursing services and the employment of at least one full-time registered nurse. However, Medicaid standards were different. When they were finally adopted in 1967, they did not require the presence of a registered nurse on any shift and permitted practical nurses, licensed on the basis of experience, to be in charge of nursing care.[16]

With amendments introduced by Senator Frank Moss in 1969, regulations became more stringent and required the establishment of standards for record keeping, medical care, environment, dietary, drug dispensing, and sanitation. A companion amendment introduced by Senator Edward Kennedy required the licensing of administrators. All of this was done, in part, in a response to discoveries by the Senate Subcommittee on Long Term Care, chaired by Senator Moss. Extensive hearings in 1965 had uncovered serious problems in sanitation, services, and basic care in America's nursing homes; but despite various legislative attempts, conditions did not improve markedly during the 1960s. When, in the early 1970s, many more negative reports on nursing homes appeared, the Nixon Administration established the Office of Nursing Home Affairs for the enforcement of existing laws and regulations. The lifting of price controls on health care facilities in 1974 caused Medicaid expenditures for nursing homes to skyrocket. Antifraud and abuse legislation passed in 1977 was, in part, an attempt to control these expenses.[17] No amount of money, however, can change the fact that nursing homes operate as part of the federal welfare system. In contrast to this, the hospice concept continues to be carried by a wave of public enthusiasm and, until recently, was not part of a government-sponsored general financing program.[18]

NURSING HOMES TODAY

Two recent and well-known books on nursing homes, *Too Old, Too Sick, Too Bad* (1977) by Senator Frank Moss and Val Halamandaris, and *Unloving Care* (1980) by Bruce Vladeck, review the organization and quality of care in American nursing homes. Both books describe inadequate conditions, find fault with public policy, and seek ways of making improvements.

Moss and Halamandaris, in a search for solutions, describe what they call "America's finest nursing homes." They are characterized by a spirit of co-operation among staff, a concern for the individualized treatment of residents, and a basic respect for human dignity. In describing testimony before the Senate Subcommittee on Long Term Care, the authors write,

> Witnesses before the subcommittee said again and again that good nursing homes are a matter of motivation. Of paramount importance to the quality of care is the administrator's ability to inspire his staff, to create the kind of harmony, unity of purpose, and spirit which makes a great symphony orchestra.[19]

In a chapter entitled "Doing Better," Bruce Vladeck examines current public policies and regulations and how they affect the nursing home industry. While he feels that incremental improvement can be expected through "the development of more flexible regulatory sanctions,"[20] other changes are necessary. In particular, he suggests rethinking the role of physicians in nursing homes with an eye toward improving the quality of medical services. Geriatric training programs, nurse practitioners, and clinical ties to universities are all seen as potential vehicles for upgrading the quality of medical care in nursing homes. The idea that physicians might also become involved in providing direction to nursing and social services within nursing homes may, according to Vladeck, be too much to expect.

Another potential avenue for reform involves "further mobilization of third parties, notably community groups, general-purpose agencies for the aging, and charitable organizations."[21] Outside sources of voluntary support can help reduce residents' isolation and simultaneously provide community residents with a greater stake in the care of elderly citizens.

The suggestions for improving nursing home care reflect the heart of the hospice movement. Good quality medical care and symptom assessment, a team approach to individualized treatment, respect for people's dignity, and the recruitment and use of volunteer services are all part of the hospice philosophy. If these ideas are compatible with better nursing home care, then the hospice concept may offer a much-needed course correction that can benefit not only the dying, but all nursing home residents. But what form might hospice care take within long-term care settings? How should a concerned manager or administrator attempt to realize hospice objectives? What are the potential funding sources? What does the community need? What services are required? What specific goals should be sought? What problems might be anticipated? And what has been accomplished already?

THE NEED FOR HOSPICE CARE IN NURSING HOMES: THREE SURVEYS

A recent statewide survey of 89 nursing homes, conducted by the Minnesota Coalition for Terminal Care, examined methods of care for dying residents and interest in the hospice concept.[22] The study respondents, who were primarily directors of nursing, characterized nearly 60 percent of all deaths in their facilities as being preceded by a period of "known terminal illness." Moreover, when asked to describe staff problems in providing care to dying residents, approximately 75 percent indicated problems in providing supportive care, relieving the discomfort of caregivers, and communicating adequately with patients and families. The majority of facilities (63 percent) spent between one and four hours a year on inservice education related to terminal care. Seventy-four percent of the respondents felt that additional inservice educational programs on terminal care would be helpful and indicated a need for information concerning (1) comfort care, (2) communications with residents and families about death, (3) how to help with grief and bereavement, and (4) the relief of symptoms.

Almost half (46 percent) of the respondents felt that they were already providing some aspects of hospice care, and a comparable proportion (45 percent) felt that most hospice principles could be implemented in long-term care facilities. Only 27 percent of the nursing directors felt that state or federal policies inhibited their ability to provide appropriate care to the terminally ill.

A similar study conducted in Alberta, Canada, in 1983 surveyed nursing directors and administrators in 83 (86 percent) of Alberta's extended care facilities.[23] Questions focused on care of the dying, including control of pain and symptoms, adequacy of meeting patient and staff needs, terminal care policies, and preferences for different models of care. The study found that most facilities did not have any specific policies regarding the care of dying residents, although a number indicated that they were currently in the process of developing palliative care policies or hospice programs. The majority of respondents felt that terminal care was distinct from other forms, citing that it was "more individualized" or "one-to-one" and often required increased attention to physical and psychosocial needs.[24] Although pain control did not emerge as a major unmet need in this study, more than half of the respondents felt that the resources available to provide emotional support to patients and families were less than adequate.[25] Educational resources for staff were also rated as less than adequate by nearly half (47 percent) of the respondents.[26] Overall, every facility except one believed that modifications could be made to enhance the palliative care provided in extended care institutions.

The surveys lend support to the idea that nursing home caregivers see a role for hospice care in their facilities. It also indicates that inservice education in the area of terminal care may be inadequate.

Another study, completed in 1981, examined the quality of care for the dying in Ramsey County, Minnesota (including the city of St. Paul and surrounding suburbs).[27] The study utilized a random sample of all county death certificate records and enlisted the services of attending physicians to identify which deaths were preceded by a period of terminal illness. Following the identification of cases by physicians, family members (N = 150) were asked to participate in an interview designed to provide a portrait of care during the last year of the decedent's life.

The study found that 36 percent of all deaths that were preceded by a terminal illness occurred in nursing homes. Moreover, nearly half (47 percent) of all respondents whose relatives had received nursing home care (N = 73) expressed dissatisfaction with the quality of care following the patient's first admission. The most frequent dissatisfactions focused on inappropriate treatment, lack of respect for the patient and family, and poor quality care. Less than one-third of the respondents could recall an offer of emotional support from nursing home caregivers. In general, both patients and family members considered nursing home care to be the least satisfactory form of care for terminally ill persons.

Taken together, the results of the three surveys suggest that nursing home staff members, as well as residents and their families, might benefit from the incorporation of hospice principles and the provision of hospice services in long-term care settings.

COMPONENTS OF HOSPICE IN LONG-TERM CARE

Pain and Symptom Control

Hospice programs focus on the control or elimination of pain in order to increase patient comfort and reduce the family's anxiety. While autonomous hospice programs with active medical direction may rely heavily on physicians to assess and adjust pain medications, hospice programs in nursing homes rely, to a greater extent, on nursing staff assessments, standing pain control protocols, and telephone requests for appropriate medication orders from attending physicians.

Some nursing home hospice programs have employed consulting pharmacists to provide pain control recommendations and inservice education for staff. Protocols may emphasize the use of pain control cocktails (oral morphine and cherry syrup in a water and alcohol base), routine administration of medication every 4 or 6 hours (not PRN), and titrated dosages that can be reduced daily until a minimum effective dosage is achieved. Other comfort measures, including the use of tricyclic antidepressants, drugs to control nausea, whirlpool baths, heat, rubs, waterbed mattresses, and patients' favorite remedies, are also employed.

Pain and symptom control is an important element of hospice services. Administrators and planners should take measures to ensure that this focus is adequately developed in a nursing home hospice program. The identification of pain control as a primary program objective can be reinforced through inservice education, the creation of a symptom control library or resource center, consultation with other hospice programs or pain control clinics, as well as the acknowledgment and reward of staff expertise in this area. Consulting pharmacists and geriatric nurse practitioners with experience in comprehensive patient assessment are particularly helpful.

Resuscitation and Supportive Care

Hospice care is appropriate when recovery is unlikely and death is expected. However, not all hospice providers agree on exactly what separates palliative and supportive care from other forms of care. Admission to some programs depends on the patient's willingness to forgo life-sustaining measures such as cardio-pulmonary resuscitation and intubation. Other programs accept patients with or without such orders. Typically, nursing home hospice programs maintain a policy of discussing potential orders for DNR (Do Not Resuscitate), DNI (Do Not Intubate), SCO (Supportive Care Only), and/or JUCTO (Justified Use of Conservative Treatment Only) with families and patients upon admission to the hospice program. While the precise implications of these orders vary among facilities, they generally mean that extraordinary measures will not be used to prolong a patient's life.

The policy of discussing these orders with potential hospice patients and families has been useful in clarifying the intent of the hospice program. Patients and families are given the opportunity to alter such orders at some future time. Occasionally, discussion of these issues results in disagreement among patients and family members concerning the appropriateness and desirability of resuscitation and supportive care. When conflicts can't be resolved, the decision of a competent patient should be followed. For more information on the ethics and legality of code orders see Chapters 10 and 13.

Another issue in the area of supportive care concerns feeding and hydration. Because of the social and symbolic nature of the feeding act, it is an issue that often sparks controversy. While the ethics of feeding and hydration are discussed in later chapters, certain technologies—for example, the use of nasogastric tubes—may create conflicts among patients, families, and staff. When death is near, families may insist that feeding continue, despite its total ineffectiveness. Hydration can also pose problems. It is not unusual in British hospices to provide fluids while the patient sleeps using rectal infusion much like an intravenous drip. However, this practice is uncommon in the United States. Fluids given by mouth may be adequate until swallowing becomes difficult, at which point smaller amounts provided at more regular intervals are necessary.

Toward the last, after even a few drops would cause choking, if a gauze wicking, one end of which is held in a cup of ice water, is put into the patient's mouth it often will be gratefully sucked. Except for drawing in the breath, sucking is the body's last, as it is the first instinctive action. Thirst is our first and last craving. The complaint just before death on the cross was, "I thirst." And then the sponge dipped in vinegar was the kindest possible offering.[28]

Staffing

Staffing is an area in which long-term care administrators are justifiably sensitive. Intermediate and skilled care facilities alike have difficulty providing necessary care without exceeding the staffing hours for which they are paid. With the advent of hospital reimbursement based on Medicare's Diagnostic Related Groups, adequate staffing may prove to be even more difficult. Patients are discharged from hospitals sooner and may place heavy demands on the staff of the facilities to which they are discharged. For this reason, nursing home hospice programs typically cannot hire a specialized hospice staff.

Hospice care in a nursing home, according to one administrator, must be " . . . entirely incorporated into the existing service delivery program."[29] This means that the hospice coordinator must also serve nonhospice patients and that hospice inservice education must be available to all employees. This situation has benefits as well as disadvantages. On the one hand, inservice education exposes all staff to the hospice philosophy while enhancing caregiving skills in the area of terminal care. It can also mean that hospice-type caregiving "rubs off" on nonhospice patients and may contribute to overall staff and resident morale. On the other hand, a greater awareness of the hospice concept among residents and staff can place additional burdens on caregivers. This occurs when nonhospice patients seek some of the same privileges offered to terminally ill residents. Increased requests for special foods, overnight visiting, or staff time by residents who are not terminally ill may seem unreasonable. These considerations can have implications for where the program is located in a facility (private rooms versus multiple-bed rooms) and how services are delivered (within a special unit or throughout the facility). These choices can, in part, be determined by how the program is viewed by nonhospice residents who see themselves either as adversaries excluded from the program or allies potentially benefiting from hospice care.

Volunteers play an important role in communicating the intent of a hospice program to long-term care residents. As in traditional hospice services, nursing home hospice programs work best when supported by volunteers. But volunteers need to work with both hospice and nonhospice residents in order that they not be seen as exclusive envoys to the dying. Volunteers who are trained in working with the dying and their families can ease staff burden, promote personal relationships, and deal more easily with nonterminally ill residents who have similar, but less immediate, concerns. Volunteers also provide community visibility for programs while encouraging other residents to actively help those receiving hospice care.

Inservice education and the formation of a team approach to residents' needs must go hand in hand in a nursing home hospice program. Staff members need to feel they have something to contribute. Inservice education should focus on the specific roles and responsibilities of nursing, social services, dietary, chaplaincy, occupational, physical, and recreational therapy, housekeeping, and volunteers. In some facilities, this can be a difficult task, particularly if there are many part-time staff. For this reason, staff development programs in the area of hospice care should be deliberate, persistent, and offered at various times during the work day. Many opportunities exist for drawing on community resources, such as local home hospice programs, American Cancer Society educational films and speakers, local physicians with special skills in the area of terminal care, consulting pharmacists, chaplains, funeral directors, and families of former hospice patients.

Family Involvement

In-home hospice programs rely, to a great extent, on family members who are willing to assume caregiving responsibilities. When patients are cared for at home, spouses, children, in-laws, and other relatives can contribute to overall patient care. Under these circumstances nurses or nurse clinicians visit the home once or twice weekly and rely on family members to provide for most of the patient's care needs.[30] In nursing homes, however, there is a general expectation that all care is performed by paid staff. Family members may groom the patient, launder clothes, or even help with feeding, but beyond that, paid staff assume most caregiving functions. In fact, staff may be resentful of families who try to do "too much" and administrators may fear liability in the event of an accident. Fostering family involvement under these circumstances can be difficult.

One solution to this problem is to offer educational programs for family members. A skilled care facility in St. Paul, Minnesota, conducted a family interest survey that included questions about visiting patterns, quality of visits, and interest in educational and social programs.[31] The study found that approximately half of the family members interviewed ($N = 190$) wanted to learn more about confusion and memory loss, as well as how visits could be made more rewarding. Other popular topics included coping with stress, Medicare and Medicaid reimbursement, understanding levels of care, and dealing with the seriously ill. Such a survey demonstrates a facility's interest in family involvement and provides direction for program planning and implementation.

Two recent studies of factors affecting family involvement in nursing homes found that families were often unfamiliar with their relatives' situations, felt frustrated about visiting, and desired meetings with staff and counselors on care plans and therapy.[32,33] Confusion and disorientation of residents was found to be especially troubling to family members and often affected the quality of their visits. Administrators of nursing home hospice programs may find that regularly scheduled family meetings can relieve frustration and promote family involvement by defining potential roles and functions. One program manager recommended informal "pot luck" suppers for the families of confused residents as an alternative to support groups or formal meetings.

In general, program administrators need to create an environment that encourages families to become involved and stay involved. The delineation of specific roles and activities for families may help with this, particularly if nursing staff reinforce these ideas in their daily contact with visitors. Finding legitimate ways for families to be involved by providing workshops on creative visiting or by listing and describing potential family-resident activities is an important first step. This alliance can also be beneficial to staff. It supplements the work force and alerts staff to occasions when families need support.

ONE MODEL

Saint Anthony Health Center is a two-story, 154-bed skilled and intermediate care facility located in a suburb of a Midwestern city. In 1982, the facility implemented a hospice program founded on the belief that "providers of health care have an obligation to direct their efforts towards meeting individual needs."[34] The program is incorporated entirely within the existing service delivery program without separate or unique staff functions. Inservice education programs provided by a nurse clinician and a consulting pharmacist ensure that all nursing staff are familiar with pain control drugs and palliative nursing care techniques.

Hospice services are seen as appropriate when the health of a resident begins to fail and recovery appears unlikely. Patients and families are offered an opportunity to participate in the hospice program and, if they agree, all medical intervention from that point on is palliative. The mandate is to provide "supportive care only," including orders not to resuscitate the patient. These issues are discussed at an initial care conference with the patient and family prior to entering the program.

The program's medical director (who also serves as the medical director of the entire facility) maintains appropriate standards of hospice care and develops policies related to the relief of pain and other symptoms. The medical director also serves as the liaison to attending physicians who may have patients in need of hospice care. While the medical director consults with attending physicians, he does not care for individual patients unless requested. The promotion of hospice care in the facility and the general community is also the medical director's responsibility.

The charge nurse on the floor where hospice patients are located (seldom more than two or three at one time) serves as the hospice coordinator. It is her responsibility to implement the hospice plan for each patient, including the pain control program, daily nursing evaluation, patient/family conferences, and involvement of other disciplines. She also works with area programs in securing educational resources and training materials.

Hospice patients are usually located in one or two rooms near the second floor nursing station, but may be cared for in other locations throughout the facility. Other than the assignment of an aide to work specifically with hospice patients, no special staffing occurs. The interdisciplinary team, in addition to the physician, nurses, and aides, is made up of social services, dietary, physical and occupational therapy, family members (if desired), and any significant others. Other resources available to the team include local clergy, mental health workers, and volunteers. Patient and family concerns are addressed in regular care conferences where pain control, comfort needs, emotional and spiritual needs, special dietary requests, family needs, and medical and nursing activities are discussed. Both patients and family members are encouraged to attend care conferences.

Social workers are responsible for conducting preadmission family assessments and for orienting and welcoming families to the facility. Families are advised of the resident's condition, palliative care efforts, and ways to work as part of the care team. They are encouraged to visit at any time, stay in the resident's room overnight, bring pets to visit, and share meals with the resident.

Following the death of a resident, the family may hold a memorial service in the facility. A social worker contacts family members within a few months of a resident's death in order to assess the need for support during bereavement. Some support can be provided by the social worker, and additional counseling can be arranged if needed.

POTENTIAL PROBLEMS ON THE ROAD TO PROVIDING HOSPICE SERVICES

Long-term care facilities, by their very nature, pose a challenge to those who wish to implement hospice programs within them. Potential stumbling blocks include the number of available nursing hours, the offering of special privileges to dying residents, the need for active medical direction, and the costs associated with hospice care.

With respect to nursing hours, hospice care is often described as "labor intensive." As noted in Chapter 10, studies of hospice care have found that dying patients require anywhere from 2 to 9 hours of nursing care daily. In hospice units affiliated with cancer programs, the number of nursing hours needed tends to be high. In home care programs family caregivers provide a good deal of daily care; therefore, the number of professional nursing hours required can be greatly reduced. It is important to keep in mind that most studies of hospice nursing hours have been conducted within programs in which 90 percent or more of the hospice patients are dying as a result of some form of cancer. Nursing home patients, however, are a mixed population and include a significant proportion of patients with cardiovascular diseases. While hospice patients may make somewhat greater demands on long-term care nursing staff than those who are not dying, it is unrealistic to suggest that any nursing home hospice program would fail simply as a result of the nursing hours required. In facilities that have adopted some form of hospice program this has not occurred.

As discussed in other chapters, special privileges pose another kind of problem that results in questions of equity and fairness. A patient in one nursing home hospice program requested special foods at each meal. Her roommate, who was not dying but who frequently sought attention from staff, wondered why she also was not afforded such luxuries. The question is not an easy one. Granting unique privileges in any setting where others are not accorded the same privileges sets up the potential for confrontation. While it may be avoided for a time with the use of a private room and/or closed doors, there is inevitably the question, "Why not me, too?" One approach to this problem is to recognize the potential within other residents to become part of the hospice team. In some facilities where educational efforts extend to residents as well as staff, the aid of other residents is enlisted to provide friendly visiting, companionship, and diversion. These peer relationships may, for some hospice patients, be more satisfying than staff relationships, particularly in the areas of emotional and spiritual support. This approach, however, cannot eliminate the fundamental problem that special privileges create and some very specific definitions of what hospice care can and cannot include may be required.

Active medical direction is a critical element in the development of a hospice program and long-term care administrators need to ensure adequate symptom assessment and control. In some nursing homes, physician service is scanty and inadequate. In other homes, it is marked by a large number of marginally involved physicians each managing the care of one or a few residents. While federal law now requires that a physician be designated as the medical director of a skilled care facility, relations with other physicians who have resident patients in the same facility are not always clear.

The designation of a hospice medical director should include an effort to inform attending physicians about the program and to identify ways in which the medical director can work with other physicians who have patients eligible for hospice care. It is also important for a hospice medical director to be trained to care for the dying and to be committed to the assessment of problems as they arise. When it appears that nonmedical care is most appropriate, the physician must be sensitive to ways in which others on the care team can contribute to the comfort of the resident and he or she must encourage them to do so.

When the level of physician involvement within a facility cannot be increased or when direction of a nursing home hospice program by a physician is impractical, the employment of a geriatric nurse practitioner (GNP) may be a reasonable alternative. GNPs are trained in assessment, diagnosis, therapy, and preventative health care and may perform complete physical examinations, manage minor illnesses, and, with established protocols, treat the symptoms of major chronic diseases.[35] The GNP can also serve as a role model for nursing staff in the care of dying patients. Studies of the GNP's roles in long-term care have demonstrated several benefits, including reductions in transfers to acute care facilities, less use of physical restraints, increased patient and family satisfaction, and higher staff morale.[36-39]

Some states are now reimbursing GNPs directly with Medicaid funds. Moreover, the Health Care Financing Administration has requested proposals to study the cost effectiveness of GNPs in long-term care, indicating an interest in future reimbursement mechanisms. A nursing home hospice program is an ideal setting for utilizing the skills of a geriatric nurse practitioner.

In the final analysis, however, no manager, planner, or administrator can avoid the question of costs. What effect will a nursing home hospice program have on expenses and revenues? Given the newness of such programs, a complete answer to this question is not yet available. Nonetheless, certain facts are clear.

First, nursing homes that have implemented hospice programs have been intent on keeping costs down. The incorporation of hospice services within existing job descriptions and staffing patterns has been a high priority for most administrators. Staff education and adequate volunteer program management require initial expenditures, as do consultation arrangements with consulting pharmacists or hospice educators. While these initial expenses are difficult to avoid, it is likely that they will decrease over time. The expense of employing a new staff member, such as a geriatric nurse practitioner, a hospice coordinator, or a volunteer supervisor, can more easily be supported if job descriptions include tasks that relate to all nursing home residents. A GNP may be involved in employee physicals and/or a staff and resident wellness program.

Second, new legislation enacted in 1982 and made effective in 1984 has enabled persons eligible for Medicare benefits to elect a hospice option, which will pay for up to seven months of hospice care in an approved hospice program.[40] While organizations with certified home health agencies are best able to benefit from the legislation, nursing homes and home health agencies can cooperate so that inpatient beds are provided by the nursing home while home care services are delivered by the home health agency. The nursing home is able, under such an arrangement, to provide respite care for hospice home care patients when family caregivers need time off.

Third, hospice care is a gift-generating program. The provision of high-quality care at the end of a resident's life is a service that is often greatly appreciated. While hospice programs cannot be expected to survive on gifts alone, some communities have found other local agencies such as the United Way and various volunteer service associations to provide financial support. In addition, several insurance companies, including Prudential, American Family, and Trans-America, now offer some hospice benefits.

SUMMARY

New program ideas such as the offering of hospice services must be adapted to the unique characteristics of varied institutional settings.

Some nursing homes currently provide excellent care to the dying. One respondent in the Ramsey County study described earlier said, "I think that God privileged him beyond all, taking him to be in a place like that."[41] To presume that one can do better by forming a hospice program may be an affront to staff members. Nonetheless, an administrator can hold up the hospice yardstick and ask, "How do we look? Are we doing as well as we might? Could we do better? Is it worth doing better? Can we generate the resources, make the commitment, and find the interest and resolve within our own organization and the community to improve the quality of care we provide to the dying and their families?"

There is little question that hospice principles can contribute to long-term care environments in many ways. They have the potential to provide a focus for individual efforts, promote team interaction, encourage family involvement, improve community relations, and offer residents and families a more complete continuum of care.

NOTES

1. J. Albin Yokie, "Hospice Care in Nursing Homes," *Nursing Homes*, May/June 1981, 26.

2. Ibid., 27.

3. Good Samaritan Village, *Hospice: A Program of Care for Dying Persons and Their Families* (Moscow, Idaho: Good Samaritan Village, 1981), 2–3.

4. National Center for Health Statistics: Advance Report, Final Mortality Statistics, 1980, *Monthly Vital Statistics Report* 32, no. 4, Supp. DHHS Pub. No. (PHS) 83-1120 (Hyattsville, Md.: Public Health Service, August, 1983), 10.

5. Peter Thoreen, "Care of the Dying Among Friends," in *Creative Long-Term Care Administration*, ed. George Kenneth Gordon and Ruth Stryker (Springfield, Ill.: Charles C Thomas, 1983), 242–268.

6. E. Rosenberg and C. Short, "Issues of Institutionalization: Five Percent Fallacies and Terminal Care," *International Journal of Aging and Human Development* 17 (1983), 43-55.

7. *National Center for Health Statistics:* A. Sirrocco; "An Overview of the 1980 National Master Facility Inventory Survey of Nursing and Related Care Homes," *Advance Data from Vital and Health Statistics*, Number 91, DHHS Pub. No. (PHS) 83-1250. August 11, 1983, 2. Public Health Service, Hyattsville, Md.

8. Cicely Saunders, *St. Christopher's Hospice Annual Report, 1977-1978*, 16.

9. Ethel McClure, *More Than a Roof: The Development of Minnesota Poor Farms and Homes for the Aged* (St. Paul: Minnesota Historical Society, 1968), 18–35.

10. Bruce C. Vladeck, *Unloving Care* (New York: Basic Books, 1980), 33.

11. Ruth Stryker, "Historical Obstacles to Management of Nursing Homes," in *Creative Long Term Care Administration*, ed. George Kenneth Gordon and Ruth Stryker (Springfield, Ill.: Charles C Thomas, 1983), 10.

12. Vladeck, *Unloving Care*, 39.

13. Medicare is a 1965 amendment to the Social Security Act (Title XVIII) that provides a national system of health insurance for those over 65. It provides partial coverage of hospital and nursing home costs and includes a voluntary provision for medical care coverage. It is financed primarily by a payroll tax on earnings paid by employers and employees.

14. Medicaid, another 1965 amendment to the Social Security Act (Title XIX), is a means-tested program of medical assistance for low-income persons of all ages. It is administered by individual states and supported by both federal and state revenues.

15. Vladeck, *Unloving Care*, 50.

16. Ibid., 59.

17. Ibid., 59–70.

18. The new hospice benefit included in the Tax Equity and Fiscal Responsibility Act of 1982 provides for a hospice Medicare option that can be elected by persons who are certified as terminally ill by two physicians. If the option is elected, other Medicare benefits are not available unless the hospice option is revoked. The hospice option includes three election periods totaling 210 days and the stipulation that inpatient hospice care must be short term and that 80 percent of all patient care days (in aggregate) must be home care days. Benefits include 24-hour nursing coverage, home care, respite care, homemakers, home health aides, 90 percent of all medication costs, and durable medical equipment. A total cap on hospice care reimbursement is set at $6,500.

19. Frank Moss and Val Halamandaris, *Too Old, Too Sick, Too Bad* (Rockville, Md.: Aspen Systems, 1977), 202.

20. Vladeck, *Unloving Care*, 211.

21. Ibid., 214.

22. Thoreen, "Care of the Dying Among Friends."

23. Carolyn C. Gotay, *Hospice Care in Alberta Extended Care Institutions: A Needs Assessment* (Calgary, Alberta, Canada: Faculty of Medicine, 1984).

24. Ibid., 22.

25. Ibid., 26.

26. Ibid., 28.

27. Greg Owen, *Care for the Dying: A Study of the Need for Hospice in Ramsey County, Minnesota* (St. Paul: A.H. Wilder Foundation, 1981).

28. Alfred Worcester, *The Care of the Aged, the Dying, and the Dead* (Springfield, Ill.: Charles C Thomas, 1935), 37–38.

29. *St. Anthony Health Center Hospice Program Guide* (Minneapolis, Minn.: St. Anthony Health Center, January 1, 1983), 1.

30. Owen, *Care for the Dying*. This study found that most home caregiving functions were performed by family members. Women outnumbered men as caregivers 2 to 1.

31. Greg Owen, "Families of Nursing Home Residents Want To Know More About Long-Term Care," *Figuratively Speaking* (St. Paul: Wilder Foundation, January 31, 1984), 4–5.

32. Johnathan York and Robert Calsyn, "Family Involvement in Nursing Homes," *The Gerontologist* 17, no. 6 (1977): 500–505.

33. Don Sands and Larry Bjorklund, "Fighting a Myth: Families in Need of Support," *The Journal of Long Term Care Administration* (Spring 1982): 29–35.

34. *St. Anthony Health Center Hospice Program* (Minneapolis, Minn.: St. Anthony Health Center, 1983), 1.

35. P.P. Ebersole, "Geriatric Nurse Practitioners," *Long-Term Care Currents* 6, no. 3 (July–September 1983): 11–14.

36. "Improving Quality Care in the Skilled Nursing Facility in the Rural Mountain West," Mountain States Health Corporation Project report submitted to the W.K. Kellogg Foundation, June 1979.

37. G.L. Jean, S.R. Brovender, R. Freeland, B. Otto, "Impact of Geriatric Nurse Practitioners on Long-Term Care" (Paper presented at the Twelfth International Congress of Gerontology, Hamburg, Germany, July 12–17, 1981).

38. D. Kremser, *Advancement in Health Care* (Greeley, Colo.: Western Division ARA Living Center, 1983).

39. P.A. Prescott and L. Driscoll, "Evaluating Nurse Practitioner Performance." *Nurse Practitioner*, July/August 1980, 28, 29, 31, 32, 53.

40. Guidelines and other assistance in setting up qualified programs are available from the National Hospice Organization, 1901 North Fort Myer Dr., Suite 402, Arlington, Va. 22209.

41. Owen, *Care for the Dying*, 99.

Chapter 5

Management of the Hospital Inpatient Hospice Unit

Karen H. May McArdle

As we have seen, the American hospice movement has begun shifting its focus from a community-based, predominately volunteer model to one that is institutionally based (e.g., located at a hospital or home health agency) and staffed by paid employees. In the hospital, this trend has been more pronounced since cost containment efforts have forced hospitals to close beds or reorganize services. The development of a hospice program provides an excellent opportunity for a hospital to divert some inpatient beds as well as to develop home health care options.

An inpatient hospice unit represents a commitment made by hospital administration. A hospital must decide if there is sufficient value (social as well as economic) to initiating a hospice program. The hospital administration must begin by carefully considering the advantages and disadvantages of establishing an inpatient unit.

A hospice program can do much to promote the image of the hospital and expand patient care options. The benefits of the hospice program can spill over into other areas of the hospital and enrich the staff and services provided, as well as potentially increase the number of filled beds. This chapter examines the advantages and disadvantages of hospital-based hospice programs, describes management and organizational issues, and identifies hospital staff training and education needs.

THE PROS AND CONS OF HOSPICE PROGRAMMING

Administrators and managers can show hospital boards and funding agencies numerous advantages to be gained from the development of hospice programming. The benefits vary depending on the model of hospice care employed, the organizational structure of the hospital, and the commitment on the part of personnel involved. On the positive side, hospice programs can publicly enhance the hospital's image as a place of help and service to the aged, the ill, and the dying. This may result in increased public funding and patient referrals. In addition to public benefits, hospice programs have been used to improve morale and staff education. The attention to the needs of the dying and their families, as exemplified in hospice, can be translated into a general hospital attitude. The expertise of hospice staff in pain and symptom control can be taught to other hospital staff, who can employ the techniques with nonterminal patients. Furthermore, for hospitals with declining daily census, creation of a hospice inpatient unit can fill beds that otherwise may remain empty.

While there are many positive aspects associated with hospice care, administrators and planners must consider negative ones as well. Availability of staff, added budgetary factors, and costs in staffing and furnishing inpatient units restrict some administrations from making a hospice commitment. Space may also present a problem. Not only patient rooms are needed but also areas for family, visitor, and staff use. A hospital may not have resources or the physical ability to expand facilities.

Federal and state regulations impose restrictions on getting started. Certificate of Need laws, reviews by health systems agencies, requirements for state licensure all create roadblocks to hospice development. In addition, availability of medical staff also poses problems for obtaining a hospice medical director and for developing sufficient client referrals.

If the hospital believes the positive components outweigh those that are negative, then attention must be directed toward long-term continuing administrative support. Ideally, the hospice concept is an extension of the hospital's philosophy. Because a hospice unit within a hospital may challenge long-standing practices and rituals, administrative approval and support of changes is necessary. Will the hospital agree to staffing patterns that resemble those of an intensive care unit in patient-staff ratios? How will the hospital handle unrestricted visiting or the hospice patient who asks for a drink of whiskey? Will there be a way to allow pets to come to the inpatient unit? How will the hospital view the practice of allowing the body of the patient to remain in the room, perhaps for hours, while family members begin their post-death grieving?

Without support from hospital administration, hospice care is no different from general hospital care. If hospice staff must fight for approval of every break with hospital tradition, the enthusiasm and sensitivity required for their work is diluted. The results of this may be an increased attrition rate or a less than desirable psychosocial atmosphere within the hospice unit. Therefore, before the first hospice bed is allotted, hospital administration must understand the positive and negative aspects of a hospice program, express a commitment to the hospice philosophy, and be willing to challenge long-standing hospital traditions that negatively impact hospice programming.

DECIDING UPON THE SETTING

Chapter 2 described three alternatives for implementing hospice care within a hospital: a separate hospice unit, hospice beds as part of a patient floor, or scatter beds. Alternatives always contain elements of positive and negative components. Table 5-1 provides a review of the major advantages and disadvantages associated with each alternative.

Each administrator must weigh the pros and cons varied settings offer and decide on an approach meeting both the needs of the organization and the hospice program. For example, if beds within a unit are chosen, high priority must be given to staff support so that staff does not become frustrated making choices about patient priorities, between critical dying patients and critical patients who will survive.

If a scattered bed approach is selected, then additional resources should be devoted to internal program coordination so that staff and families can share information and experiences. The loss of a communication network is common in a scatter-bed hospice facility.

DEVELOPING THE ORGANIZATIONAL STRUCTURE

The structure of an organization is important. It serves as a guidepost for carrying out organizational goals and objectives, promoting organizational priorities, and identifying individuals responsible for organizational productivity. In relation to the larger hospital structure, the hospice administrator should serve as a unit director with input into general hospital administration. He or she should have responsibility for hospice staff hiring, recruitment, and assignment.

To best implement the hospice philosophy, the organizational structure of the hospice should be as independent as possible from the general hospital structure: that is, a separate board should be created, a distinct budget, and so on. An independent structure has important advantages. It allows the staff flexibility to break from hospital tradition and implement innovative hospice care techniques. It provides an opportunity for greater community linkages through board and volunteer contacts. It allows the hospice to take on its own identity, which is especially important in promotional, educational, and fund-raising activities. Finally, a distinct organizational structure expresses a strong commitment on the part of the hospital to promoting and encouraging the development of hospice in the community.

Just as the organizational structure of the hospice should allow the hospice administrator easy access to hospital administration, the internal organization of the hospice should allow staff an opportunity for open and easy communication.

Table 5-1 Advantages and Disadvantages To Consider in Choosing the Setting

Setting	Advantages	Disadvantages
Scatter beds	Little, if any, change in space resources.	Distinction for patients and families between hospice and hospital care may not exist.
	Few, if any, changes in state licensure requirements; i.e., a certificate of need may not be necessary.	
	Little, if any, change in staffing resources.	Staff may experience problems providing the varied and intensive care needed by hospice patients.
	Beds are free for other patients during low hospice census.	Variety of locations with staff who may not understand, support, or feel comfortable with hospice philosophy.
	Staff may have option to care for terminal patients and experience the hospice philosophy.	If hospice patient or families are treated differently, other patients in the area may feel discriminated against, e.g., and demand more liberal family visiting.
	Nonhospice patients may be positively affected by the hospice care philosophy— a potential spillover effect exists.	Guidance and control of quality hospice care is difficult.
		Staff support and education may be insufficient.
		Education and guidance of hospice staff caregivers is difficult.
		The family-centered approach and the feeling of togetherness of patient, family, and hospice team is hard to achieve and/or easily lost when contact is intermittent.
		Mutual patient-family support is impossible when there is no central meeting area.

Table 5-1 continued

Setting	Advantages	Disadvantages
Beds as part of a patient floor.	Staff is centrally located making support, guidance, education, and control of quality hospice care easier to accomplish.	If hospice patient or families are treated differently, other patients in the area may feel discriminated against, e.g., and demand more liberal family visiting.
	A homelike atmosphere can be more easily created when part of a nursing unit is set aside for hospice care.	It may be difficult for staff to change their perspectives about patient care if they are assigned to care for hospice and nonhospice patients during the same work day.
	Few changes in staffing resources are required if hospice staff also care for the other patients in the unit.	During periods of high census, it is likely that a busy nurse will devote her or his time to the critical rather than to the critical hospice patient who will die.
	Reduced burnout of experienced staff, and staffing options are expanded.	Hospice patients may be treated no differently than the dying located elsewhere in the hospital.
	Nonhospice patients may experience the positive effects of hospice care.	
Separate unit	Hospice care becomes a visible alternative in care for the dying.	Space is used to produce a homelike setting and may not be used for other, more traditional curative hospital functions.
	A separate staff can be guided and trained more proficiently.	Additional costs are involved in staffing and maintaining a unit. Empty beds are a liability if unavailable for general hospital patients.
	With an adequate selection process, all staff can be assigned to hospice because	The misconception of hospice as the "death house" is perpetuated. This may be

(continued)

Table 5-1 Continued

Setting	Advantages	Disadvantages
	of their belief in the concept.	avoided through active ongoing education.
	Quality assurance is more easily accomplished and ongoing monitoring of hospice care is more thorough when hospice patients are segregated.	The more isolated the hospice within the hospital, the longer it takes to achieve acceptance. Totally separate units will take longer to become accepted than will units in which beds are scattered or part of another hospital area.
	Modifying or changing common hospital practices is less upsetting to general hospital staff and more easily accomplished to fit the needs of hospice patients and families.	Additional regulatory standards may be required, e.g., a special certificate of need, which will create increased administrative costs.
	A reduced sense of discrimination exists among nonhospice patients when the unit is segregated and outside the mainstream of hospital care.	
	Patients and families mutually supporting each other is frequent and encouraged.	
	Staff, working from similar patient care perspectives, are more likely to support each other and attend to collective needs.	

Because the team approach is basic to all hospice care, the organizational chart of an inpatient unit should have as flat an administrative hierarchy as possible, to promote team interaction.

This process can begin in early planning stages. Each staff discipline needs a clear understanding of each member's capabilities. In this way, staff can find the most appropriate resources from among team members to care for patients and family members. At the same time, care should be taken to avoid assigning staff strictly on the basis of titles and current job functions. The more administrators view staff, and volunteers, in terms of what they offer because of their interests, motivations, life experiences, education, and creative talents, the richer the patient's care. When the organizational hierarchy is developed in terms of a "my job-your job" mentality, hospice care suffers. Staff lose their opportunity to grow and to develop in ways that enhance hospice care. If the occupational therapist feels comfortable saying a prayer with the patient, if the social worker is in the patient's room when the nurse needs help making a bed, if the chaplain plays the guitar and the patient wants a song—why not? Whoever said that only chaplains pray, that nurses alone are responsible for making beds, or that only music therapists play music? Whatever the patient needs should be provided by someone able and comfortable doing it. This important point should be considered by hospice planners early in program development.

STAFFING RATIOS

The nursing staff is the largest staff in any hospital unit. A conscious administrative decision should be made regarding the integration or segregation of hospice nursing staff from hospital nursing service departments. Continuity and quality of care are important and likely to be achieved if regularly assigned, distinct nursing staff provide care to hospice patients.

Primary factors to consider in deciding if and how hospice nurses should be separated from general staff include (1) staff selection, (2) training requirements, and (3) a staff floating policy. Effective hospice nursing staff display certain attitudes, beliefs, and skills. Although staff selection process is addressed later in this chapter, it is important to note that random assignment of nursing staff to hospice patients or families is not beneficial. Not everyone feels comfortable working with the terminally ill. Assigning nurses who are uncomfortable in this area hampers the quality of care. It is crucial for hospice program administrators to have control over staff selection.

Comprehensive staff orientation and training programs are essential. All nursing staff do not have the same degree of clinical and psychosocial skills. When hospice staff are provided distinct hospice training and inservice programs, their skills can be improved, and their motivation increased. Hospice nursing staff should have initial and ongoing educational programs beyond those educational programs provided by the hospital's nursing service department.

Hospice planners and administrators should avoid using a floating practice as a way of hospice staffing. Floating a nurse into a hospice unit who does not understand the goals or purpose of palliative care, or who disagrees with hospice philosophy, or who is uncomfortable with dying patients and grieving families, is unfair to both the nurse and the patient and family.

Nurse-patient ratios are determined, to a great degree, by administrative philosophy. The more personalized and individualized the value of patient care is, the smaller the patient-to-staff ratio. As we shall see in Chapter 10, hospice care is intensive nursing care. The determination of ratios resembles those of an intensive care unit. "Because dying persons and their families have needs that go beyond basic physical care, additional staff members are required. . . . The desired ratio of patients to staff in hospice work is generally cited as one nurse per shift for every three patients . . . (or one to one over the 24 hour day)."[1] Hospice care requires that tasks be performed; however, hospice care is not task oriented. Staff distribution by shift should be equalized. Since the patient-family is the focus of care, the evening hours may be as busy as the morning hours, when there are numerous family members or significant others with whom to deal. A nurse's work load should be determined not only by the number of patients cared for but also by the number of family members or significant others requiring attention.

To meet complex needs in complex situations, primary nursing, or some modification of it, is best suited to the hospice setting. Identification of the patient with a professional primary caregiver does much to allay the symptom of anxiety and often the symptom of pain. There are times when the primary nurse feels overwhelmed with a particularly burdensome situation. In this case, the hospice manager can build a staff assignment system that relieves the nurse for a time.

In addition to nursing staff, there are professionals that need to be considered in any developing hospice, including social workers, clergy, therapists, dieticians, pharmacists, a volunteer director/chief administrator and appropriate medical records/secretarial support. As noted in Chapters 2 and 10, Medicare and other third-party insurers are fairly specific in terms of the number and type of staff required to service hospice patients. A physician is needed to serve as the program's medical director, along with a social worker, clergy member, volunteer coordinator, and an administrator.

Hospital administrators are encouraged to consult other hospitals and discuss their hospice staffing experiences. The demands on nurses will be greatest, followed by those on volunteers, social workers, and other staff, depending on the program model employed. Planners and managers should consider potential patient loads, availability of existing staff to perform hospice functions, and the ability of the organization to recruit and train volunteers in the development of a staffing plan.

POLICY DEVELOPMENT

Policy development is a guide to creating an inpatient unit and serves as a method of problem solving. Developing policies for an inpatient hospice unit has become easier over time. The National Hospice Organization (NHO) and the Joint Commission on Accreditation of Hospitals (JCAH) have developed comprehensive guidelines for hospice care providers. These guidelines are useful and have been successfully employed by several hospital based hospice programs.

The Hospice Standards Manual,[2] published in 1983 by the Joint Commission on Accreditation of Hospitals, contains guides for decision making in policy planning and development. The JCAH criteria specify that written policies and procedures should include areas such as treatment modalities and a position on patient resuscitation. Also required are specifications for patient privacy, visiting, and overnight accommodations.

The National Hospice Organization has also developed standards for a hospice program of care.[3] These standards include guidelines in the areas of administration, continuity of care, inclusion of the patient-family as the unit of care, personnel, symptom control, bereavement, quality assurance, records, and the inpatient unit.

The American Medical Records Association, as part of a Kellogg Foundation Grant, field tested a standardized hospice record in 1984. The chart forms used cover the gamut of record keeping from a history and a physical to bereavement records.[4] In addition, the Medicare reimbursement regulations provide guidelines for hospice managers regarding the development, organizational structure, and service delivery of hospice care.[5] In short, there are more resources available today than just a few years ago to guide managers and planners in developing an inpatient unit.

SERVICE CONSIDERATIONS

Integrating and coordinating the services of many hospital departments is one of the managerial functions of the hospice planner and administrator. Breaks with hospital tradition or rituals occur when activities are centered around the needs of the patient rather than around hospital organizational priorities. In most hospitals, changes in practice patterns are possible. However, because almost all departments are affected by a hospice program, it is important to have widespread involvement in hospice planning. A few examples illustrate techniques for interdepartmental planning.

When the hospice patient comes to the hospital for admission, he or she presents symptoms that are "out of control." The patient and the family are distraught. If the patient enters the hospital through an emergency room (ER) admission, consideration should be given regarding appropriate treatment. Since the patient came for symptom control or because death is imminent, treatment may not be a necessary part of his or her care. The hospice manager should consider arrangements that allow hospice patients to be admitted directly to the hospice unit without the need for ER care. This spares the patient and family an additional financial burden and allows their psychological-emotional needs to be addressed more quickly because unnecessary testing or treatment is not initiated by staff unfamiliar with the patient's circumstances. Palliative care experts in the hospice unit can more quickly initiate appropriate treatment to comfort the patient and the family.

Admission procedures normally begin in an office where forms are filled out, information is collected, and signatures are obtained. Administrators should consider procedures that allow hospice patients in crisis to be directly admitted to the hospice unit. The suffering of the patient and family is quickly addressed and necessary paperwork can be completed by hospice staff.

A dietician should be assigned to the hospice unit to deal with anorexia and other common problems of cancer patients. He or she can offer a range of nutritional resources to improve the patient's condition. For some patients, the goal is food intake of any sort rather than consumption of a nutritionally balanced meal.

Palliative occupational therapy and physical therapy have a different focus. Hospice patients are not candidates for rehabilitation in the conventional sense. Skills of occupational and physical therapists should focus on activities that encourage reminiscing and life review and, most important, pain control.

Medical records is another department to include in the planning and education process. Hospice patient records may differ from the standard hospital record. Psychosocial assessments or bereavement notes may need to be incorporated into the chart.

It is the ability to individualize the care for unique patient and family needs that ultimately improves quality. In some situations, the appropriate use of technology or treatment may be the key factor in the patient-family's satisfaction. In other circumstances, a quiet, listening volunteer may fill the biggest need. On the other hand, a party to celebrate a life event may be the key to meeting a primary need of the patient-family. This kind of individualizing from other clinical departments is part of the groundwork that must be laid in development of the organizational structure of the hospice inpatient unit.

FINANCIAL CONSIDERATIONS

Patients' financial resources are often severely limited or depleted by the time hospice care is sought. The hospice manager should know if hospice patients are billed differently from others in the hospital. Will there be a daily rate or flat fee? Will the hospital be willing to accept what insurance covers? What about patients who need inpatient care and have no insurance or ability to pay privately? These and other financial, philosophical, and ethical questions need to be considered.

Financial considerations vary as a function of the hospice model employed. When determining the charges for hospice care, home care staff support, inpatient services, and costs for volunteer recruitment and training must be considered. Medicare provides a flat fee for each hospice patient, and it is incumbent upon the administrator to be sure that the capitation fee sufficiently covers the patient's needs. Research has shown that hospital hospices are slightly more expensive than home-based programs. This is largely due to increased institutional costs.[6] Therefore, administrators should consider a mix of patients to cover overhead costs. Membership drives, funding campaigns, and support from private philanthropy may be initiated to supplement the hospice's budget. Hospice fund-raising projects are often successful and should be conducted apart from larger hospital campaigns. Often, hospice board members assist in fund-raising efforts.

THE TASK OF EDUCATING

Physicians affect the success or failure of a hospice inpatient unit. In this respect, physician hospice education should begin while the inpatient unit is being planned. A questionnaire to physicians provides hospice planners information regarding medical staff views toward terminal illness, palliative care, and hospice philosophy. Presentations about hospice care can be made at medical staff meetings. Video materials and other media can be used to explore issues surrounding care for terminal patients.[7] Generally, the training focuses on a small group of staff physicians expressing interest in the hospice philosophy. During the planning process, hospice administrators should concentrate organizational energies on this group rather than on the entire medical staff.

Once the inpatient unit is established, continuing and ongoing informal education must be followed up with all physicians who refer and care for hospice patients. For some physicians, brief, polite questioning concerning the use of a test or treatment is necessary to provide the physician with options for doing something for the patient. In other circumstances, hospice staff need to be strong patient advocates, promoting a patient's rights to know the truth or to refuse prescribed therapies. In other cases, a well-informed hospice staff can suggest a different approach in dealing with pain control or the family's anticipatory grief. These interactions promote the team concept and begin the process of reeducating physician practitioners.

General hospital staff are usually curious about a new hospital area. The more adequately the hospital staff understand the hospice structure within their institution, the more likely they are to support it. Institutions with identified hospice programs must educate staff about the hospice philosophy. Printed materials should be distributed to staff. Audiovisual programs and presentations by hospice staff should follow up the distribution of printed materials. Because new hospital staff are frequently employed, including an explanation of hospice care as part of their orientation is necessary.

In addition to physician and hospital staff, community education is also important. Hospice administrators can accomplish this in various ways. First, a brief description of the hospice concept in the general information materials provided to all hospital patients is helpful. A second step involves public media. Local radio shows can be enlisted to sponsor hospice representatives to discuss the concept for listeners. Articles in local newspapers reach another segment of the population. Providing educational programs for the community at large is also beneficial.

One of the best ways to educate the community is through a speakers bureau. The speakers should be informed staff and volunteers, available for presentations to civic, social, religious, and other local groups. Speakers can address public misconceptions about hospice care and use questions to assess the public's attitude toward this type of care. In some cases, hospice speakers have been able to dispel notions that the hospice unit is a hospital death ward.

The education process never ends. There are always new hospital staff, new physicians, and new community groups to reach. Because the topics of death and dying and hospice may be uncomfortable for many, they often do not hear the information presented. The opportune learning moment for many may not come until they have a personal need for hospice information. To present one educational session to the hospital staff or to the public is not the end; it is the beginning.

ACCEPTANCE WITHIN THE HOSPITAL

Acceptance of hospice and hospice staff within the institution depends on several factors. New ideas and changes in delivery of services are often viewed skeptically. One way to encourage acceptance is to prove the value of hospice care to others. Suspicion of hospice care providers by hospital staff occurs in most settings. "I could never do that kind of work" may mean "What attracts you to such a morbid situation?" or "What is wrong with you that you want to work with terminal patients?" or "Don't you think you will burn out fast in that kind of work?" To overcome this problem, hospice staff must support each other and demonstrate to critics that hospice is a realistic and important approach to patient care. The "what is wrong with you" attitude sometimes conveyed to hospice workers requires that they have strongly grounded personal views and feelings that can withstand skepticism and challenge by other staff members.

Administrators have often voiced concerns over "alleged" hospice burnout. The "burnout" question assumes that there is extraordinary stress. With sound management practices the degree of stress among hospice staff is generally lower than in other hospital areas. Stress is decreased when staff share philosophies and goals, choose their work, have adequate support systems, and are allotted time to obtain satisfaction.

Acceptance by and integration into the hospital will be a time of testing, teaching, and trials. It is a task that hospice staff can accomplish. The ultimate success in achieving these goals depends upon the effort of management to persevere and achieve a united staff.

STAFF SELECTION, ORIENTATION, AND CONTINUING EDUCATION

The employee or volunteer interview is the first step in creating an appropriate staff. Hospice staff require special characteristics. There are a number of factors managers should consider during an interview. These factors include motivations and past life experiences as well as clinical or related expertise. Appropriate motivators are evidenced from such statements as "I was very frustrated working in intensive care and having to do things to patients I couldn't agree with"; "I was very stressed because I didn't have enough time to give patients the extra care they needed"; "I have worked with the dying before and found it very satisfying." Exploring these kinds of comments reveals the "giving" quality of hospice workers.

Inappropriate motivations are discovered through comments such as "I know dying can be a beautiful experience for everyone"; "All people need is faith and their dying will not be difficult at all"; "I have had experience in moving people through each stage of dying." These comments often reveal an inflexible personality and an individual who believes he or she holds the answer to the patient's problems. This person is inclined to impose his or her views on others.

Previous experiences influence motivation and needs of potential staff. Managers should ask questions that determine if the applicant is currently working through a grief experience and inappropriately sees hospice as a source of self-healing rather than as an atmosphere where the giving of oneself to others is required.

Inpatient hospice care requires clinical expertise. However, it is also important for those with clinical skills to be willing to learn and to translate those skills to a hospice care philosophy. For example, a nurse knowledgeable in progressive muscle relaxation techniques or imagery techniques provides additional pain control resources. The nurse with group therapy or communication skills experience is a valuable resource in patient-family conferences.

Nonwork interests and hobbies should be explored. When stress does exist in hospice work, one way individuals cope is by having other areas of involvement besides their work. A workaholic does not belong on a hospice staff.

Quality hospice care must always be individualized to the patient-family. Managers must recruit flexible staff. During the interview, administrators should consider the applicant's appreciation and use of humor as well. Laughter is a healthy activity. It is something to be shared with patients and families. A person who rarely smiles and laughs does not belong in a hospice inpatient unit.

Once staff are selected, an orientation to the inpatient unit establishes initial standards, expectations, and goals. During the first orientation meeting managers should identify those caring philosophies they feel must be expressed by staff. Review of clinical skills should also be accomplished at this time.

Managers should avoid the temptation to utilize the orientee for service before the learner has acquired some degree of comfort and competency. The learning experiences should be structured so that goals and objectives are clear, yet loose enough to promote individualized learning. By this process the philosophy of "individualized" learning can also be translated later into the philosophy of "individualized" care.

In addition to inservice orientation, the effective manager encourages hospice inpatient staff to expand their horizons and talents. Pain and symptom control are growing fields. Skillful interpersonal communications, effective conferences with patient-families, and caring assistance with grief require continued learning. Awareness of the ethics and legal ramifications of some hospice situations is also important so that staff interventions are appropriate.

PLANNING PHYSICAL-PSYCHOSOCIAL SPACE

Careful attention should be paid to the environment created in the inpatient unit. The addition of color is important in setting a feeling tone. Harsh colors may negatively affect patients. Some patients are jaundiced, many are pale. Color should be used to make patients feel and look better.

Light also sets a mood. Floor or table lamps in patient rooms provide a warmer feeling than standard fluorescent wall lights. Outside light and sunshine should be utilized to the fullest. Sensory deprivation occurs more easily in darkened environments and pain, anxiety, restlessness, and confusion are exacerbated. Proper light and sunshine can assist in counteracting this problem.

Kitchen facilities are essential. In our culture social activity and relaxation revolve around eating and drinking. Coffee and tea pots are essential items for the inpatient unit. An atmosphere of relaxation and sharing can be much more easily initiated when a cup of tea or coffee sits between the staff and patient-family. The atmosphere created by this amenity enhances therapy and encourages input and social interaction.

A microwave oven is the next most versatile appliance for the inpatient kitchen. Food from home can be cooked or reheated in the microwave. Patients have the flexibility of eating when they feel hungry and not when food trays are delivered.

Third on the list of environmental items is a space used as a family room. The family room provides a common meeting place for patients to interact as well as a space for family breaks. A family room is also ideal for parties. Celebration of life events should be encouraged in the inpatient unit. If possible, the unit should also provide accommodations for pet visits.

Planning is required for space and resources for overnight family stays. Such accommodations are very important, especially when the patient is actively dying. On the other hand, administrators may want to consider a flexible no visiting day policy. Establishing this concept allows the patient a day of rest and, equally important, allows family to stay home without feeling guilty. If a family feels compelled to visit on a no visiting day, the right should not be denied.

Space for staff use only is critical in the inpatient unit. Because hospice inpatient care includes intense involvement in personal situations, staff need space away from patient-families where they can laugh, cry, or be angry, out of sight from those for whom they care. Availability of staff space is a great stress reducer.

The physical environment is important. Pictures on the wall should be encouraged so that patients can reflect on life events. Time and date orientation in every patient's room is provided by clocks and calendars. Music is a source of stimulation and relaxation. The availability of TV, radios, phonographs, or tape recorders offers many possible avenues of recreation and relaxation for patients.

Provision for privacy for patient-family is essential. Included in this concept is the need for privacy between patient and spouse, parent and child, or for the grieving family when death occurs. Staff must be sensitive and know when they are needed and when they should allow patients privacy.

In addition to the accoutrements comprising the physical surroundings, attention must also be given to the psychosocial environment. Inpatient staff (paid and volunteer) create and maintain the psychosocial environment. Communications among staff and patients should reflect a position of compassionate honesty and an acceptance and support of emotions expressed. Patient-family participation in care is encouraged and enhanced by openness and honesty. The finest interior decorating work in a hospice is of little value if staff fails to create and maintain a warm, caring, and supportive feeling within the unit.

PATIENT CARE

Nursing staff provide the bulk of hands-on involvement in the care of hospice patients. Ideally, the nurse and physician should have a collegial relationship in which ideas are shared rather than a one-way relationship in which orders are given. The chaplain, or the patient's own pastor, sharing knowledge with the team provide a broader picture of the patient, which facilitates individualized care. The pharmacist, occupational therapist, physical therapist, unit secretary, social worker, housekeeper, and volunteer all may have knowledge, ideas, or skills that benefit a patient's care. Hospice managers must encourage team interaction to utilize all staff resources.

Motivation is more likely to occur when an individual has a personal investment in established goals. Goal setting and planning become most efficient and effective when the goals and plans result from joint efforts among patients, family members, and staff.

A potential source of effective communication and planning is the clinical care conference. A regularly scheduled, interdisciplinary care conference provides two primary outcomes. First, team input facilitates comprehensive care for a patient's physical, spiritual, psychosocial, and family-related problems and symptoms. Second, regularly held clinical conferences ensure that team members are informed of the current status of the patient-family. The more informed the staff, the more timely and appropriate are patient and family interventions.

Nursing staff play a primary role in symptom control. The patient who has unresolved physical symptoms and is in great distress cannot benefit from spiritual, psychosocial, and other supportive interventions. Nursing staff must become clinical experts in observing important cues in symptoms so that the cause of these symptoms can be determined. Without accurate diagnosis of causative factors, treatment will be inaccurate and ineffective. Nursing staff must become clinical experts in hospice treatment modalities.

Specific pain medication, for example, needs to be given in the correct dosage, at the correct time interval, by the most appropriate route. Decisions about dose, time, and route require nurses to know about duration, action, side effects, and interactions with other drugs. Clinical knowledge and nursing skill supplement physician expertise and allow for ongoing nurse and physician interactions.

The medical community at large demonstrates a lack of expertise in some areas of terminal care. Nursing staff must be assertive and function as patient advocates. When a patient is undermedicated for pain and continues to be distressed by this symptom, the nurse must be able to rationally recommend a different, more appropriate approach. To do this, the nurse needs to be confident and operate from a well-grounded knowledge base. The hospice manager must be supportive of staff and encourage and expect staff to expand their knowledge and clinical skills so that the best interests of patients are served.

A great deal of a hospice manager's energy is devoted to evaluation. When results are less than desirable, the nursing process needs to be revised. Perhaps the initial assessment was incorrect, the plan inappropriate, or patient intervention incomplete. As noted in Chapter 3, continual evaluation and planning are part of the hospice administrator's role and daily function.

Statistics are one way to measure achievements or to discover deficiencies. Formal research in the inpatient unit may be ideal but not always realistic. The hospice manager can, however, promote less formal studies and encourage staff to do this according to their areas of special interest. Utilization review and quality assurance are ongoing processes, required by many states and federal reimbursement programs. Surveys and collection of statistics can provide a good reporting system over a long-term period. Comprehensive record keeping also provides tools to measure hospice effects and benefits. Measurement of quality hospice care is sorely needed.

UTILIZATION OF VOLUNTEERS

Volunteers have varied functions in the hospice unit. They can perform administrative as well as clinical care tasks. In terms of administrative functions, volunteers are used to serve as receptionists or to perform clerical tasks.

A family's first impression of an inpatient unit is an important one and creates the environment that will either encourage or discourage interactions during the patient's stay. The initial welcome to the hospice unit is extremely important and is an area in which a volunteer can play an important role. Before volunteers are employed in clinical care activities, hospice managers must address issues regarding organizational liability. This is discussed more fully in Chapter 9; however, it is important for administrators to assess potential liability problems that could result in lawsuits.

Volunteers with appropriate training and supervision can assist with uncomplicated direct patient care. Assisting the nursing staff with bathing, feeding, dressing, and bedmaking are functions volunteers can and often do assume.

Socializing with families encourages therapeutic interactions and forms a support network. Volunteers are valuable in this function, especially when staff focus on patient clinical needs. While children are encouraged to visit in the unit, there may be times when it is more helpful to families to have some privacy with the patient without children present. Having the volunteer available to keep young children occupied is important to families. The sensitive volunteer can explore the child's perceptions and provide appropriate support or information. He or she provides valuable resources and can expand a program's ability to offer new services and to serve patient and family needs.

STAFF SUPPORT

It is unrealistic for the hospice manager to expect that a well-functioning hospice unit has no tension. The manager's role is to reduce stress. Setting aside specific time for support group meetings is important but requires that staff also have support sources in their daily activities.

At some point, hospice staff may feel it is time to learn a different type of work. If the hospice manager creates an environment that views this as a failure to cope with hospice care, that stress will be present with staff in their daily work. If the manager views staff moving out of hospice and into new work as a choice to seek new opportunities and challenges, the burden of the guilt of failure will not hang over the heads of staff members. The daily function of the hospice manager is communication. Effective communication is the prime source of staff support.

Support groups are a valuable adjunct to the ongoing support staff within the unit. Meetings should be open and held when staff attending are not on duty. The group leader should be skilled in group communication techniques and not directly involved in the day-to-day operations of the hospice unit. An outside leader is more easily able to retain objectivity and to encourage divergent views for effectively solving problems. If the group leader is part of the hospice staff and is involved in the issues and problems raised, the probability of the group leader using the staff for his or her own support needs increases.

SUMMARY

Development of an inpatient unit is a challenging, exciting, and satisfying task. Because hospice has consequences for most hospital areas, planning should be interdisciplinary and multidepartment focused at the onset. The inpatient unit ideally is structured as a distinct alternative in care rather than as another traditional hospital unit. To accomplish this distinction may require changes in attitudes, routines, and rituals, approaches to patients and staff, and methods of delivery of services.

An inpatient hospice unit can have a positive impact on the hospital. Once the unit is set up, the work to educate and inform must be ongoing. Hospital staff, physicians, and the community at large require continuing education and reinforcement or reeducation. Hospice inpatient workers require ongoing sources for personal and professional development and support. Organizing and maintaining a productive team effort requires a manager's constant energy and attention. Maintenance of a cohesive team is one role the manager plays in the delivery of quality services.

An inpatient unit is a challenge to persistence and creativity. The effective administrator must be familiar with varied approaches to hospice care, understand staff needs and volunteer requirements, and have a flexible attitude toward program development.

NOTES

1. Charles A. Corr and Donna M. Corr, *Hospice Care Principles and Practice* (New York: Springer, 1983), 301.

2. Joint Commission on Accreditation of Hospitals, 875 N. Michigan Ave., Chicago, IL 60611.

3. *Standards of a Hospice Program of Care*. National Hospice Organization, 1901 N. Fort Meyer Dr., Suite 402, Arlington, VA 22209.

4. American Medical Records Association Foundation of Record Education, 875 N. Michigan Ave., Suite 1850, Chicago, IL 60611.

5. "Rules and Regulations," *Federal Register* 48, no. 243, December 16, 1983, 56008–56036.

6. David Greer, Vincent Mor, Howard Burnbaum, Sylvia Sherwood, and John Morris, National Hospice Study Preliminary Final Report (Providence: Brown University, November 1983).

7. "From Both Ends of the Stethoscope," Scripps Memorial Hospital Cancer Center, 9888 Genesee Avenue, LaJolla, CA 92037.

Chapter 6

Developing a Pediatric Hospice: Organizational Dynamics*

Kenneth H. Lazarus

We all die sometime. Unfortunately, some die before they have a chance to experience life. A child's death is as difficult to bear if not more difficult than the death of a spouse or other loved one. While adult hospice care is developing widespread acceptance, the concept of pediatric hospice care is new and largely unexplored.

Adults have a difficult time thinking about a child's death, much less trying to build programs to handle such cases. Physicians, nurses, social workers, parents, and relatives find it much harder to give up finding a cure for a child and allowing the natural death process to occur than they do for a 70-year old man with a cancer reoccurrence. In our medically sophisticated society, children are not supposed to die. For this reason, hospice planners and managers have been reluctant to build programs and services to care for terminally ill children.

This chapter describes the process of creating a pediatric hospice program. Using the example of one small, well-established program in a Texas community, issues related to the organization and development of a pediatric hospice are discussed.

THE PEDIATRIC HOSPICE AND THE ADULT HOSPICE

A pediatric hospice can be defined as a program designed to meet the unique medical, emotional, and spiritual needs of terminally ill children and their fam-

* Opinions expressed herein are those of the author and do not necessarily reflect opinions of the United States Air Force.

The author wishes to acknowledge the enormous support provided by Major Patricia Damler and by Mrs. Marjorie Jacks in the establishment and running of our hospice. Thanks also are due to Mrs. Velma Grantham and Ms. Mary Lou O'Connor for their editorial and secretarial assistance and to Dr. Lonnie Zeltzer for providing me this opportunity. Finally, a world of gratitude is owed to my wife, Marian, for her support and encouragement.

ilies. The pediatric hospice differs significantly from the adult hospice in three important ways: societal acceptance, legal rights of the minor, and psychological factors.

First, it is extremely difficult to acknowledge that a child may die before his or her parents. Parents, friends, relatives, and medical staff find it hard, both emotionally and psychologically, to accept the fact that their child or a child they know is dying. The dying child is not a subject of widespread discussion or research. Most investigations explore how a child deals with the death of a loved one rather than how a child handles his or her own impending death. Because the hospice philosophy is based on an acceptance of the inevitability of the approaching death, the concept of pediatric death is difficult to present.

Second, children are minors and are not legally capable of deciding to enter hospice. This is a significant problem for pediatric hospice managers, especially in light of several recent highly publicized cases questioning who has the right to make medical decisions for a dying child. The issue is more than just academic. The government and the courts have ruled that critically ill neonates must undergo therapy even after the parents have refused.[1] Such outside interventions could easily be extended to the child entering hospice care.

Finally, the psychology of death and dying in children differs according to the age, maturity, intelligence, and sensitivity of the child, and the beliefs and structure of the family. Recognition of the child's attitudes and those of other children affected by the child's death, such as siblings, is crucial to a successful hospice experience.

CHOOSING A PEDIATRIC HOSPICE MODEL

Once hospice planners and managers understand and accept these important differences, selection of a pediatric hospice model should be the first priority. Just like its adult counterpart, pediatric hospice care can be provided in the child's home, in a hospital, or in a free-standing hospice. There are four basic hospice models that can be employed. A pediatric hospice could be established as a free-standing entity. A second model places the pediatric hospice under the auspices of an adult hospice. The third model, the guideline model, develops instructions for running a pediatric program but activates the guidelines only as needed. A fourth possibility utilizes inpatient facilities, such as oncology units or parent-care wards, to provide in-hospital hospice care. Variations and combinations of these models can be used by pediatric hospice planners and managers to develop a pediatric hospice. There are few pediatric programs in the country responsible for sufficient numbers of terminally ill children to warrant a totally independent full-time pediatric hospice. Therefore, pediatric hospice organizers are encouraged to explore the three other models.

Placing the pediatric hospice under the auspices of an established adult hospice has the advantage of providing knowledgeable, trained personnel whose sole interest is hospice care. Organizational details including costs and equipment for the pediatric section could be smoothly handled within the larger framework of the operating adult hospice.

A major drawback of this model is its focus on the dying adult. Few who work with terminally ill adults are comfortable or trained to deal with the dying child. Another disadvantage is that hospice personnel may be different from those who had cared for the child during earlier phases of treatment. There may be an inability or unwillingness of the dying child or parents to accept strangers at a time when support is crucial.

The guideline model provides protocols or instructions for operating a pediatric hospice program but activates those protocols only when a child is in need. This model offers the advantage of individualizing care for each child/family unit. Since the personnel who cared for the child in earlier phases are often the ones who provide the hospice care, the transition is less abrupt and better accepted than with the former model. However, personnel funding and administrative machinery must be reestablished for each hospice patient. Thus, there might be greater difficulty obtaining trained hospice personnel, reduced knowledge and availability of community resources, and insufficient program funding.

The model that calls for the use of private rooms on oncology or parent-care wards allows for utilization of established facilities, resources, and personnel. It reduces duplication of effort and thereby decreases costs. There are many disadvantages, however, to this model. Hospital personnel who normally work in the area but who are not hospice workers may feel uncomfortable around the family and child. Other parents and children may have difficulty dealing with their own feelings about death and dying, which are exacerbated by the nearby hospice situation. The in-hospital hospice experience also forces the family to remain away from home in a different and less comfortable environment. The financial burden brought on by hospice care in a hospital setting may be quite high.[2] In addition, physicians and nurses not involved with the hospice program may perform medical actions such as resuscitation if not properly informed of the hospice concept and intent.

Each administrator and planner of a pediatric hospice must select a model that addresses a variety of organizational issues including the type of children to be served, the development of the hospice team, the sources of reimbursement, and an array of ethical and legal questions.

Most pediatric hospices will be operated under the auspices of an established hospital or adult hospice. Hospital and hospice administration commitment to the concept is crucial to development of a successful pediatric hospice program. In the hospital setting, the chief hospice administrator needs strong ties to the main hospital administration so that resources and funding can be made available.

There must be close communication with departments that may play important roles in the management of terminally ill children, such as nursing, physical therapy, occupational therapy, pharmacy, dietary, and respiratory therapy. If the pediatric hospice is established within the control of an adult hospice, the chief administrator of the pediatric hospice must be directly responsible to the adult hospice administrator so that specific needs and concerns can be addressed expeditiously. Many hospitals, while verbally supportive, limit resources at the hospice staff's discretion, which complicates delivery of services.

DETERMINING THE POPULATION BASE

An important consideration prior to selecting a hospice care model is to determine the population base. There are approximately 6,000-7,000 newly diagnosed cases of pediatric cancer in the United States annually.[3] About 40 percent of these children will die of their disease.[4] If one assumes that 60 percent of these terminally ill children will be hospice candidates, then there should be about 1,500 children with cancer who require hospice care each year. Even if 10-20 percent more children with nononcologic diseases become hospice candidates, the available patient population in any one area will be relatively small. The model of pediatric hospice care chosen should accommodate the potential population. However, the small number of hospice candidates may further decrease a hospital's commitment to the program.

Criteria by which children will be selected for hospice care must be determined by the hospice administration before any planning is initiated. Most hospices deal mainly with oncology patients for several reasons. Once a patient with a malignancy relapses, the duration of survival is fairly predictable, and the period of time for which intensive, in-home care is required is limited. Children with other chronic diseases frequently considered terminal, such as cystic fibrosis, degenerative neurologic diseases, cardiac diseases, etc., may survive for protracted periods. The ability of medical personnel to provide intensive emotional support for a prolonged period is limited. Also, oncologists, unlike most general pediatricians, are educated in concepts of death and dying and feel more comfortable dealing with such patients. Regardless of what disease the child has, his or her primary physician needs to be actively involved in the hospice program.

THE HOSPICE TEAM

After selecting a model and identifying a patient population, administrators must determine who will serve on the hospice team. If the hospice team is allied with an adult hospice, the personnel who deal with children could be selected from those employees who volunteer to work with children. If the guideline model is selected, then procedures for the hospice team must be delineated.

The hospice team is multidisciplinary, including physicians, nurses, social workers, child psychologists, clergymen, dieticians, teachers, and lay parents who have had a hospice experience of their own. The individuals on the pediatric team differ only slightly from those on an adult hospice team. The pediatric team must be prepared to deal with the developmental and intellectual status of the child.

The pediatrician serves as the overall director and coordinator of care. He or she is usually seen by the family as the main member of the team—the person with all the answers. Therefore, there is great need for his or her active and frequent involvement. Despite this viewpoint, nurses serve as the focal point providing the majority of the patient care. The chief hospice nurse should be directly responsible to the pediatrician so that care is coordinated and not duplicated.

Nurses can be hired from agencies as needed or recruited from a volunteer pool within the hospital or clinic where the child has previously received treatment. Volunteer nurses familiar with the child and family offer an advantage over nurses hired solely to provide hospice service. Children who are ill generally fear strangers and change. Introduction of new nurses for hospice care is traumatic and may be poorly received. In addition, parents are protective of their children and may be reluctant to invite unfamiliar persons into their home. This protective attitude may lead to fewer requests for hospice team visits, even if the need for such visits exists.

Obtaining volunteer nurses is usually simple once the concept of the hospice program and their role in it have been explained. Professionals can often be recruited from volunteers in the community. The inclusion of a lay parent should be approved by the other members of the team. The lay parent should have had a positive hospice experience and express a desire to help. As is pointed out in Chapter 13 on bereavement, volunteers who need to ease personal grief should not be selected in this situation.

REIMBURSEMENT

Administrators and planners of pediatric hospices also must contend with reimbursement questions. The suggestions for dealing with financial issues discussed in other chapters are generally applicable only to the adult hospice situation. Pediatric hospices are rare, and third-party and government agency involvement is poorly defined.[5] Many pediatric oncology patients receive support from Medicaid or Crippled Children's Services but most of the payments are for inpatient care. Whether these programs, as well as third-party medical insurance programs, can provide payment for pediatric hospice and terminal care is unexplored. Recently, some third-party payers have agreed to fund pediatric hospice care similar to adult hospice care.

The use of volunteer personnel substantially decreases costs. Yet, there are issues regarding the ability of these volunteers to provide clinical services and to adequately meet patient and family needs. The question of payment is important. Administrators and planners should explore funding possibilities prior to establishing pediatric hospice care.

CONSENT AND MINORS' RIGHTS

Issues regarding minors and minors' rights vis-a-vis medical care have only recently been tested. Legally, some children have the understanding, maturity, and ability to make decisions regarding their treatment, and even about whether to enter hospice care or not.[6]

Many hospitals now have ethics committees composed of physicians, nurses, chaplains, psychologists, lawyers, and lay persons to help decide difficult moral and ethical questions regarding medical care of children.[7] If the hospice is based in a hospital where such a committee exists, the hospice administrator should consider obtaining committee advice regarding selection of individual pediatric candidates. Those actively involved in hospice care may have difficulty realizing that parents or other family members may not share their viewpoint. This may lead to confusion and misunderstanding between the family and the medical staff. The ethics committee can prevent miscommunication by providing a non-biased forum for discussion of the child's illness and available treatment options including hospice care. The committee also may recognize potential areas of conflict between parents and medical staff, thereby defusing potentially explosive situations. For example, one parent of a dying child may strongly support the hospice concept but the other parent may oppose it. Hospice members may not recognize the opposing parent's views. An ethics committee could explore the parents' conflicting desires and help the medical staff deal more appropriately with the parents and the child.

On most consent forms, assent must be obtained from children the attending physician feels can make a reasoned decision. Assent differs from consent in that it indicates agreement, but by itself it is not adequate to allow the treatment to proceed. Consent from parents or guardians is still necessary in order for treatment to be provided. Difficulty arises when the child does not give assent but parents give consent. Generally, the decision to enter the hospice is made jointly by parents and their child. If the parents are hesitant, the desire of their child to be at home is often enough to sway them in that direction. The hospice philosophy does not presuppose that the parents are making a decision between life and death, but that they are choosing the option that will provide the greatest comfort and support for themselves and their child at an extremely difficult and painful time. The preservation of the rights of minors is extremely important. Hospice does not represent a new treatment. What it offers is an alternative to inpatient hospital care.

In many programs the parents sign a trust agreement (consent form) that defines hospice care, their role as parents, and the program's role in treating the disease symptoms and family needs (see Exhibit 6-1). This trust agreement forces the medical staff to be unequivocal about what is happening to the child, which greatly minimizes the risk of miscommunication.

Exhibit 6-1 Hospice Trust Agreement

I understand that my child _____ has _____. Conventional medical therapy designed to produce a remission or cure for this disease has to date been unsuccessful. My child's physician has completely informed me of all options available for effective therapy at the present time. I realize that the only therapy available for prolonging the life of my child would be untried or unproven experimental treatments. I do not choose to place my child in an experimental treatment program.

In order to carry out this choice I elect to participate in the Wilford Hall Medical Center Pediatric Hospice Program. I understand this program is designed to provide my family, my child, and myself with medical, emotional, and spiritual support during and after this very trying period.

While this program is designed to allow my child to be at home during this period, I realize that I may request that my child return to the hospital at any time. I also realize that entry into the hospice program does not remove my right to elect for an experimental treatment program in the future. I also understand that refusal to participate in the hospice program will in no way jeopardize my child's care.

_____

SIGNED

_____

WITNESS

_____

WITNESS

_____

DATE

ESTABLISHING A PEDIATRIC HOSPICE

Hospice X is a small, exclusively pediatric hospice established in a large military hospital in Texas. This hospice utilized the guidelines model for management of children during the terminal phases of their illness. The hospice team is brought together when a child requires hospice care. Approximately 7 to 10 children require hospice support each year. The personnel are all volunteers and except for the physician, chief hospice nurse, and social worker vary among patients. Each hospice experience has utilized as few as 5 and as many as 12 persons, depending on the family's needs and the number of volunteers. The program is administered by the pediatrician. Because Hospice X is established in a military hospital, it utilizes the facilities and resources of that hospital and therefore does not have a separate budget. Hospice X will serve as an example of techniques and ideas to be utilized in setting up a pediatric hospice. A flow chart of occurrences at Hospice X once a potential patient is identified can be found in Figure 6-1.

Hospice X was developed by a multidisciplinary team consisting of a pediatric hematologist/oncologist, four pediatric nurses, a social worker, a marriage counselor, a child psychologist, a chaplain, and a lawyer. Although they were not directly involved in establishing this program, advice from a pharmacist, a dietician, and/or a public health nurse should be considered. Five committees were defined in order to facilitate program development and management: (1) support for decision making, (2) medical management, (3) actual events surrounding the child's death, (4) bereavement and follow-up, and (5) education.

Support for Decision Making

Initially, an intake interview is conducted with parents when their child is diagnosed as having the possibility of a terminal disease. The interview is conducted by a social worker and lasts approximately 60 minutes. Intake information is obtained at the time of diagnosis rather than upon entering the hospice program because of the difficulty of asking such intimate and sensitive questions at a time when the parents are marshalling all their energies to deal with the impending death of their child. Information in the intake interview is used to identify sources of stress other than those produced by the child's illness and is updated by the social worker as events and conditions change. This information is kept in a separate social file and is not made available to those seeking access to the child's medical file without the permission of the parents. When hospice care becomes a selected option, the information in the file is passed on to the hospice team members.

Key questions addressed during the interview include:

Figure 6-1 Flow Chart of Activities at Hospice X Once a Potential Patient Is Identified

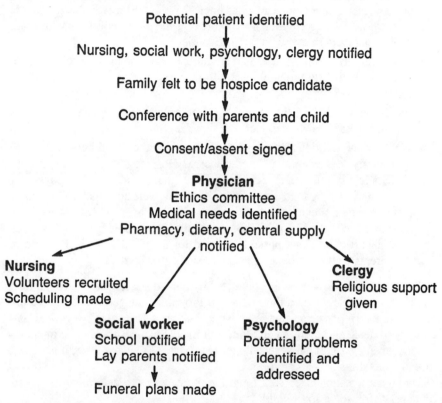

Potential patient identified

Nursing, social work, psychology, clergy notified

Family felt to be hospice candidate

Conference with parents and child

Consent/assent signed

Physician
Ethics committee
Medical needs identified
Pharmacy, dietary, central supply notified

Nursing
Volunteers recruited
Scheduling made

Social worker
School notified
Lay parents notified

Funeral plans made

Psychology
Potential problems
identified and
addressed

Clergy
Religious support
given

- Are these parents the natural parents? If the mother or father are stepparents, what role does the biological mother or father play in the child's life? Do we need to include them in the discussion or decision making?

- Are there financial burdens that will be worsened by the child's illness? For example, if both parents work how will care for the child be provided? Will the parents be able to arrange adequate time off to care for their child?

- Are their prior problems with emotional instability, drugs, alcohol, etc., that may affect this child's care or that may recur because of the enormous stress? One must know how the family has handled the underlying disease. If there have been problems with alcohol or drug abuse, child or spouse abuse, noncompliance with protocols, marriage difficulties, or even marked personality conflicts with members of the hospice team, there may be reasons to reconsider offering the hospice option.

- What is the relationship with other nonimmediate family members? In cases of single parents or where both parents work outside the home, how supportive are grandparents, aunts, and uncles? Will they be available to provide physical as well as emotional support? Are there any conflicts with other family members that may create difficulties?
- How strong is this marriage? Is there an open communicating relationship, or are there already problems that will be compounded by the stress of the child's illness?
- What is the ability of the family to comprehend the full meaning of their child's illness? How compliant will they be with the medical program?
- What are the religious beliefs of the family? Do they hold beliefs that will be contrary to the goals of medical care? Hospice X had the experience where a family joined a church that believed their child would be physically healed only if they held a positive faith. They were told that any negative thoughts would prevent the child's cure. Since the hospice team would have presented the reality of the child's death, the team would have been viewed as a negative force and possibly blamed for the child's death. Because of the parents' religious beliefs, hospice was not offered.

The intake interview must be conducted by trained staff, sensitive to the fears and concerns of parents and their children. Program managers must be sure that staff assigned to perform interviews have background in social work and psychology of death and dying in children. For many hospices this intake interview is done when the child has reached a terminal state. At such a time, it is helpful to know the stresses shaping the family.

Two other questions assist staff and family members to determine the appropriateness of hospice for a child:

- Can the family arrange to have someone available to provide care around the clock? Few patients require such constant care as the pediatric hospice patient. Even if both parents plan to continue to work, hospice care can still be offered if other family members are willing to take on the responsibility.
- How far does the family live from the hospital? Do transportation considerations preclude visitations by hospital personnel? For patients who live great distances from the treatment center, local public health nurses and the local pediatrician might be enlisted to provide hospice care. However, this option is not optimal. The nurses will be strangers to the family and child, and they are usually unable and sometimes unwilling to provide the type of care the child needs. Local pediatricians, even if willing, are frequently unable to give the child the necessary time. Still, this option is generally preferable to the child dying in a hospital far from home.

The decision to offer hospice care should be made by the entire hospice team. It should be based on whether the child and family can tolerate the stresses and whether the hospice experience will be a positive one. Once the patient and family are considered as candidates for hospice, the physician should confer with the parents or guardians. The decision to include the child in the discussion should be left to the parents' discretion. Administrators should be sure that the conference is tape recorded or is attended by a nurse and/or a social worker to ensure an accurate account of the presentation. Options for therapy should not be directed by the physician's wishes. The family may be considering care specifically because it requires the family to play an active participant role.

Many families are reluctant to choose hospice. First, they are afraid they will be unable to care for their child at home. Reassurance from all members of the hospice team may be necessary on multiple occasions to convince the parents that they are capable and that the hospice team will be available whenever the family needs them. Second, parents need to know they have done everything possible for their child. Any doubt or guilt will make the grieving process after death more severe and difficult. For some families, this overwhelming need will not permit them to participate in a hospice program.

It is important that the hospice option be presented as a positive therapeutic decision and not as a loss of hope for the child's survival. The parents should be told that hospice is a positive choice and that other therapies would only prolong the child's suffering. This reassurance must be ongoing, frequently extending into the bereavement period.

Once the family opts for hospice, administrators should ask parents to sign the hospice trust agreement form. A written report of this conference should be made by the physician and a hospice file established. Written documentation is necessary to ensure that an accurate account of events is maintained. Despite all precautions and care, misunderstandings do occur. The written record also helps the hospice team review positive and negative experiences.

Medical Management

Medical management of pediatric hospice service is best conceptualized as a dichotomous action that involves providing for the medical needs of the family and arranging for and scheduling the hospice team.

Providing for Medical Needs

There are four major areas of medical management that produce the greatest anxiety in parents and that may lead to a poor hospice experience, or abandonment of hospice. First, medical staff must be prepared to deal with the pain brought on by the spread of disease. Relaxation and hypnosis techniques may prove valuable in decreasing the need for pain medication.[8] Oral medications, including acetaminophen, codeine, oxycodone, meperidine, and hydromorphone are excellent agents. Methadone offers the major advantage of pain management with minimal sedation. The child remains alert but is comfortable. A good starting dose of 0.07 mg/kg/d followed by six-hour doses works well. This can be changed or "scheduled" as needed. Antidepressants such as amitriptyline and anxiolytic agents such as valium or hydroxyzine may potentiate the effects of some of the narcotic medications. Physical techniques to decrease pain include providing hospital beds, or encouraging the parents to obtain a water bed. Egg-shell mattresses and sheepskin may provide softer, less abrasive surfaces and decrease pain and bed sores. With judicious and responsive medical management and support, parents, and even the children themselves, can become quite adept at managing pain.

A second complication is bleeding. Bleeding is a feared event but is generally rare and easily controllable. Serious bleeding such as gastrointestinal or intracranial bleeding is unusual, although it may be the terminal event. In such cases, supportive care for the child continues and reassurances are given to the parent that little would be done differently if the child were in the hospital. Topical bleeding, especially of the nose and/or mouth, is usually managed with local pressure and topical anticoagulants. Aminocaproic acid can frequently decrease minor bleeding in a patient who is thrombocytopenic.

Infections and fevers represent a third area of concern to parents. Local infections can usually be treated with topical or oral antibiotics. It is important to emphasize skin care to the parents so that skin breakdown does not produce additional sites of pain and discomfort. Fevers can be treated with acetaminophen and cool baths or towels.

Respiratory distress is probably the most feared complication. Home oxygen frequently is adequate to help reduce anxiety and perhaps decrease agitation in children who are developing hypoxia. When hypoxia and dyspnea are due to infiltration of the lungs by metastatic tumor, oxygen is only a temporary solution. Reassurance to the parents that they are doing everything that could be done in the hospital short of endotracheal intubation will frequently allow the family to continue in hospice. Severe dyspnea is usually followed shortly by death.

Everything that is done at home is geared to comfort. Poor intake of fluids or food may be of concern to the parents and institution of nasogastric or intravenous feedings may be appropriate.

Arranging for and Scheduling the Hospice Team

An essential and difficult job of the hospice planner is arranging home visitation and phone call schedules of various participants. One person, either the chief hospice nurse or a patient care coordinator, should be responsible for scheduling available nurses. It is possible to change this person among several patients, but using the same person lends stability and experience to an important position and is preferable.

At Hospice X, the chief hospice nurse recruits three or four volunteer nurses from those pediatric nurses who have worked with the terminally ill child and who feel close to the family from prior hospitalization or clinic visits. If the hospice planner chooses to use commercial agency nurses, three or four nurses will most likely be necessary to decrease enormous emotional and time demands on any one person. Because it is expensive to hire an agency nurse to make phone calls or to be available as needed, it is most practical to use one person for all care needs until the patient requires daily visits.

Currently, there are many companies providing home nursing care. Many also provide hospice care. Using commercial agencies simplifies nursing care scheduling but pediatric hospice planners must recognize that there are perils inherent in using these services. The nurses are unfamiliar with the family or child and could produce unnecessary anxieties. In addition, those who have worked closely with the family previously may feel uncomfortable with their decreased involvement and the family may view their decreased involvement as abandonment. In some hospices, however, agency nurses have been routinely used with excellent results.

If the patient lives far from the place of treatment, the chief hospice nurse or hospice administrator coordinates home care through public health or commercial agency nurses or through an established hospice in the family's home town. The primary physician also arranges for medical care with a local pediatrician.

Once hospice nurses are available, the hospice administrator or the chief hospice nurse should use a rotating schedule so that minimally one nurse is available daily. Some families may not need or want a daily visit. Regardless of how well a child is doing, however, the hospice nurse should make a phone call to the home at least once a day and a home visit at least once a week, as is pointed out in Chapter 10. Documentation is important and managers should require that all phone calls and visits are recorded in the child's hospice file. This enables the hospice team to keep track of the child's and family's progress. Ideally, the doctor should call the family daily or on alternate days and visit the home as needed.

Visitations by clergy members, social workers, dieticians, psychologists, and others are also made as needed. Visitations should be made only at the invitation of the family. Many parents will respond negatively when asked if they need help.They may feel that they would be burdening the medical staff or causing inconvenience by requesting a visit. Therefore, it is important for the medical staff to give specific times for visitation and to ask if such times are convenient for the family.

A home visit by the nurse, doctor, volunteer, or other hospice staff member serves several purposes: First, the visit is designed to assess the medical condition of the child. Should a change in pain medication or fluid management be needed this should be communicated to the physician. The visit is also made to evaluate how well the family is handling the enormous pressure of hospice. If signs of fatigue or stress are noticed, the family can be offered respite and the child readmitted to the hospital, where the same hospice principles are applied. An order not to resuscitate must be placed on the chart and the permission of the parents documented.

A third purpose of the medical visit is social. It actively demonstrates that the team cares about the child and will be available when needed. It also reassures the parents and the child that they have made the right decision and helps the family resolve the doubts that continuously arise. Two outstanding resources, by Martinson and Martinson and Moldow,[9] contain much useful information.

It is important that the child be encouraged to remain as active as possible. Activities should be geared to the child's age and ability to participate. A trip to Disney World is wonderful, but if a child is too young to comprehend what is happening or too ill or in too much pain to appreciate the surroundings, it can become a disaster. Short trips to nearby favorite areas are to be encouraged. For the older child, it is wisest to find out what the child would enjoy. New organizations have been established in many areas of the country that grant requests to dying children. One child at Hospice X with recurrent neuroblastoma wished to go with her family to Disney World. A local program paid for the child and her immediate family to go for four days free of charge. Another child wished to be a Dallas Cowgirl. She and her family were flown to Dallas to meet with the Dallas Cowgirls and join in their practice sessions. Such programs, if available, represent excellent resources.

Events Surrounding the Child's Death

Generally, hospice programs assist the family in making funeral arrangements prior to death. This is also the case in pediatric care. Because of the difficulty of acknowledging that a child may die, making funeral arrangements may be viewed by the family as an end to hope for the child's survival. At Hospice X, parents are told that making funeral plans is like buying life insurance or making a will. Such actions do not mean that death will definitely occur but that one is prepared for it when (or if) it does. It is best if a lay parent or one of the team who has prior hospice experience takes the family to the funeral home. Making such plans prior to death allows for more rational decisions regarding funeral arrangements. Some adolescents (admittedly, very few) have even wanted to be involved in the planning of the funeral service.

The family must be advised as to what to expect as death approaches. There usually is a gradual withdrawal from outside involvement until virtual nonresponsiveness or coma occurs. Often within a short period before death (as long as a week or as short as a few minutes), there may be a period of increased lucidity. If the process has been one associated with pain (especially bone involvement), this period may be marked by great agitation and severe pain. The patient may act as if all narcotic analgesics had suddenly worn off or been neutralized. The period may last from a few minutes to a few hours and is usually followed by a calm period leading to a peaceful death. These events should be described to parents before they happen so that if they occur, they will not be frightened. The agitation is extremely difficult on the parents, and it is virtually nonresponsive to pain medications. Physicians should recommend that parents try to comfort the child as much as possible and continue or increase pain medication if possible.

Many parents are afraid that death will be an ugly time—a time of struggle and suffering—for their child. In fact, death usually, though not always, is very peaceful. The parents may need frequent support regarding their fears about death, as may the medical staff.

Psychology of Death and Dying

Managers and planners must be sure their staff understand the psychology of death and dying. This is important because all hospice participants are at varying stages of the grieving process. Moreover, as discussed in previous chapters, hospice care must be unique and individualized. Regardless of the underlying disease, symptoms, or reaction to pain therapies, no two deaths are alike. In addition, conveying the concept of death to a child is much different and often more difficult than with an adult. Comprehension of death for the child depends on his or her age, maturity, intelligence, family background, and to some extent on the openness of the parents and physician.

The Preschool-Age Child

Prior to age two or three, the child has few if any reference points for death. In addition, the child is unable to adequately communicate his or her feelings. It would appear that these children do not fear death, but rather separation from parents. They are quite capable of understanding the feelings of sadness they see and hear around them, so that even very young infants may become depressed and withdrawn. Support for children of this age requires a great deal of patience and loving. For the very young child, time spent reading, drawing, playing simple word games, or just watching television together may serve as a great source of comfort. Short absences by the parents may be poorly tolerated. Trusted and loved nurses, doctors, family relatives, or friends may, however, give parents the opportunity to get occasional breaks.

The child between ages three and six usually has had some exposure to death. This may have been the loss of a grandparent, a close friend, another patient in the same clinic, a pet, or even such losses as a favorite toy or a move to another neighborhood. The irreversibility of death, however, is poorly understood and is not completely formulated until adolescence. In addition, religious teachings at this age, in many families, refer to a benign, beautiful heaven. Death is not feared by the preschool-age child.

Preschool children indulge in fantasy thinking and often believe that their thoughts become facts. This belief may lead to a feeling that they are being punished for bad thoughts, or that they are responsible for the sadness occurring in the family. Because of this, the child may withdraw or display anger toward his or her family. A child of this age also fears separation and abandonment, so again, a patient, loving attitude must be adopted.

Some children ask questions about their condition. Long answers are boring and tedious for this age child. Short direct answers, honest and to the point, are best. The timing of the child's questions may often seem strange, but questions are asked when the child needs an answer. A promise by the parents that they will always remain with the child and that they will be together again in heaven will often relieve the child's anxiety at the impending separation.

The Grade-School Age Child

The school-age child has usually developed a wider range of security sources. The parents no longer represent the only source of acceptance by the world. He or she can understand the seriousness of his or her condition, and time begins to take on meaning. In addition, the permanence of death is becoming an understandable concept. Still, the child has less fear of death than of being different and isolated. The child of this age may only have one or two people with whom he or she is willing to share feelings.

The school-age child may have difficulty with the changes in body image produced by marked weight loss, tumor growth, or inability to control excretions. The use of diapers, which make management of defecation and urination far easier, may be a major source of embarrassment. Allowing only immediate family or medical personnel to see the diapers and patient explanations of the need and usefulness of such items may greatly facilitate the patient's emotional comfort.

Often, a sense of continuity provides a great sense of security. Having the child involved in family events as much as possible provides the child with a feeling that all is right with his or her world, even though the child knows it is not. Having the child continue with schooling, if at all possible, or having homebound instruction or work brought home from school provides a link with a normal environment. Continued schooling also serves as a means of taking the child's mind off what is happening.

Frequently, this age child will become resigned to death before the family does. In such cases, the child may take on a comforting role and try to assure the parents that he or she is not afraid to die. The strength and maturity of these children is often remarkable. Some parents have been greatly comforted after their child's death by this acceptance.

Adolescents

Adolescents also fear loss of independence and being different probably more than they fear death. The loss of independence forced on them by disease may lead to power struggles with parents and become a source of antagonism during a very trying period. Allowing the adolescent as much autonomy as possible may improve the relationship and communication. Examples would be allowing the teenager to choose clothes, foods, dressing change times, and the timing of pain medications. Even allowing the teenager to be the final arbiter of the choice between hospice and experimental treatment usually provides a great sense of control. The realization of death may overtax the teenager's ability to cope with his or her anxieties and may result in withdrawal or a regression to an earlier, more dependent stage.[10]

It is very important to be honest. Dishonesty will limit communication and further isolate the adolescent. Discussions of disease progression should be held directly with the adolescent and parents. The adolescent who has an adult outlook on life and death (although with more fantasy thoughts about immortality) needs to feel there is some purpose to his or her life. One way is to allow the adolescent to divide up possessions and to arrange for their dispersal after death. Helping other children, writing a story or poem, keeping a diary, painting a picture, or making a videotape are all ways that an adolescent has of providing some purpose to his or her life. One 15-year-old boy who was dying of a recurrent lymphoma, and whose mother was pregnant, was quite depressed for he felt he had nothing to leave the soon-to-be-born baby. He was able to make a videotape in which he told the baby who he was and what he would have liked to teach him or her. Following the videotaping, he was far calmer and happier. Such ideas are to be encouraged and promoted.

The adolescent is usually very sensitive to the effects of his or her illness on parents and siblings. This may lead to attempts to protect the family. One 19-year-old boy dying with Ewing's sarcoma said he was not afraid to die but was very concerned about the effect of his death on his family. Here is where communication lines must be kept open between parents and teenager. It is interesting that, despite feelings of depression, isolation, and even worthlessness, suicide is relatively rare in this group. Perhaps this is because they are so closely watched by family and medical personnel. It also may be that in contemplating their own death, these teenagers come to appreciate the value of life.[11]

Coping Responses

There are several psychological ramifications that may affect parents' reactions to the death of their child. Guilt is a major problem and arises out of feelings of failure, anger, and relief. Parents sometimes feel that they must be towers of strength and cannot be weak in front of the child. Inside they may feel they are failing the child because they are not always strong. They may feel they have caused the illness or failed to prevent its recurrence. They may feel they have not adequately tried for full treatment. The mother may feel she has failed the dying child's siblings, which further adds to her feelings of guilt and inadequacy. Parents may feel quite angry at the child for the inconvenience and hardships he or she has caused and then feel guilty and ashamed for having such feelings. They may also reach a point where the death of their child would be a relief and this feeling can also produce feelings of guilt. Despite the fact that this desire for relief is very common and the parents usually have access to narcotics which could end their child's life, they almost never deliberately administer an overdose. The ambivalence over a desire to shorten the child's suffering and the desire to have the child with them for as long as possible is clearly evident. The father may feel inadequate if the illness has brought financial hardships on the family, which will also exacerbate feelings of guilt. The knowledge that these feelings are normal may be very comforting to the parents.

Feelings engendered by the care of a dying child are often not expressed and may lead to marital problems. Despite this, Oakley and Patterson[12] and Stehbens and Lascar[13] did not find any evidence of divorce or separation in 15 and 20 families, respectively, 6 months to 3 years after a child's death. Lansky and associates[14] reported that the person-year divorce rate (the number of divorces occurring for each year of marriage) for parents of 191 children treated for cancer was slightly lower than the general population as a whole.

The parents who have been through Hospice X generally have seemed to grow closer. This probably has occurred because of the involvement of the entire family in the hospice program. If the child is in the hospital, it is usually the mother who stays with the child while the father works. The father then sees the child infrequently and may not be actively involved in the care. This may lead to miscommunication between the parents, with the father not being able to understand the wife's fatigue and grief and the mother angry about being left alone to shoulder the entire burden of care. While the father may still work during hospice care, when he is home the child is there and the situation cannot be avoided. As a result, both parents must participate and communication between mother and father is facilitated.

Stepparents have a more difficult role to play than real parents. They often are expected to shoulder the full responsibility for the child's care, yet may not have the desire to do so, nor may they be fully accepted by their spouse or by the child. In addition, poor relationships with the natural parent may exist. Hospice X includes the stepparents actively in the program. If a natural parent is not living in the home, the consent of the parents/guardians who are living with the child is obtained before including that natural parent.

Siblings represent a group with potentially major psychological difficulties. Again, the age and maturity of these children are important in assessing the reaction. Very young siblings notice only the absence or decreased attention of the parents. Attention-getting behaviors may frequently be disruptive and cause further stress to the parents. Removing the very young child from the environment may improve the situation. Removing older preschool and school-age children only serves to increase their grief reaction. Four-to-seven-year-olds may develop a great deal of resentment and anger toward the sick sibling because of loss of attention from the parents and because the illness allows the sick child more freedom. There may be fantasy feelings that thoughts of anger or resentment were what caused their sibling to get ill, and this may produce strong feelings of guilt. Frequently, these may manifest themselves as difficulty with peer relationships, restlessness, disobedience, temper tantrums, soiling, enuresis, or school problems. These reactions may arise shortly after the death or even several years later.[15]

There may also be feelings that the siblings too will get some disease and die. This is particularly true if the dying child was a twin. Cairns and associates[16] examined school-age patients and healthy siblings from 71 families on a battery of psychological tests. Siblings and patients both experienced similar levels of stress and anxiety. An important statement in this study is that these siblings "are essentially normal children." It is important to recognize, in the midst of our concern for the patient and his or her parents, that the siblings suffer too. After the child dies, the sibling may suffer from guilt because he or she has survived. In addition, there may be new pressures placed on the sibling by the parents who may expect the sibling to take on the dreams and aspirations and successes of the dead child.

It is most important that the hospice staff become adept at recognizing the anger, frustration, and guilt feelings brought on by the death of a child. These feelings are occurring not only in the family but also in the medical personnel as well. If unrecognized in the staff, they can lead to excessive identification with the family with prolonged grief and burnout or to open hostility with the family. The references by Gyulay, Easson, and Bluebond-Langer contain further information about the psychology of death and dying with respect to children.[17]

The Death Itself

At the time the hospice experience is started, a list of important phone numbers is given to the family. This should include:

- Doctor
- Chaplain
- Hospital wards
- Hospice team members
- Funeral home
- Police

- Mortuary affairs
- Health benefits
- Relatives

It should be placed right by the telephone so it is readily available. If the physician is not present when the child dies, the parents or any person in attendance calls him or her to tell of the death. Hospice administrators should advise program physicians that upon arriving at the home, his or her first action is to confirm the death, to note the time, and then to call the local police department. The police are told that a physician is in attendance and emergency medical assistance is not required. The police will obtain information regarding the death. In most cases, they will call the medical examiner's office to obtain permission to release the body to the funeral home. If the family desires an autopsy, the doctor will phone the funeral home that the family had previously selected. Usually, the funeral home arranges for transportation of the body to the morgue so the autopsy can be performed. Few families request or grant permission for an autopsy, and the medical examiner's office rarely demands that one be performed.

While waiting for the police, other important phone calls can be made. The family usually has a list of individuals they would like called. Many hospices designate one volunteer to make all phone calls. The members of the hospice team should also be called; however, it is not appropriate for all members of the team to descend on the home at the same time. If the family has a good relationship with a clergy member, it might be wise to call him or her.

Bereavement

In formulating a pediatric hospice, it is important to plan bereavement and follow-up programming that addresses the needs of parents, siblings, the extended family, and the medical staff. At Hospice X, a rotating hospice file has been developed by the social worker so that the family is contacted either by letter, card, phone call, or home visit one week, one month, three months, six months, and one year after the child's death. The family also is reached yearly on the child's birthday, at Christmas or Hanukkah, and on the anniversary date of the death. After two to three years, a follow-up card is sent on the anniversary date of the child's death. Feedback from the families on this follow-up program has been positive. The family realizes that affection and support given during hospice was genuine and extended beyond the hospice itself. They appreciate the idea that their child is remembered and is important to someone other than themselves. The social worker has also established a bereavement group for parents who have lost children at Hospice X. This group meets once a month or every other month at a member's home to discuss issues common to each of them.

As is pointed out in Chapter 13, it is important to recognize that grieving does not have a specified time for completion. It is clear that the first few months usually are marked by numbness which then gives way to stunning reality. Most parents have their greatest difficulties six months to one year after their child's death. Unless grieving appears to be pathological, it is important not to interfere with the process.

Siblings often have severe problems with the death of their brother or sister. Feelings of guilt are common and frequently relate to the child's belief that he or she caused the brother or sister's illness. The sibling may be resentful of the attention given to the sick child and feel guilty because of that resentment. Finally, the child may feel that he or she somehow caused the sadness and grief and this will produce additional feelings of guilt. Unless directly addressed (and even if addressed), the long-term effects of this guilt mixed with sadness and feelings of loss may lead to several problems. Behavior problems, school difficulties, and drug and alcohol abuse are all problems that have been observed in siblings of dying children. The hospice process may decrease these reactions as long as the dying child's brother or sister are involved. Dishonesty or total involvement by the parent with the dying child to the exclusion of the brother or sister only serve to make the grieving process more difficult. It is important to recognize problems with siblings before they occur and offer support and counseling as needed.

Grandparents, uncles, aunts, cousins, and friends are also affected by a child's death and must be allowed to grieve. At Hospice X there is no formal program for recognizing problems that may occur in the extended family; however, hospice personnel are prepared to help such individuals as needed.

One group that may be extremely affected by a child's death are those children being cared for by the same doctor, or who have the same disease and who knew the dead child. The amount of contact with the dead child may have been minimal, but the effect of that death may be profound. Bereavement follow-up must be an active ongoing program.

At Hospice X, hospice members are not required to attend the child's funeral and hospice members should not feel obligated to attend. One family at Hospice X even requested that nonfamily members not attend. Occasionally, some hospice members may feel that the funeral would be too painful. For most hospice members, some closure is necessary. Hospice administrators should plan a final post-death meeting of the hospice team one or two weeks after the funeral in order to provide for a summation and discussion of the events of the preceding days and weeks. Staff members experiencing difficulties should be identified and steered to appropriate resources for help. One common feeling often generated is guilt that more could have been done for the child or for the family. It is important to allow staff members to verbalize this feeling in order to decrease long-term depression. Participation in hospice care, however, is usually an extremely positive experience for the staff members.

Education

There are three major goals of the hospice education program: (1) to train medical personnel in concepts of dealing with death and dying in general and with the terminally ill child specifically, (2) to teach family members what is happening to their child and to themselves and how to deal with those changes, and (3) to inform the general public about the concepts, goals, and needs of a pediatric hospice.

Many medical and nursing schools now provide courses and seminars in death and dying that help young nurses and doctors deal with hospice issues. Hospice administrators might consider establishing death and dying seminars and workshops in area hospitals, community centers, universities, etc., for those interested in pediatric hospice. These workshops educate professionals about age-related concepts of death and help hospice team members deal with their own fears and misconceptions about death and dying. Prior to beginning hospice care for a child, the hospice administrator should hold one or two sessions informing the participants about the child's and family's individual needs and problems. Hospice planners and managers must recognize that learning about death and dying with respect to children is ongoing and largely experiential.

The education of the family and the dying child is central to the hospice concept. Parents and children need to be taught about the events that are occurring so that death is less frightening. Visits to the home may serve no medical purpose but are important to provide comfort and support. Hospice personnel should be informed that honest communication about daily changes as well as what the family and child may expect on a long-term basis is crucial to the education process.

Informing the public about the goals and aims of pediatric hospice care through use of television, radio, and newspapers demystifies the process. Education of the public begins at a young age. Several books are available for young children to introduce them to the concepts of death and dying.[18] Conferences, seminars, and courses in high schools and junior high discussing death and dying can go a long way to eliminating unreasonable fears in the young. It also helps to have members of the hospice team talk with school teachers. Increasing educators' knowledge of what is happening to the children eases their own anxieties. Medical personnel who are not involved with hospice care also need to be taught about the goals and purpose of a hospice program. Knowledge of the hospice concept increases its acceptance and makes it easier to get funding and support.

THE GOALS AND FUTURE OF PEDIATRIC HOSPICE

Pediatric hospice programs should be available in all major pediatric treatment centers or at least in all large cities. If the personnel or funding are not available at any one center, then a combination of resources among the various pediatric programs in a close geographic area could result in a successful pediatric hospice for all the local programs. A combined effort often is not undertaken because of lack of sufficient interest or professional jealousies. Education and cooperation among organizations and professionals increases the acceptance and success of the pediatric hospice concept.

Economic support for pediatric patients is generally poor. Cuts in federal and state spending for child care greatly affect the ability to provide quality care to children, much less allow for hospice care. In addition, hospice is not a glamorous concept like the cure for cancer or muscular dystrophy, and thus receives low priority during budget development. It is important for those active in pediatric hospice care to lobby in legislatures and hospitals for better support. New lines of funding, such as through United Way agencies, need to be developed. Hospice care not only is less expensive than in-hospital care but it is more supportive and loving. It is a concept that must be encouraged to grow and flourish.

Finally, education of the public and medical personnel about the realities of death and dying in childhood must be a high priority. We are inundated daily in the newspapers and on television and radio about miracle cures and marvelous breakthroughs. Our television doctors are always right and never lose a patient. Talk shows, conferences, and forums about medical realities, the facts of death and dying, and the need for hospice care must be encouraged and expanded. In this way dying children and their families will have the chance to realistically deal with death in a supportive and loving environment.

SUMMARY

The recognition that a child may die is a difficult concept for all who come in contact with that child. The desire to escape or to try experimental, dangerous, or painful procedures in the hope that the child may be salvaged is strong and pervasive. Hospice helps provide the emotional, psychological, medical, and spiritual support systems to help the family and child deal with dying and death. Pediatric hospice succeeds only when it is supported by the medical establishment. This support is sometimes unavailable because hospice connotes a reality of death in an atmosphere of fantasy about the child's curability. Hospice planners and managers must recognize that those closest to a dying child may be unable to accept that he or she is dying.

When establishing a pediatric hospice, managers and planners have four models from which to choose. Regardless of the model selected, certain issues must be addressed. These include how to deal with ethical, legal, and consent problems, where to obtain funding and personnel, and what sorts of patients to include in the hospice. The hospice manager must develop means of evaluating the family and establishing guidelines to select those who are hospice candidates.

Plans for medical, emotional, and spiritual support must be developed. Personnel scheduling programs and ideas for control of the various medical problems need to be prepared.

It is advisable to plan some program of bereavement follow-up so that contact with the family does not end with the death of the child. Finally, an education program for medical personnel, family members, and the public should be developed. Pediatric hospice requires active participation by physicians, nurses, social workers, psychologists, chaplains, and others in order to be successful.

NOTES

1. George J. Annas, "The Case of Baby Jane Doe; Child Abuse or Unlawful Federal Intervention?" *American Journal of Public Health* 74 (1984): 727-729.

2. Howard G. Birnbaum and David Kidder, "What Does Hospice Cost?" *American Journal of Public Health* 74 (1984):689-697.

3. John Z. Young, Herman W. Heise, Edwin Silverberg, and Max Myers, *Cancer Incidence, Survival, and Mortality for Children under 15 Years of Age* (New York: American Cancer Society, 1978).

4. Ibid.

5. Glenn Austin, "Child Health-Care Financing and Competition," *New England Journal of Medicine* 311 (1984):1117-1119.

6. Rubrecht Nitschke et al., "Therapeutic Choices Made by Patients with End-Stage Cancer," *Journal of Pediatrics* 101 (1982): 471-476.

7. Ruth B. Purklo, "Ethics Consultations in the Hospital," *New England Journal of Medicine* 311 (1984): 983-986.

8. Lonnie Zeltzer and Samuel LeBaron, "Hypnosis and Nonhypnotic Technique for Reduction of Pain and Anxiety during Painful Procedures in Children and Adolescents with Cancer," *Journal of Pediatrics* 101 (1982): 1032-1035.

9. Ida M. Martinson, *Home Care. A Manual for Implementation of Home Care for Children Dying of Cancer* (Minneapolis: University of Minnesota, 1978); D. Gay Moldow and Ida M. Martinson, *Home Care. A Manual for Parents* (Minneapolis: University of Minnesota, 1979).

10. Daniel C. Moore, Charlene P. Holton, and George W. Marten, "Psychologic Problems in the Management of Adolescents with Malignancy. Experiences with 182 Patients," *Clinical Pediatrics* 8 (1969): 464.

11. Myron Karon, "The Physician and the Adolescent with Cancer," *Pediatric Clinics of North America* 20 (1973): 965.

12. Godfrey P. Oakley and Richard B. Patterson, "The Psychologic Management of Leukemic Children and Their Families," *North Carolina Medical Journal* 27 (1966): 186.

13. James A. Stehbens and Andre D. Lascar, "Psychological Follow-Up of Families with Childhood Leukemia," *Journal of Clinical Psychology* 30 (1974): 394.

14. Shirley B. Lansky et al., "Childhood Cancer: Parent Discord and Divorce," *Pediatrics* 62 (1978):184.

15. Gilman D. Grave, "The Impact of Chronic Childhood Illness on Sibling Development," in *Chronic Children Illness. Assessment of Outcome*, ed. Gilman D. Grave and I. Barry Pless, DHEW Pub. No. (NIH)76-877 (1974): 225-232.

16. Nancy U. Cairns et al., "Adaptation of Siblings to Childhood Malignancy," *Journal of Pediatrics* 95 (1979): 484.

17. Jo Eileen Gyulay, *The Dying Child* (New York: McGraw-Hill, 1978); William M. Easson, *The Management of the Child or Adolescent Who Is Dying* (Springfield, Ill.: Charles C Thomas, 1970); Myra Bluebond-Langer, *The Private Worlds of Dying Children* (Princeton, NJ: Princeton University Press, 1978).

18. John B. Coburn, *Anne and the Sand Dobbies* (New York, Seabury Press, 1964); Gerald G. Jampolsky and Pat Taylor, *There Is a Rainbow Behind Every Dark Cloud* (Millbrae, Calif.: The Center for Attitudinal Healing, 1978); Jonathan B. Tucker, *Ellie, a Child's Fight Against Leukemia* (New York: Holt, Rinehart and Winston, 1982); Judith Viorst, *The Tenth Good Thing About Barney* (New York: Atheneum, 1971).

Chapter 7

Management of the Hospice Home Care Program

Linda Proffitt

Patients who are in active treatment until they die have a certain philosophy about the care they receive. It is future oriented with hope for cure. Patients who know their treatment is no longer effective begin seeing their lives with a different perspective. They find themselves feeling restless and uneasy as well as rejected by an environment oriented toward cure rather than comfort and acceptance of death. For patients who wish to acknowledge death, a hospice system of care offers great support.

The home is considered a place of comfort and support. Increasingly, terminally ill patients prefer to die at home surrounded by family and friends. However, the family, friends, and relatives who provide most of the home care for the dying patient face several hardships. Frequently they lack the required expertise to treat the patient and relieve chronic pain. They are frustrated and unsure of how and where to find help at a price they can afford. Consequently, the terminal patient and the family are forced to use an institutional system that increases physical, emotional, and financial burdens and results in elevated fear and anxiety.

Hospice represents an alternative way of providing care for terminal patients. As discussed in earlier chapters, it emphasizes death with dignity in a familiar and comfortable environment. The hospice addresses the special needs of the patient and family, without imposing on their privacy and independence. The total needs of the terminally ill patient are identified and medical, social, nursing, and other appropriate services are organized to meet these needs. The hospice program packages these services for the family, helping them to avail themselves of needed resources.

Care in the home is the backbone of the American hospice movement. Data from hospice programs in Cleveland, Ohio, show that hospice patients spend approximately 80 to 85 percent of their days at home and only 15 percent in an inpatient setting.[1] The development of home care services is critical to the overall success of a hospice program. Historically, in the United States hospice programs provided home care as the primary and at times sole option. It is only recently that hospice programs were expected to coordinate home, inpatient, and bereavement care as part of an organized service delivery system. However, even though a complete system of services is essential, the first priority is to establish the home care component. This chapter describes the principles of planning hospice home care.

PLANNING HOME CARE

Once the hospice care concept is understood and an administrative commitment is made to develop the program, planning can begin. As Chapter 2 explained, a series of questions must first be answered. These include:

- How many potential hospice patients are there in the community?
- Will this hospice program be designed to serve all of these patients?
- What admission criteria will be established?
- What staffing pattern is needed to serve these families adequately?
- How many beds will be needed to complete the system of services?
- How will the program operate?
- What is the line of authority among staff members?
- How will the hospice be reimbursed for the services it provides?

Community Needs Assessment

A community needs assessment is particularly important for a home care program. First, the hospice patient must be identified and described. Although hospice patients generally suffer from some form of cancer, individuals with other progressively debilitating, fatal conditions can also benefit from hospice care. These patients include persons with cardiovascular disease or renal failure.

According to generally accepted criteria, hospice care is appropriate for certain patients. First, the patient is in the final or terminal phase of the disease. The physician has decided recovery is no longer a realistic expectation, and further attempts to arrest or reverse the disease are futile. The patient's prognosis is six months or less to live.

The second criterion for identifying hospice patients is that they themselves have decided they no longer want a treatment regimen intended to cure. Instead, these patients have accepted the imminence of their death and want to spend the remaining time in a comfortable and satisfying setting. The hospice philosophy will not succeed if the patient's expectation is a "medical miracle."

Reports on hospice patients in the Cleveland study exemplify a typical hospice population.[2] Over 95 percent of the patients have a diagnosis of cancer and less than 5 percent have some other disease. Approximately 64 percent are 65 or older; 56 percent are male and 44 percent are female. Specific populations may differ slightly and can be assessed through an examination of past area death certificates. Death statistics are critical in planning services and anticipating reimbursement patterns.

Hospice program planners must determine the number and type of patients to be served. Will the program provide care for 500 or 20 patients yearly? Will most of them be over or under 65 years of age? Will they live in a concentrated geographic area or be dispersed throughout a large region? The answers to these and other questions will assist in determining staffing, financing, and organizational needs.

The actual projected hospice program caseload is based on the number of patients who die of cancer in a specified area per year. First, the service area must be determined. Is it a county or metropolitan area? If the hospice is part of another organization (for example, a hospital or nursing home), will referrals come strictly from the parent institution or from other sources? If the entire community is the service area, how large a district can be reasonably served? Long driving distances between patients' homes are time consuming. A 30-minute driving time from a hospice office to a home is considered reasonable for a hospice team service area. If more than one team operates in the hospice program, the service area can be much larger. Are other groups planning to offer this service? If so, what part of the population will they serve?

After identifying the service area, a review of county death certificates is useful in calculating the number of potential hospice patients. Reviewing past cancer death trends helps to identify whether the incidence is rising, stable, or decreasing. The percentage of increase or decrease can be applied to identify a potential patient load several years into the future.

Not every dying patient agrees with the hospice philosophy of care. Recent data from programs in operation indicate a saturation level of approximately 35 percent of all dying cancer patients being served by their programs.[3] Thus, 35 percent of all terminally ill cancer patients in a service area represents 95 percent of an expected yearly hospice caseload. Because patients without cancer will be referred, a factor of 5 percent of the cancer caseload should be added to project potential hospice patients to be served by the program to be implemented.

A word of caution! In most programs during the first years of operation only 20 to 25 percent of all terminally ill cancer patients are referred for hospice care. There is a start-up, as well as a community awareness, period. Thus, during the first years the projected caseload will be smaller than in later years.

Finally, consideration must be given to admission criteria. This could severely limit or expand a program's caseload. Although these criteria may eliminate potential patients, it is necessary for program administrators to identify the population to be served. A hospice program cannot expect to serve everyone. Lack of family support, inadequate living arrangements, and legal issues may reduce the caseload. Each criterion should be weighed and related to available resources. The following admission criteria are utilized by programs around the country.

- Patient has an incurable disease and receives palliation only. (Note: Some programs restrict to cancer only. Others allow some treatment and do not restrict patient to palliation only.)
- Patient and family are aware of the diagnosis and prognosis. (Hospice can only be effective in an honest and open environment.)
- Patient, family, and attending physician understand the hospice philosophy and agree to work cooperatively with the team. (Without this understanding conflicts will arise.)
- The prognosis of life is six months or less. (Premature preparation for death can be difficult for patient and family.)
- The patient lives within the boundaries of the specified county, city, state. (Team members must be able to get to the patient/family within reasonable time limits.)
- The patient is an adult. (Some programs accept children.)
- There is a competent caregiver available who cares for the patient while in the home. This person may be a family member, a friend, or a paid caregiver (Without a caregiver many more services will be required by the patient. The program would need the ability to have staff or volunteers in the home, around-the-clock. This is costly and demanding with respect to staff resources.)
- The patient is not comatose with a prognosis of less than 48 hours. (The hospice team needs time to work with patient and family to be effective.)

Home Care Program Services

Once the number of patients has been determined, the next step is developing program services. There are several precepts upon which all hospice programs are based. These precepts, having evolved over time, distinguish hospice care from other programs.

Hospice care is:

- exclusively for the terminally ill
- for patients for whom a cure is no longer possible
- patient *and* family focused

- provided through the bereavement period
- provided by an interdisciplinary team
- medically directed
- available 24 hours a day, 7 days a week
- a service using volunteers as an integral part of the program

While these precepts are generic to any hospice program they must be translated into services. The three major components are well known: home care, inpatient care, and bereavement care. The actual services provided within each of these components must reflect individual patient and family needs.

The trauma of terminal illness affects every aspect of one's life pattern. Family members undergo severe stress that can adversely affect the patient. Since the hospice program seeks to care for the total patient, services are often made available to family members as needed. Thus, the case becomes the patient and his or her family unit.

With such diverse needs of both patient and family, a hospice home care program must be prepared to arrange for and to coordinate a wide array of services. Almost all cases will require the basic types of services discussed in the following sections.

Physician Care

The patient's referring physician is responsible for medical direction of patient care and treatment. The physician orders all medical treatments and prescribes medication. In addition, the hospice medical director is available for consultation and serves as a liaison between the hospice team and the referring physician.

Nursing Care

Home nursing care is provided on an intermittent basis by registered nurses. It focuses on pain and other symptomatic problems. Nurses monitor the patient's condition and report the patient's status to the physician. The nurse teaches the patient and the family how to care and treat symptoms. In addition, hospice nurses supervise home health aides and provide regular assessment of the patient's condition. Since the hospice home care team is on-call 24 hours a day, 7 days a week, nurses generally fill this role. Home care nurses make on-call home visits as appropriate to meet the needs of patients and families.

Home Health Aide Care

Home health aide care is provided to patients requiring personal care with such tasks as bathing, skin, hair and teeth care, linen change, and exercises under the direction of appropriate personnel. In addition to these services, the aide promotes as much independence and activities of daily living as feasible for the patient.

Social Work Services

Social work services are available to provide counseling and guidance for the patient and his or her family. Social workers make home visits and assist the family to use community resources as necessary. They also provide bereavement counseling for the family up to one year after the patient's death.

Spiritual Care

Pastoral caregivers are available to the patient and/or family for spiritual and psychological support.

Volunteer Services

Volunteers are available at the request of the patient and family and are supervised by the director of volunteers. In cooperation with the hospice team, they provide the following services: companionship, assistance with errands, transportation, some light housekeeping tasks, and child care. In addition, volunteers can be trained to provide bereavement counseling for family members and/or caregivers. Some programs add legal services as an additional volunteer component.

Other Services

A home hospice program must be able to provide these six basic services. In addition, the program should be able to arrange for other services that the patient/family needs. These services may include, but are not limited to, physical therapy, occupational therapy, speech therapy, nutritional counseling, transportation, medications, sick room supplies, and equipment.

When the patient enters a hospice program a plan of care is developed by the physician as well as other members of the hospice team, the patient, and the family. As the patient's condition deteriorates, it is likely that his or her needs and those of the family will change. Therefore, an important component of hospice care is periodic reassessment and modification of the care program as necessary.

Staffing Hospice Home Care

Staffing for hospice care is determined by two factors: (1) patients' average length of stay (LOS) in the hospice program and (2) intensity of services required by the patients.

Length of Stay Projections

While the definition of a patient for whom hospice care is appropriate is one whose prognosis is six months or less to live, the typical hospice patient is referred with only four to eight weeks left to live.

In a 1981 study of hospice patients served in Cleveland, Ohio, the average length of stay (LOS) in hospice care was 48.3 days for 152 hospice patients evaluated.[4] However, the median LOS was only 27.0 days. Thus, it is critical to realize that many patients may be in the program less than one month. Table 7-1 shows the distribution of those 152 patients by length of stay in hospice care. These data were taken from programs that had only been operational for one year. The experience of other programs indicates that after three to four years of operation, the community becomes well versed and familiar with the hospice concept and services and the average length of stay increases.

Intensity of Services Required

Staffing requirements are determined, in part, by the patient's location during the hospice stay. Summary data from ten hospices across the nation show that, based on a 60-day length of stay, patients can be expected to use:

Table 7-1 Length of Service in Hospice Care among 152 Cancer Decedents

	Hospice Cancer Decedents		
	N	%	
Less than 2 weeks	33	22	1 to 13 days
2 to 4 weeks	44	29	14 to 27 days
To 8 weeks	28	18	28 to 55 days
To 12 weeks	12	8	56 to 83 days
12 to 24 weeks	32	21	84 to 167 days
More than 24 weeks	3	2	More than 168 days
Total	152	100	Total
6.9 weeks	=	Mean	=	48.3 days
3.9 weeks	=	Median	=	27.0 days

Source: Reprinted from "Cost Savings of Hospice Home Care to Third-Party Insurers," with permission of The Hospice Council for Northern Ohio, Blue Cross of Northeast Ohio and Case Western Reserve University, © 1984.

- 51 days at home—85%
- 8.4 days in in-patient—15%
- .6 continuous care days—0%[5]

Although the greatest portion of care is provided for the patient at home, most patients can expect to die in an institution.[6]

The actual number of visits into the home varies per patient according to LOS and available family support. The Cleveland analysis provides useful managerial information. Results showed that before hospice home care begins, one standard home care visit is made every 42.6 days. However, once hospice care begins, a home visit is made every 4.1 days.[7] This represents a ninefold increase in home care use.

Similarly, hospice patients, compared with nonhospice terminally ill patients, show higher use of home care services.[8] During the last two weeks of care before death, hospice patients average 5.3 home care visits, compared with only .4 visits for nonhospice patients.

The number of home visits intensifies as patients approach death. For example, during the last 12 weeks of life, a home care hospice visit is made every 4.1 days. During the last eight weeks of life, a visit is made every 3.6 days. A 2.9-day lapse exists between visits when the patient is four weeks from death. During the last two weeks of life a hospice visit is required every 2.6 days.

A manager can quickly see that patients referred very close to death require a great deal of staff time. It is important, therefore, to balance patient prognoses for each staff caseload (patients with longer and shorter lengths of stay) to effectively provide care.

Nurse Staffing Patterns

Just as home care is the backbone of the hospice system in the U.S., nursing care is the backbone of hospice home care. All other staffing ratios are developed once the need for nursing care is calculated.

It is expected that one nurse can handle a *maximum* of 10 to 12 patients living in reasonable geographic proximity. The steps below provide managers with a guide for calculating the total number of nurses needed per year.

Step 1: Take 365 days per year and divide it by the anticipated length of stay per patient. This number represents the yearly caseload turnover.

Step 2: Use the yearly projected caseload and divide it by the number calculated in Step 1 above. This number represents the average daily census.

Step 3: Divide the number calculated in Step 2 by 12, the maximum caseload per nurse. This number represents the minimum number of nurses needed per year. For every four nurses, a new team should be established.

Table 7-2 shows how the change in length of stay and number of patients served can affect the staffing pattern.

Other Hospice Home Care Staffing

Data from the National Hospice Organization (NHO) indicate that for programs whose patients have an average length of stay of 60 days, approximately 34.5 home visits are provided.[9] This number is higher and shows more frequent home visits than the Cleveland data. The discrepancy may be because NHO programs had been operating at least three years or more, while the Cleveland programs were in service one year when the data were collected. In addition, some programs reporting to the NHO were in federal pilot programs and received reimbursement, while the Cleveland programs received no such reimbursement.

According to the NHO findings, the 34.5 hospice home visits were distributed as follows:

- Registered nurses make 49% or 17 visits,
- Physicians make 3% or 1.1 visits,
- Home health aides provide 26% of all visits representing 9 of the 34.5 visits,
- Social workers make 12% of all visits, an average of 4.2 visits to each family,
- Clergy, under the direct management of the hospice program, provide 1% of all visits,
- Volunteers provide approximately 4%, and
- Therapists (PT, OT, Speech and Nutrition) provide 4% of all visits, or 1.4 visits per patient.[10]

Table 7-2 Hospice Nurse Staffing Pattern, Affected by LOS and Numbers of Patients Served per Year

Average Length of Stay	Patients Served per Year		Number of Nurses Needed	
	A	B	A	B
28 days	120	300	.8	1.9
42 days	120	300	1.2	2.9
60 days	120	300	1.6	4.1

To complete the team, for every four nurses, add ⅛ of a physician's time, 2½ to 3 home health aides, one social worker, approximately ⅛ of a full-time clergy, and at least one home care volunteer per patient.

Inpatient Hospice Bed Projections

Inpatient beds required for respite and pain/symptom control can be easily calculated. The use of beds varies according to the length of stay (LOS) in hospice. On average, hospice patients use six inpatient days during their hospice care. It takes approximately 60 patients per year to fill one hospice bed at 100 percent occupancy. This number is obtained by dividing 365 days by 6. Using Cleveland data, Table 7-3 shows frequency of inpatient LOS in a hospice program.[11]

PROGRAM OPERATIONS

After thorough planning, the hospice home care program can be implemented. The manager must address areas such as the referral and team process, budgets and reimbursements, and regulatory mechanisms.

Referrals

Patients are referred to the hospice program through various sources including physicians, discharge planners, friends and family members, social service agencies, clergy, and community organizations. Patients can enter the program directly from a hospital, a home health agency, or a nursing home, or from home. Managers should establish a centralized intake service to assess the appropriateness for admission. A director of clinical services, usually a nurse, should discuss the program with family members to determine their understanding and acceptance of the hospice care philosophy.

Table 7-3 Use of Inpatient Care According to LOS on Hospice

LOS on Hospice Care	Frequency of Use of Inpatient Care
12 weeks	Every 7.2 days
8 weeks	Every 6.0 days
4 weeks	Every 4.8 days
2 weeks	Every 4.5 days

Team Process

Once a patient is admitted, the hospice team develops a care plan. The team is interdisciplinary and consists of physicians, nurses, social workers, home health aides, clergy, therapists, and volunteers. Usually, a nurse or a social worker is the case manager. Each team member offers suggestions for meeting the needs of the family. Visits are scheduled intermittently as needed. If the patient is admitted for inpatient care, the team continues its services to the patient until death or until the patient chooses to discontinue the hospice program. Generally, team services continue with the family for one year after the patient's death. Figure 7-1 shows the movement of patients from acute care into the hospice system of service.

Exhibit 7-1 describes steps in this continuum.

An individual patient chart is needed in order to record patient progress. The chart includes an initial patient/family assessment and medical information obtained from the physician. A format to record visits by each discipline is established as well as a system to record hospice team coordination. The record should show team discussion of the patient to demonstrate the interdisciplinary team planning process.

Budget Development

Hospice managers should develop a yearly budget that includes staff salaries, fringe benefits, equipment, and supplies. (See Chapter 2 for a detailed budget example.) Space for employee recordkeeping and dictation is necessary and must

---

Figure 7-1 Hospice Care Continuum

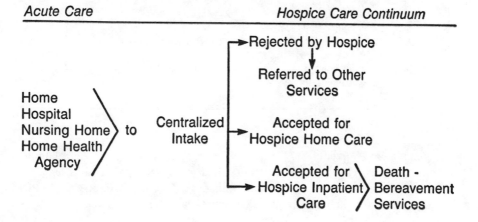

Exhibit 7-1 Hospice Program Patient Care Flow Chart

  I. Intake
     A. Referral from:
        a. Hospital/Nursing Home/Home Health Agency
        b. M.D.
        c. Family/friends/patient
        d. Community agency
     B. Criteria for Admission:
        a. Diagnosis of terminal illness
        b. Prognosis of 6 months or less
        c. Patient/family want hospice care
        d. M.D. agrees to philosophy
        e. Caregiver available when necessary in the home
     C. Alternative:
        a. Referral
        b. Waiting list
        c. Hold for discharge from institution
 II. Contact with patient/family (if not direct) (Director of Clinical Services or designee)
     A. Obtain verbal consent to contact M.D.
     B. Explain hospice care concept to patient/family
III. Contact M.D. (Director of Clinical Services)
     A. Obtain confirmation diagnosis/prognosis; preliminary orders received
     B. Obtain consent to hospice philosophy *or* discuss possible transfer to Hospice Medical
        Director (or other physician)
 IV. Assign case manager for assessment visit
  V. Home Visit or Inpatient Admission
     A. Hospice acceptance obtained
     B. Services initiated
 VI. Care Conference (Team)
     A. Formalization/completion of care plan
     B. Institute volunteer and other services as indicated (Volunteer Director)
     C. Change case manager if indicated by assessment
VII. Continuity of Care (Team and Case Manager)
     A. Accomplished through a weekly care conference
VIII. Bereavement Follow-Up (Team)
     A. Initial assessment by staff, secondarily and/or simultaneously through volunteers as
        necessary and indicated
 IX. Documentation (Team)
     A. Ongoing in clinical record
  X. Case Closed (Team and Case Manager)

be included in indirect costs. Additional indirect costs include public relations, fund-raising activities, travel, education and training of staff and volunteers, volunteer recruitment, and program evaluation. A program director, whether paid or volunteer, along with adequate secretarial support is crucial.

Reimbursement

Once the budget is established, reimbursement can be projected. For most patients over 65 years of age Medicare can be utilized. Cleveland data indicate that approximately 70 percent of hospice costs can be paid for under the regular Medicare reimbursement system.[12] An evaluation of the new Medicare reimbursement law for hospice care as it relates to the program budget is necessary. Chapter 8 identifies the major components of the Medicare law.

For populations under 65 years an assessment of the home care or hospice benefits available through local insurers is required. Blue Cross plans may include a hospice benefit. Other insurers nationwide are beginning to add varying types of hospice benefits.

After assessing policy options, the administration can identify those services that cannot be reimbursed and are potential budgetary problems. If there is a deficit, community fund raising may be initiated. Many local United Way agencies have funded unreimbursed expenses of hospice care so that this service may be made available in their communities.

Regulatory Processes

As described in Chapter 2, various regulatory activities must be undertaken to meet national, state, and local requirements for operation and reimbursement. A review of things to consider includes:

1. *Certificate of Need (CON)*—CON is required for most new health care services. Eligibility to apply for reimbursement may depend on having a CON. Many states require a home care program to obtain a CON. If new beds are being considered, a CON is required. In most states, the state health department determines whether a certificate of need is required. If a CON is required, application should be made promptly so that hospice programs are eligible for reimbursement as early as possible.
2. *Certification of Home Care Agency and/or Hospice*—To receive Medicare funds from either the traditional reimbursement system or under the new hospice reimbursement option, certification is necessary. In most states the state health department conducts a survey to determine whether all of the conditions of participation have been met. Services must be provided for a two-month period before the program can be certified.
3. *Accreditation*—The Joint Commission on the Accreditation of Hospitals (JCAH) now accredits hospice programs. This accreditation is *voluntary*. Since JCAH does not have "deemed status" this process cannot substitute for the above "certification" process. However, some private insurers may eventually reimburse programs based on accreditation. If a hospital has a

hospice program it will be surveyed at the next JCAH hospital accreditation review as a part of the total hospital review.

4. *Licensure*—Many states have passed licensing laws for hospice programs. In a state with such a law, a license to operate will be required.

CONTEMPORARY FORCES SHAPING HOSPICE HOME CARE

In ten short years, hospice has become established in America as a significant service in the total health care system. However, hospice has come of age in a period of great change and turmoil in the health care industry. Thus, hospice has been forced to change and respond to the times. Some changes have been beneficial and some have adversely affected the original hospice concept of care.

Reimbursement Constraints

While hospice care is perceived as a valuable service by many, it is evolving at a time when the costs of hospital and other medical services in the U.S. are skyrocketing. In the zeal to have hospice care reimbursed, hospice providers argue that hospice care saves money and is cost effective because of the heavy home care emphasis. On the basis of this premise, some health insurers, including Medicare, added hospice as a benefit to their insurance programs.

The current method of reimbursement by Medicare may restrict hospice care to a select few. Originally, hospice care was for anyone terminally ill. Now many programs restrict admission to those with a primary caregiver living in the home. What about the elderly, widowed, or single person who lives alone? These patients are often automatically eliminated from hospice care because they require "too much care" to maintain them in their own homes.

Select terminal patients, those with reduced comorbidity, are being sought by program managers. These clients require fewer services and are less demanding. Because many regulations require that a program continue services even if a patient exhausts insurance coverage, patients who will require fewest resources are most likely to be admitted. The limited time frame ensures that money will not be lost, but do the patient and family receive the full benefit of the program? Since the prognosis for other diseases is difficult to predict, patients with diagnoses other than cancer will have a difficult time getting accepted into the hospice program. As discussed in Chapter 12, significant moral and ethical issues arise when care is restricted to a preferred few. Is this fair to patients who need these services?

Program Service Constraints

The formalization of hospice care has also put constraints on program development. One of the original reasons for hospice care was that the needs of patients' families did not or could not fit into a formalized, bureaucratic system. Hospice programs, through the use of volunteers, did many things now being offered and provided by paid staff. However, because of the high cost of individualizing services, the hospice system is becoming less flexible and offering fewer services. Hospices are beginning to provide only those services reimbursed by third-party payers.

The hospice philosophy is being restructured as hospice becomes a part of the health care system. Licensing, accreditation, certification, and other regulatory processes are time consuming and expensive and have made hospice a business first and a commitment and dedication of the caregivers second. Small community hospice programs, or those that are all-volunteer, may not be able to exist in an environment requiring sophisticated and concerted management. As a program, hospice is less individualized because it must address costly rules and regulations. To survive, managers must increase patient volume to cover administrative expenses; thus, programs are less able to respond to the unique needs of each patient—the original reason behind the establishment of hospice care.

Over the past years, fewer volunteers have been involved in hospice programs. Volunteers must be trained and supervised, and this demands a great deal of staff time. These costs are generally not reimbursable by third-party payers. It is easier to let the volunteer program diminish than to keep it vital. Emphasis on *quality* of life was the original focus of hospice care. Volunteer services add to quality of life. Has hospice lost its emphasis on quality because it now provides only the profitable services?

Another change facing hospice programs is the movement back to the medical model of care and away from a comprehensive system approach to care. More and more emphasis is on the medical/physical problems of the patient, with fewer and fewer resources going toward counseling, spiritual care, and family support. It is less expensive to have a home health aide do physical care than to provide several hours of social work support to a spouse who may be anxious and fearful. Care to the spouse or children is generally not a reimbursable service.

In its effort to control the cost of hospice care, the federal government has also severely altered the complexion of hospice care. For example, the 80-20 rule, requiring that patients, on average, spend at least 80 percent of all hospice days in the home and no more than 20 percent in an institution, strengthens and legitimizes the decision to reject patients lacking primary caregivers. It renders very ill patients, who need extensive inpatient care, ineligible for care. The rules established by the federal government eliminate those patients who may need hospice care the most, the elderly who live alone.

The need to fill empty beds in acute and long-term care facilities might also negatively influence the development of hospice care. Will hospice patients be used to fill beds? Will they even be referred for hospice care? By not billing under the new hospice-specific program, terminally ill patients could remain in a hospital. Will patients be admitted and discharged without consideration of their need for pain and symptom control?

Competition among Hospice Providers

Today's health care system is competitive. The demands for cost containment and the desire for control over patient care have led to a proliferation of home care and hospice programs. To retain a market share many home health agencies have gone into the hospice "business." How does this affect the delivery of hospice care? Can more than one hospice program survive in a community? Even as hospice programs struggle to retain their identity and independence, representatives of the home care industry contend there is no difference between home care and hospice home care.

Finn Paradis and her colleagues have examined these conflicts, as well as the advantages and disadvantages of a home care agency establishing a hospice program.[13] Advantages for the patient include continuity of care as the illness progresses from curative to palliative and improved symptom control. For home health agencies, opportunities for more reimbursement and funding alternatives are available. Moreover, if the hospice improves the image of an agency, patient referrals are likely to increase. Finally, establishing a program means that some other agency or community group is less likely to start a hospice program and operate in direct competition.

There are disadvantages, also, of having both home and hospice care provided by the same agency. First, the hospice program requires a set of operating procedures that are distinct from those used for routine home care. Second, hospice staff are on call. They must be specially trained and oriented in their approach to patient care. Third, hospice staff members have other professionals available to them not usually available to home care staff including volunteers, clergy, lawyers, and social workers. Fourth, much more time must be devoted to hospice team meetings, planning, and follow-up than is necessary for home care. As a result, fewer daily visits are made by hospice staff than by regular home care staff. These differences often result in friction between the two staffs.

Hospice staff may take on a feeling of exclusiveness or specialness. In response, home care staff claim that hospice staff do not "carry their load." In addition, recognition of the hospice staff's "service to the community," to the neglect of the services provided by home care staff, is also a source of stress. Hospice care receives widespread public recognition for humane treatment of the dying. Because hospice is a relatively new concept within the framework of traditional medical care, it stands out in its importance and receives accolades from varied community groups, the media, and financial institutions. In the case of financial institutions, support is received in both praise and monetary assistance. Thus, hospice staff members are more likely to hear about the "positive" value of their work than are home care staff.

While the hospice and home care programs are separate, hospice and home care directors must strive to have everyone work in tandem for the overall good of the patient. Joint team meetings, discussions of sources of conflict, and joint training and continuing education seminars are a few ways to build cooperative working relations. The successful administrator must be astute to the potential problems and use his or her imagination in facilitating a good working environment.

CONCLUSIONS

Establishing a hospice home care program requires a detailed analysis of community needs and in-depth planning and preparation before services can begin. The program must be comprehensive to meet an array of patient and family needs. Yet it must be flexible since changes and crises occur daily, sometimes hour by hour.

Implementing a hospice home care program also takes commitment. Developing a working, effective team of professional staff and volunteers takes time, guidance, and skill. Since reimbursement is not adequate to cover all required services, a commitment to finding additional resources must exist. Services should not be denied, but rather resources must be sought.

Managers must be prepared for the volumes of required paperwork to meet regulations, some seemingly detrimental to delivering quality hospice care. They must also hire dedicated staff who will make more visits a day and likely not complete paperwork on time. Finally, a hospice program manager must be willing to face a constantly changing health care environment. It is this environment that makes the development of a hospice program both challenging and rewarding.

NOTES

1. Quarterly Utilization Reports from local hospice programs submitted to The Hospice Council for Northern Ohio, 1980–1983.

2. Ibid.

3. Quarterly Utilization Reports from Hospice of Lake County, Inc., submitted to The Hospice Council for Northern Ohio, 1983.

4. Charles H. Brooks and Kathleen Smyth-Staruch, *Cost Savings of Hospice Home Care to Third-Party Insurers*. Final Report of the Hospice Evaluation Project (Cleveland, Ohio: Hospice Council for Northern Ohio, Blue Cross of Northeast Ohio and Case Western Reserve University School of Medicine, September 1983), 31.

5. Data presented by Don Gaetz and Hugh Westbrook, National Hospice Organization Northeast-Central Regional Meeting, Indianapolis, Indiana, 1983.

6. Brooks and Smyth-Staruch, *Cost Savings*, 29.

7. Ibid., 45.

8. Ibid., 33.

9. Data presented by Don Gaetz and Hugh Westbrook, National Hospice Organization Northeast-Central Regional Meeting, Indianapolis, Indiana, 1983.

10. Ibid.

11. Brooks and Smyth-Staruch, *Cost Savings*, 33.

12. Quarterly Utilization Reports from local hospice programs submitted to the Hospice Council of Northern Ohio, 1980–1983.

13. Lenora Finn Paradis, Jill Schultz, Kay Hollers, and Keith Markstrom, "Home Health Agency and Hospice Mergers. Will the Marriage Bells Ever Sound?" *Nursing and Health Care* (in press).

BIBLIOGRAPHY

Brooks, Charles H., and Kathleen Smyth-Staruch. *Cost Savings of Hospice Home Care to Third-Party Insurers*. Final Report of the Hospice Evaluation Project. Cleveland, Ohio: Hospice Council for Northern Ohio, Blue Cross of Northeast Ohio, and Case Western Reserve University School of Medicine, September 1983.

Finn Paradis, Lenora, Jill Schultz, Kay Hollers, and Keith Markstrom. "Home Health Agency and Hospice Mergers. Will the Marriage Bells Ever Sound?" *Nursing and Health Care* (in press).

Kaff, Theodore H. *Hospice: A Caring Community*. Cambridge, Mass.: Winthrop, 1980.

Plan for a Hospice System of Care for Cuyahoga, Geauga, Lake, Lorain, and Medina Counties. Cleveland, Ohio: Metropolitan Health Planning Corporation, 1979.

Part III

Hospice Care: Financing and Reimbursement

The Development of Reimbursement and Regulation for Hospice Programs: A Historical Perspective

Michael Rosen

When the General Accounting Office (GAO) reported to Congress in March 1979 on the topic of the growing hospice movement in America, the Office concluded that the scope and cost of hospice services would have a profound impact on the future direction of hospice care. "There is presently no standard definition of what a hospice is or what services an organization must provide to be considered a hospice," wrote the GAO.[1] The report continued, "we were unable to obtain detailed information on the quantity of services provided to the average patient and family or the costs of specific services. Thus, we could not determine what the cost of hospice care for a 'typical' patient would be."[2]

These problems were not news to the leaders of hospice programs. It was widely known that there were almost as many models of hospice care as there were groups using the term. A survey published by the National Hospice Organization (NHO) in September 1979 listed 20 different delivery models.[3] (The major models are discussed in Chapter 2.) Freestanding hospices provided either comprehensive professional and support services or solely resource referral. They provided some direct services and arranged for other services to be delivered by other providers. They offered only limited services and left the patient/family on their own to find the rest of the required care. Hospital-based programs fit these divergent patterns with the addition that some had organized hospice units while others scattered hospice patients throughout the institution.

Home health agencies operated hospices. Some of these had designated hospice home care professionals, others spread hospice visits over the entire staff. Skilled nursing facilities and health maintenance organizations also fostered the development of divergent hospice program models.

Note: Lettered superscripts in text refer to textual notes listed at the end of the chapter.

Just as program types varied, so did medical involvement. Some hospices were directed by physicians; others were openly antiphysician. Some hospices were greatly dependent on hospitals; others perceived dehumanizing terminal care practices of hospitals as a primary motivation for the development of the hospice movement and shunned hospital affiliation.

Given the great variety of service patterns and organizational models, it was not surprising that the GAO could not determine the cost of hospice care. As discussed later in this and other chapters, a number of studies, demonstrations, and surveys have attempted to document the cost of hospice care. However, it is unlikely there will be a firm identification of actual care costs until cost report data from Medicare-certified hospices have been analyzed. Even then, the data will show only the cost of hospice care provided according to the standards established by the Medicare program.

The diversity uncovered by the 1979 GAO report, which counted 59 organizations identifying themselves as hospices, did not diminish three years later when a survey by the Joint Commission on the Accreditation of Hospitals (JCAH) found some 1,145 hospices.[4] This variety of hospice models represented a virtually unparalleled demonstration of administrative creativity. These programs managed to find a niche, however precarious, in the health care delivery system without formal reimbursement mechanisms, licensure structures, or defined standards. Furthermore, programs survived in an atmosphere of competition and suspicion from many health care providers and in an environment of meager public knowledge of the purpose or existence of hospice care.

Some hospice leaders recognized, however, that this niche could not be maintained indefinitely without standards, licensure and reimbursement. The question was, Is hospice a concept or a health care provider? Should the term be used primarily as an adjective or as a noun? Many hospice caregivers felt it was a concept of care that could be implemented in any health care setting. In this sense, hospice was identified not only as a specialized form of care for the terminally ill but, in a broader context, as a more humane approach to all health care practice. These early organizers believed that when the hospice concept had fully pervaded the care of the dying, the philosophy would spread to medicine, surgery, obstetrics, pediatrics, and psychiatry, among other disciplines. Ideally, hospice would be so successful there would no longer be a need to identify it as a special program.

Those who saw hospice as a provider of services took a different approach. Arguing that the mission and goals of a hospice and those of other health providers, such as hospitals, were intrinsically different, they worked toward separate reimbursement and licensure for hospices. These advocates pushed to identify the costs of hospice as distinct from conventional forms of care for the terminally ill. They worked to pass state licensure and certificate-of-need legislation and to obtain insurance benefits; they lobbied to convince Congress to include hospice as an identified provider in the Medicare program.

While both points of view continue to exist within the hospice movement, by now hospice is clearly established as a distinct type of provider. Furthermore, the success or failure of the concept is largely tied to the performance of these newly recognized participants in the health care delivery system. While the journey from concept to provider has not been without controversy, hospice administrators and caregivers must now deal with the realities of reimbursement and regulation that confront them.

DEMONSTRATIONS, STUDIES, AND SURVEYS

At the time the GAO did its research on hospice care in the summer and fall of 1978, there had been little credible research on the costs of hospice care. Since then there have been four major attempts to systematically compare the costs of hospice care with those of traditional modes of terminal care. Two of these have been summaries of existing literature, one a statistical research project, and the fourth a large demonstration project. In addition, two studies estimated the cost of care in the absence of hospice services.[A]

The HPA Study

The earliest study was commissioned by the Warner-Lambert Foundation at the request of the National Hospice Education Project (NHEP) and conducted by Health Policy Alternatives, Inc. (HPA). Completed in November 1981, it was used to promote the passage of Medicare hospice legislation. The study examined costs from the perspective of the potential impact on the Medicare trust fund. Thus, it defined the costs associated with providing the type of comprehensive services contemplated under the proposed Medicare bill. To estimate cost savings, HPA looked at three variables: the number of Medicare beneficiaries who would be eligible for the new benefit, the number of those eligible who would use the benefit, and the average cost of the benefit compared with other forms of care.

HPA reviewed nine hospices and/or hospice studies which revealed that about 90 percent of hospice patients had cancer diagnoses. Cancer mortality statistics from the National Center for Health Statistics, the American Cancer Society, and Georgetown University's Public Services Laboratory were used to project cancer deaths from 1975 through the year 2000. HPA then cited data from a National Cancer Institute study which found that 93 percent of cancer patients over the age of 65 and 1 percent of cancer patients under 65 were Medicare beneficiaries. When these data were combined—1 percent of the projected cancer deaths of persons under 65 plus 93 percent of such deaths for those over 65, plus 10 percent to cover hospice patients with noncancer diagnoses—the total number of potentially eligible Medicare beneficiaries was estimated by HPA to range from 272,000 in 1981 to 309,000 in the year 2000.

To determine the number of beneficiaries likely to use hospice services, HPA looked at six studies on the potential use of hospice services by cancer patients. The percentage of Medicare users ranged from 10 to 40 percent. Taking a medium estimate of 20 percent, potential users were put at 54,000 in 1981. Using an increase of 2,000 every five years, this estimate grew to 62,000 for the year 2000.[B]

In the area of cost comparison, HPA examined several studies reporting the average Medicare cost for patients receiving traditional terminal care. The 1980 average Medicare reimbursement for hospital care of cancer patients during the year of death was $5,981. (These patients all died in a hospital.) This was compared with a National Cancer Institute study that reported a 1980 average patient cost of hospice care at $3,660. Further, HPA suggested that, if—as reported in six studies—the per-day cost of hospital care of cancer patients was $400, the saving of some nine days of hospital costs per patient would pay for all hospice costs, not just added costs. Looking then at three studies of the substitution effect of hospice for hospital care, HPA found a range of savings from $800 to $2,600 per case. This information was used to project a potential Medicare cost savings from $13.6 million to $49.6 million in 1982 and from $29.6 million to $131.3 million in 1986. These figures represented five-year savings of between $112.8 and $462.8 million.

All this led Health Policy Alternatives to conclude that "the coverage of comprehensive hospice services may be added to Medicare as proposed by the hospice bill, without increasing the costs of the Medicare program. In fact, . . . the proposed legislation probably would result in substantial aggregate dollar savings."[5] The circulation of this study in Congress by NHEP and its introduction in evidence at a House Ways and Means Subcommittee on Health hearing in March 1982 helped persuade lawmakers that hospice could be financially, as well as philosophically, attractive.

The CBO Study

The other major study that estimated costs and associated cost savings of hospice care was released by the congressional Budget Office (CBO) in June 1982. This document was also used by NHEP and its congressional supporters to argue for the cost effectiveness of the proposed legislation. Like the HPA study, CBO's analysis indicated "sizeable savings for each new user of hospice care as a result of the substitution of that care for a more expensive mix of traditional services for the dying."[6]

CBO obtained estimates of the cost per day and the average length of stay for hospice care from sources including NCI, NHO, JCAH, and interviews with hospice administrators. These were adjusted to create the average daily cost of a hospice that delivers comprehensive services and in which inpatient care does not exceed 20 percent of total days. Translated into 1983 dollars, the result was $105 per day for an average stay of 45 days. After adding costs for services such as those provided by the attending physician, the total gross Medicare cost per hospice user was estimated to be $5,010.

Based on a study conducted by the Health Care Financing Administration (HCFA), CBO projected Medicare expenditures of $6,130 for traditional services for which hospice would provide a substitution. This produced a net savings of $1,120 per beneficiary. Using basically the same estimates of total potential users as HPA, CBO said that 15 percent would use the new benefit in 1983, 12 percent in 1984, 22 percent in 1985, 31 percent in 1986, and 41 percent in 1987.

CBO also assumed there were a number of current users who, in addition to using existing Medicare benefits to pay for some of their hospice care, would access the proposed new benefits, resulting in higher Medicare outlays for these beneficiaries. A figure of $710 was therefore multiplied by the projected number of current users and offset against the savings of $1,120 per new user (a new user meant someone using the new benefit to pay for virtually all hospice services).[c] Even so, the savings were dramatic, a total of $109 million between 1983 and 1987.

The Hospice Council of Northern Ohio Study

In September 1983, a research project was published by the Hospice Council of Northern Ohio and others that dealt with the cost savings of hospice home care to third-party payers. In this study, a retrospective analysis was conducted on about 1,500 Medicare A or Blue Cross of Northeast Ohio claims for Cleveland residents who died of cancer between April and December of 1981. Of these, 152 were recipients of hospice care and 1,397 were not. The reimbursement records were examined, and the use of various services was arrayed by hospice/nonhospice status for selected time intervals prior to death.

Total costs for these services were determined and the relative cost of hospice versus traditional care extrapolated. Dollar savings were shown to be 51 percent in the last two weeks of life, 47 percent in the last four weeks, 44 percent in the last eight weeks, and 39 percent in the final twelve weeks.

The major premise of this study was that cost savings associated with hospice care results primarily from the substitution effect of home care days for hospital days. As in the HPA and CBO studies, the authors concluded that substitution will occur, resulting in substantial savings, and that "the hospice care services provided by home health care agencies does not represent 'a layer of services

added on to those already available in the more conventional care settings' . . .
Accordingly, third-party insurers are advised to seriously consider expanding
their coverage to include hospice home care."[7]

The National Hospice Study

As early as 1976, hospice leaders met with Congress and the then Department
of Health, Education, and Welfare (DHEW) to explore the possibility of a major
government-funded hospice demonstration and evaluation project. It took until
October 1978, however, for such a project to be announced. In a speech to the
first annual convention of the National Hospice Organization, DHEW Secretary
Joseph Califano lauded the concept of hospice care but challenged hospices to
assess their cost effectiveness and to determine how abuse could be prevented
while promoting quality of care. After the speech, copies of the "Announcement
of Medicare and Medicaid Hospice Projects" were made available.

The goals of this project were ambitious. The announcement listed ten specific
objectives, everything from identifying the range of services provided by hospices
and developing standards of care to recording patient, family, and physician
attitudes toward hospice services. Not all of these objectives were included in
the final research design. In particular, the proposal to study alternative methods
of reimbursement (that is, other than cost-based) was dropped. This would later
have an impact on the debate over payment methods and rates for the legislated
Medicare hospice benefit.

By March 1979, DHEW received more than 230 applications. There had been
some 1,800 requests for information. Many in the hospice movement assumed
that the project would be underway quickly, but it was not until October that
the Department announced the selection of 26 demonstration sites. Again, despite
assurances and expectations that funding would start within three months, it was
another year before the project began. This period of delays, missed deadlines,
and postponements caused considerable disruption in the sites and resulted in
additional costs.

Essential to the usefulness of the demonstration was the data collection/eval-
uation component. However, the decision to appoint an evaluator was also
delayed. The contract finally went to Brown University in October 1980. Data
collection, expected to commence in April 1981, was delayed until August.
While some preliminary findings were announced at the November 1983 NHO
convention, the "Preliminary Final Report" was not available until May 1984.
The final report was scheduled to be released sometime in 1985.[8]

The National Hospice Study was not a grant project. Rather, coverage policies
that were seen as restrictive to effective hospice care were waived. Furthermore,
payments were made to the demonstration sites following the usual cost-based
guidelines.

The project studied the costs at 14 hospital-based (HB) and 11 home-care-based (HC) hospices. One hospice site was not included because it did not comply with the terms of the demonstration that required the provision of home care services. The cost of conventional cancer care was studied at ten sites. The preliminary report covers the first 15 months of the demonstration, utilizing data on 1,143 HB patients, 2,746 HC patients, and 334 conventional care patients with terminal illness. Cost data came from annual cost reports filed by the hospices, while information on quality and other factors was derived from various patient subsamples. Major findings included:

- The average length of stay in an HC hospice was 72 days, 62 in an HB program. HB patients spent 18.2 days as an inpatient, whereas HC patients averaged just 5.2 days.
- HC costs averaged $4,758 ($66 per day); HB patients had greater utilization of inpatient services, raising their costs to $5,890 ($95 per day).
- The costs for HC patients were below those of conventional care regardless of the length of stay. HB patient costs, however, rose above conventional costs for stays of longer than 60 days.
- The incidence of intensive medical intervention was less for hospice patients, who also received fewer blood tests and x-rays than conventional care recipients. Use of respiratory therapy was about the same for hospice and nonhospice patients. Hospice patients were more likely to receive medical social services.
- Freestanding hospices had nearly four times the level of volunteer service than did hospices based in other types of providers.
- Overall quality of life and patient satisfaction with care was not different among HC, HB, and conventional care providers.

Conventional Care Cost Studies

The two important studies that attempted to determine the cost of conventional care in the last months of life were conducted by the Health Care Financing Administration and The Blue Cross and Blue Shield Association (BCBSA).

The HCFA study[9] was available in draft form by mid-1982. Records of Medicare beneficiaries who died in 1976 were selected from the Continuous Medicare History File. This file records the continuous experience of a small sample (5 percent) of Medicare enrollees selected on the basis of their Medicare identification numbers. The data showed that 91 percent of Medicare enrollees used their benefits in the last year of life. Furthermore, of all expenses in that year, 30 percent were spent in the last 30 days. Average reimbursement for all enrollees was $3,351; an average of $6,621 was spent on behalf of beneficiaries who had at least one hospitalization with a cancer diagnosis. In the final version of this study,[10] these numbers rose, for those who died in 1978, to $4,527 per enrollee and $8,297 for hospitalized cancer patients.

The other major study of conventional care cost for terminally ill patients was available late in 1982.[11] Under a contract with the Department of Health and Human Services (DHHS), the Blue Cross and Blue Shield Association reviewed claims of relatively well-insured individuals who died of cancer in 1978 and 1979. Data were supplied by three BCBSA plans, located in Indiana, Georgia, and Michigan. Results showed that the total mean expenditure for the last six months of life was $15,836 in 1980 dollars, of which 78 percent was for inpatient care. The proportion of expenditure increased in the later months, with one half of the patient's days in the final month spent in a hospital.

Comparison of Studies

It is tempting to put all these demonstrations, surveys, and studies together in one big pot, stir well, and cook into an authoritative synthesis of the cost and value of hospice care. For a variety of reasons, however, this is not possible.

The main problem is the disparity in the range of services provided by divergent hospice models. Many hospice programs studied did not provide comprehensive services. Of these, many had only rudimentary coordination or professional management relationships with the institutions providing services—usually inpatient care—not furnished directly by the hospice. This lack of uniformity in service delivery patterns distorts not only costs but also utilization of services. For example, home-care-only hospices may selectively admit patients who are likely to be maintained at home with a primary caregiver, resulting in a patient population that uses a low number of inpatient hospital days. The amount of inpatient care may rise in those programs that institute homelike hospice inpatient care because patients have an attractive alternative to hospital admission.

Another problem in comparing these studies is that some assessed cost, some charges, and others a combination of the two. This makes comparisons of hospice costs difficult. Further, hospitals may have reported costs or charges associated with typical room and board expenses for medical-surgical patients when the staffing levels, dietary requirements, and social service/counseling time may differ for hospice patients. Home health agencies may have reported the average cost per visit on an agencywide basis when the length of time spent and the nature of services rendered on a hospice visit may make such a visit more expensive. Differences in the amount of services rendered by volunteers also contribute to the problem of consistency in cost reporting.

Fluctuating research time frames also create difficulty in achieving a synthesis. Some studies were conducted over the period of one year prior to death, others over six months, two months, or two weeks. The average length of care for patients within each hospice is another variable. Programs with a shorter length of care tend to experience higher per-day costs due to the more intense medical needs of those closer to the end of life.

Despite these problems, every study shows a substantial cost-saving potential when hospice care is compared with traditional services for the terminally ill. This was true before, during, and after the drive for expanded third-party coverage of hospice care. By the time these studies began to appear, hospice leaders realized that the grants were of fixed duration, the demonstrations limited, and the studies, while interesting and provocative, did nothing to help meet the payroll. What was needed was a breakthrough in reimbursement policy. With the elderly comprising a majority of hospice patients, the target became the Medicare program.

MEDICARE HOSPICE LEGISLATION

Inclusion of hospice care as a covered benefit of the Medicare program was under consideration by Congress as early as the summer of 1980. On July 2, Representative Leon Panetta of California introduced H.R. 7744, calling it "a bill to improve access to hospice services for the terminally ill."[12] H.R. 7744 was designed to extend coverage under Part B of Medicare to patients with a life expectancy of six months or less. It provided a broad range of covered home care and inpatient services, including up to three sessions of bereavement counseling for the family within one year of the patient's death.

Though it was the first federal legislation to specifically identify hospice as a separate provider category and to offer coverage of specific hospice services, this bill had two major flaws. First, because coverage was provided under Part B, there were coinsurance provisions that would not apply if the beneficiary chose hospital or home health care under Part A. This would have created a strong disincentive to use the hospice benefit. Second, there was no clear definition of hospice in the bill, leaving the development of standards entirely to DHHS. Many hospice advocates felt that without clear legislative direction the outcome of this process might prove harmful to developing programs.

H.R. 7744 did not gather the support necessary for passage, partly because there was no organized effort within the hospice movement to push for it. But when the new Congress convened in 1981, hospice supporters were at work on remedying that shortcoming. Hugh Westbrook, one of the founders of Hospice, Inc., in Miami, Don Gaetz, who helped organize hospices in Wisconsin and Florida, and Dennis Rezendes, organizer of the Connecticut Hospice and first executive director of the National Hospice Organization, formed the National Hospice Education Project. This ad hoc coalition eventually included more than

600 hospices and was instrumental in organizing the hospice movement to actively support the passage of a comprehensive Medicare benefit.

Hearing Issues

Nearly a year of meetings with members of Congress, Senate and House committee staff, business leaders, religious groups, and hospice administrators led to the introduction in December of hospice coverage bills in both the Senate and the House. Representative Panetta was principal sponsor in the House and Senator Robert Dole introduced companion legislation in the Senate. By February, sponsorship in the House had grown to more than 80 and a hearing was scheduled in March before the Subcommittee on Health of the Committee on Ways and Means. By the date of that hearing, March 25, 1982, there were some 200 House sponsors and 30 Senate sponsors.

The hearing set the tone for the following five months of debate on the bill. Speaking for the Reagan Administration, then HCFA Deputy Administrator Paul Willging praised the hospice concept but said the Congress should await the results of the HCFA hospice demonstration project before passing a hospice benefit. Support for Willging's position came from representatives of the Blue Cross and Blue Shield Association and the Association of Community Cancer Centers. Virtually all the rest—NHO and NHEP leaders, business groups, and those who had experienced hospice care—enthusiastically supported the proposed legislation.

Aside from the question of waiting for results from the HCFA study, two issues were raised at the hearing: the cost of hospice care and the provision of hospice as a separate provider class.

The "wait for data" argument was overcome thanks to the efforts of Representative Willis Gradison and NHEP vice-chairperson Dennis Rezendes. Without the legislation, Gradison said at the hearing, "we may see the movement developed in a way which might not be optimum from a point of view of controlling costs and offering the most appropriate means of service." In written testimony, Rezendes accused HCFA of "hiding behind the social scientist's understandable need to 'complete one more study' before making a decision which will be uninformed and too late to be effective." "At best," he continued, "the HCFA study will confirm what is already known. That will be helpful, but not significant enough to postpone action on H.R. 5180."[13] Rezendes' most telling point was that while the NHS would examine how 26 different approaches to hospice care function, this was merely studying the "round peg into the square hole," the "negative effect of the current jumble of reimbursement systems." The NHS will shed no light, he said, on "the costs or service implications of a round peg in a round hole, which is what H.R. 5180 would accomplish."[14]

Although the separate provider issue continues to be debated today, the Congress opted for a single entity that could be surveyed against standards, provide a direct audit trail for reimbursements, and give the patient a single organization to rely on for services. This accountability was judged more important than the concern over duplication of existing services, the organizational change that would be required of some hospices, or the realignment of relationships among health care providers.

The question of the cost of hospice care was addressed by the introduction into the hearing record of the Health Policy Alternatives Study. However, many members of Congress chose to await the results of the CBO study requested by the Subcommittee on Health. When the study was released on June 28, it ended weeks of speculation and anxiety. Supporters of the legislation were well aware that in the spending-conscious atmosphere of the 97th Congress there was little chance for a new benefit that would increase federal expenditures. The CBO estimates of substantial Medicare cost reductions made the hospice bill into a legislator's dream: an additional benefit that saved money.

After the CBO study, things moved quickly. On July 15, the House Ways and Means Committee approved H.R. 5180, but not before several days of intense negative lobbying by the home health care, hospital, and nursing home industries, countered by persuasive arguments of NHEP leaders Gaetz and Westbrook. There were several areas of disagreement between NHEP and the traditional providers, particularly in the area of contracting for core services and separate provider status. The legislation had always contained the provision that certain basic or "core" services should be provided directly by hospices. Originally, this included not only a number of home care services but inpatient care as well. Later, inpatient services were dropped from the core list but hospices were to be precluded from contracting with all but other Medicare-certified hospices.

Separate status and core services greatly concerned home health agencies, who saw themselves as legitimate recipients of substantial amounts of hospice contract business. Through existing referral or transfer arrangements, home health agencies delivered skilled services on behalf of hospices and billed Medicare under the home health benefit. This arrangement could be converted into a formal contract in which hospices would pay the home health agencies directly for services rendered. This would enable the agencies to convert a cost-reimbursed service to a charge-based system in which any excess over cost could be retained by the agency. Hospital, nursing home, and home health agency lobbyists also argued that their constituents should be able to render hospice care as an additional protocol in their existing provider agreement rather than through a separate hospice provider agreement.

In the end, the Ways and Means Committee agreed to allow hospices to contract with other types of Medicare-certified providers, but not for the four core services of nursing, physicians, counseling, or social work. Separate provider's agreements would be required, but home health agencies, hospitals, and nursing homes would not be surveyed against those hospice standards that duplicated requirements for existing providers. The final House version was a major victory for NHEP.

The Senate had not conducted hearings on the hospice bill and opponents, including the Reagan Administration, were confident that Senate action could be delayed or even stopped. NHEP leaders, however, had anticipated victory in the House and had been meeting quietly with key Senators, including Republicans Robert Dole, Bob Packwood, John Heinz, Mark Andrews, and Pete Domenici, as well as Democrats Lawton Chiles, John Glenn, Lloyd Bentsen, and Edward Kennedy. NHEP persuaded Heinz and Chiles to go directly to the floor of the Senate with the legislation and attach it to the Tax Equity and Fiscal Responsibility Act (TEFRA), then under consideration.

Passage

In a July 22 Senate session, literally hundreds of other attempts to amend TEFRA were being defeated on the floor as Democratic and Republican leaders united against "non-germane" amendments. However, to the surprise of virtually all observers except NHEP leaders watching from the Vice-President's Family Gallery in the Senate Chamber, the required two-thirds plus one of the Senate's membership voted to, in effect, suspend the rules and allow Heinz to introduce the hospice bill as an amendment.

Even in cynical Washington, it was a moment of high drama. The Senate halted its tax and budget debate at nearly midnight allowing Heinz, Chiles, Glenn, and other Senators to rise before a packed Senate floor and urge extraordinary parliamentary action on behalf of the terminally ill and their families. The year of methodical vote-gathering by NHEP paid off. The support was there and the legislation passed by a simple voice vote. Although the House and Senate versions differed slightly, the Senate called for a copayment on some types of home visits and an exemption from certain provisions of the bill for hospices in operation prior to January 1, 1975.[D] These details were worked out in a Conference Committee in early August. On August 19 the hospice Medicare benefit passed both the House and the Senate as Section 122 of the Tax Equity and Fiscal Responsibility Act of 1982.

The conference committee dropped copayments on home visits but retained copayments for outpatient drugs and inpatient respite care. When signed by President Reagan on September 3, hospice coverage became part of Public Law 97-248. The benefit was scheduled to commence November 1, 1983. And while many of the specifics of the new coverage were outlined in the law, several major issues were left to HCFA and the regulation process.

Development of the Regulations

About a month after the hospice benefit was signed into law, meetings began between industry representatives and HCFA officials. NHEP and NIIO sent spokespersons to Baltimore to discuss the issues confronting the regulators. Delegations from the National Association for Home Care and the American Federation of Home Health Agencies and others also had October meetings with HCFA. Opponents of the Medicare hospice benefit hoped to reclaim in the regulatory process the issues they had lost on the floor of Congress.

When the National Hospice Organization held its annual convention in November, NHEP held a one-day workshop on the provisions of the law. Congressional aides, committee staff, HCFA officials, and hospice administrators spoke to a large group of interested and, at times, confused hospice partisans. The NHO meeting that followed also presented sessions on the benefit and a number of the speakers from these and the NHEP workshop circulated at the convention, holding informal discussions with attendees. During these discussions the seriousness of HCFA's desire to move toward a prospective payment system became clear. Also apparent was the continued opposition to hospice reimbursement within the Reagan Administration and that the implementation of the law would be as difficult as its passage.

NHEP co-chair Don Gaetz, now elected as NHO's new president, saw the difficulties ahead and warned the hospice movement:

> With the passage of the Medicare hospice benefit, we have neither passed over the River Jordan into the Promised Land, as some have hoped, nor have we crossed the River Styx into Hades, as others have feared. We find ourselves, instead, less than halfway home, surrounded on all sides by the crosscurrents of change and the eddies of opposition. The passage of this bill was only the first step. The faithful implementation is the next step, but only a step, not a destination. For those who seek equitable reimbursement for hospice in America, this is not the end nor even the beginning of the end. It is, perhaps, the end of a beginning.[15]

On November 15, 1982, a roundtable discussion of the regulation development process was held in Washington. A large number of interested industry groups attended along with HCFA officials.[E] A discussion paper, circulated at this meeting, identified three basic issues in the implementation of the benefit: (1) the payment system, (2) the responsibility of the hospice to professionally manage contracted services, and (3) the acceptable site/standards for hospice inpatient care.

Reimbursement

Although cost-based reimbursement had been considered, HCFA felt this approach would lead to higher costs. Other options, such as a comprehensive prospective system, based on either a per capita, per case, or per diem basis, also were discussed. The reimbursement method favored in the discussion paper and eventually adopted proposed a prospective payment approach with separate rates by level of service.

From HCFA's perspective, an advantage of selecting a prospective payment system was that it would obviate the need for extensive regulations describing distinctions between covered and noncovered services. Under prospective pay, a set amount is reimbursed, based on an estimate of what hospice care "should" cost. As a result, the itemization of covered services would become an issue for rate setting but not for day-to-day reimbursement. With this question settled, a preliminary draft of the regulations was circulated in late December. Most hospices seemed to support the concept of prospective payment, but many worried about how equitable rates could be set without adequate cost data on such a new program. These fears proved very real.

One major problem was the calculation of the cap amount. Congress had created the cap, not as a strict per-patient limit on benefits, but rather as an aggregate overall average limit on reimbursed expenses. The cap was designed to limit Medicare's exposure for the hospice benefit to the cost of conventional care for the terminally ill in the last six months of life. This concept has been difficult for many people to grasp. Concern over losses associated with cutoffs of reimbursement after the patient's bill reaches the cap amount is often voiced. However, the cap is not based on individual utilization. The total number of a hospice's Medicare patients is multiplied by the cap amount and the product is the limit on total Medicare reimbursement to that hospice. So while Mrs. Jones' bill may be $30,000, the hospice does not face a loss of payments unless there are enough patients like Mrs. Jones to raise the average per case above the cap amount.

Early data had indicated that the average cost incurred by Medicare in the last six months of a beneficiary's life was about $7,200. With this figure in mind, first drafts of the legislation pegged the cap at 75 percent of these costs. The CBO study, however, projected that the cap amount would actually be much higher, based upon a new last-six-months estimate of $14,600. The figure appeared to be the result rather than the base of the calculation. This led Congress to replace the 75 percent factor with one of 40 percent which, it was assumed, would produce a cap of about $7,600. This amount was acceptable to most hospices. However, instead of being 75 percent of a larger amount, the $14,600 was in fact the base itself.

HCFA knew that the data used to produce the estimate included only patients with at least one hospitalization. They reasoned that some cancer patients were not hospitalized in the last six months of life and the estimated average should therefore be lowered. After this adjustment, HCFA estimated a cap of less than $4,500.

When word of this reached the hospice movement in February 1983, there was great concern. This was more than a $3,000 reduction in the expected cap. The new number was inadequate to cover the costs of care.

The Reagan Administration insisted that the downward-calculated cap couldn't be changed without congressional action. Representative Panetta responded, "If it was a B-1 bomber that they had made a mistake in terms of evaluation, I am pretty convinced that the administration would find a way to do it through regulations that would correct that problem."[16]

NHO took the Administration at its word and a campaign was undertaken to persuade Congress to establish a fixed cap in the law itself. This removed HCFA's ability to calculate the cap with its own methodologies and data. Co-sponsors were quickly recruited behind Representatives Panetta and Gradison and a hospice cap restoration bill was passed in August 1983. The cap was fixed at $6,500.

Meanwhile, in April, a second draft of the hospice regulations was circulated. The April draft contained an important difference: the addition of a fifth level of care. The December draft proposed four levels: routine (intermittent) home care, continuous (eight or more hours on the same day) home care, inpatient respite (admission for psychosocial reasons), and inpatient acute (medical admission). The new level was "general inpatient care," which fell somewhere between respite care and hospital acute care services. Inpatient acute care was to be paid under the diagnosis related groups (DRG) scheme used for Medicare hospital reimbursement. General inpatient, the new level where hospice practitioners predicted most of the inpatient days would fall, was to be paid at a per diem rate of just over $57. This was approximately $275 less than the preliminary cost estimates for hospice inpatient care reported in the National Hospice Study.

To counter this disastrous development, public and congressional pressure was required. A hearing was held on May 25 before the House Select Committee on Aging. Witnesses, including Representative Panetta, testified about the nature of hospice inpatient care and the true cost of this service. They predicted that the low rate would result in counterselection of those patients for whom the substitution of hospice home care for hospitalization holds the greatest cost-saving potential.

Partly as a response to this hearing, the expected June 1 date of *Federal Register* publication for the proposed regulations was pushed back. In early July, HCFA dropped the idea of a separate acute inpatient DRG-based rate and raised the payment for general inpatient care to $271. Publication was further delayed, however, by proposals from the Office of Management and Budget (OMB). Rejecting CBO's claim that hospice would save money, OMB director David Stockman proposed strong limitations on the hospice benefit. He suggested that patient eligibility be limited to 31,000 individuals and provider eligibility to "existing hospices" in the first year. Beneficiaries would be issued vouchers for $4,200 but existing hospices could get more based on first-year cost reports. After year one, additional hospices would be permitted and there would be open competitive bidding for patients among existing and new hospices.

These proposals were not well received by NHO, members of Congress, or even some professionals at HCFA. The NBC television network tried to arrange a debate on the issues between Gaetz and either Stockman or Health and Human Services Secretary Margaret Heckler. Gaetz readily agreed but both Stockman and Heckler refused to appear. On NBC's "Today Show," Gaetz accused the Administration of trying to "kill the hospice benefit." He promised a fight on the floor of Congress and in the courts.

Heckler met with Gaetz and other NHO leaders in late July to forge some compromises. Discussions continued into August. OMB insisted on severe provider limitations through tight conditions of participation. NHO countered that quality of care, not arbitrary exclusions, should be the only basis for the standards. Finally, the Administration withdrew Stockman's proposals and some of NHO's suggestions on quality standards were accepted. The proposed regulations were published on August 22, 1983 in the *Federal Register*.

HCFA set a 30–day comment period in order to publish final rules before the hospice benefit was scheduled to commence on November 1. Again there were delays. Hospices requesting certification were surveyed in October, November, and the first half of December for compliance with the conditions of participation in the proposed regulation. Hospices were promised a resurvey if significant changes were made in the final version.

More than 200 comments were received by HCFA in response to the August publication. A number of comments were rejected because they proposed the deletion of standards mandated by the statute. Among these required standards were: (1) no more than 20 percent of the aggregate number of hospice days may be inpatient days, (2) core services must be provided directly, (3) care must not be discontinued when hospice benefit days are exhausted, and (4) bereavement services, while required, may not be reimbursed. Other suggestions that were not accepted included the use of cost-based reimbursement, masters level credentialing of social workers, credentialing of counselors, payment exceptions, and reimbursement of bad debts.

Aside from minor and technical changes, the principal revisions accepted included permitting employees of parent provider organizations to work part-time in the hospice program, allowing a patient representative to sign for the hospice benefit on behalf of a mentally or physically incompetent beneficiary, and a requirement that volunteer services constitute at least 5 percent of the total hours of patient care provided by paid staff. Cost reporting would be required of all hospices. Further, some modifications were made to the payment method for continuous home care and some new standards were added for freestanding inpatient units.

Rebuffed on the issue of patient and hospice eligibility, OMB attempted to pressure HCFA to lower the rates. Armed with new data from the National Hospice Study, OMB suggested that $255.55 for general inpatient care—down from $271—and $36 for routine home care—instead of $53.17—were adequate. At the NHO annual meeting in Minneapolis in early November 1983, participants were shocked and outraged when HCFA Associate Administrator Lynn May announced that the Department had decided to go along with these reductions. While NHO agreed not to challenge the concept of prospective rate setting in the absence of solid data, the organization assumed that reimbursement rates would allow viable operation of hospices until true costs could be determined. Now, NHO members felt betrayed. Hugh Westbrook won a standing ovation when he thundered at May, "You will not balance the budget on the backs of dying people."

Following the annual meeting, hospice leaders went to Washington to argue for restoration of the August rates. They had a meeting on November 15 with HCFA Deputy Administrator Dan Bourque, who confirmed the cuts. A letter was prepared for distribution to members of Congress, asking for assistance in appealing to DHHS to restore the August rates. The letter, signed by Don Gaetz and NHO's new president, Carolyn Fitzpatrick, described the effect of the cuts on hospices:

> Even with the rates published in August, hospice programs would have to not only continue but also intensify community fund-raising and the use of volunteer resources in order to subsidize Medicare and provide a similar level of services to non-Medicare patients. Based upon the response of our membership, it is our judgment that no hospice in the United States will be able to render the level and extent of services mandated under the hospice legislation at the reduced rates proposed by the administration.
>
> The result, as is well-documented by both public and private studies, will be that persons who otherwise would be cared for in hospice programs will be institutionalized at much higher costs to Medicare. . . .
>
> In good faith, hospice programs throughout the country have relied upon the Congress and the Administration for faithful implementation of the hospice legislation. . . . Hospice programs have been forced by

the Department's tardiness to rely upon the rates published in August and have negotiated contracts, expanded services, hired staff, and begun rendering care. Patients with only weeks or even days to live are relying upon a level of care which the new rates will not provide.[17]

There was considerable support from members of Congress, buoyed by letters and phone calls from hospice constituents. Despite the preparations for an adjournment before Thanksgiving Day for a two-month recess, several dozen members wrote to Margaret Heckler and David Stockman, arguing that lower rates could preclude Medicare participation for many, especially smaller, hospices. Senators Paula Hawkins and Daniel Patrick Moynihan introduced a resolution in the Senate on November 18, calling the proposed reductions "shortsighted and misguided." Senator Pete Domenici, chairman of the Senate Budget Committee, and Representative Edward Roybal, chairman of the House Select Committee on Aging, both wrote particularly forceful letters, suggesting the Congress would not tolerate cuts and questioning the use of NHS data for rate setting. There was also extensive press coverage. Two articles appearing in the *Washington Post* and the *New York Times* also covered the story. The Associated Press carried three hospice stories in November and local papers across the country editorialized on the subject.[18]

In response, the general inpatient rate was restored to $271. The routine home care rate, proposed by HCFA in mid-November to be $42.17 (OMB's $36 plus an inflation factor), was raised to $46.25. With these figures, as well as an increase in the continuous home care rate and a decrease in the inpatient respite rate, the regulations were finally published in the *Federal Register* on December 16.[19]

Rate Setting

At the heart of the reimbursement controversy was the applicability of NHS data to the costs experienced by hospices providing care under the new benefit. The NHO letter also addressed this issue, citing reasons why NHS data should not be used for rate setting. NHO argued that fewer than half of the study sites provided a range and mix of services comparable to the definition of hospice in the new law. Furthermore, the costs of services proposed for coverage under the benefit were not captured in the data. For example, a primary caregiver in the home was required in the NHS but not in the benefit. The absence of a caregiver, said NHO, would require more intense and frequent services. Patients in the NHS were not required to waive other Medicare benefits, as they would be under the hospice legislation. This might lead to shorter lengths of stay as patients delayed the decision to forgo traditional care.

The issue of average length of stay in hospice programs was of paramount importance. The reduction in the per diem rate for routine home care was not based on lower service component costs but rather on a less frequent need for services. This reduced frequency was a direct result of longer average lengths of stay as hospices in the NHS began to care for patients earlier in their course of illness. Intensive service was generally not required during these early periods.

In a letter to NHO, Dr. David Greer of Brown University, principal investigator for the NHS evaluation, agreed that

> the NHS cost data is based on our observed length of stay distribution and many factors could affect it in the future. An increase in the number of patients dying from diseases other than cancer, the inclusion of patients without principal care persons, and the requirement that patients waive their other Medicare benefits under TEFRA [P.L. 97-248] are a few examples of the factors which might affect length of stay in either direction.[20]

Greer lent further support to the contention that the data were not necessarily useful in the rate setting process: "We have been quite candid concerning the applicability of this data to the conditions of the Study exclusively and have made no claims that it would accurately reflect hospice experience under the different conditions established by TEFRA."[21]

This theme was echoed by NHO after the regulations were published in December. In March 1984, Representative Tom Vandergriff introduced legislation to preclude DHHS from setting rates below the August levels. Also in the House, the two members instrumental in the passage of the original legislation, Leon Panetta and Willis Gradison, introduced a similar bill in April. Their bill put a two-year floor of $53.17 on the routine home care rate and directed DHHS to adjust all rates based on reported costs after that period. Lending support to the claim that hospice experience under the benefit would differ from the NHS, a May telephone survey by NHO found that the average length of stay in Medicare-certified hospices was only 35 days. This was about half of the length used by HCFA in determining the frequency of service. Using the 35-day figure, CBO estimated the cost of restoring the routine home care rate to $53.17 at $2 million in fiscal year (FY) 1985 and $4 million in 1986.

Participation by hospices in the new benefit began slowly. By February 1984, 39 programs were certified; the figure rose to 54 in March, 61 in April, and 77 in May. By early December, 153 hospices were certified.

In March, at the request of the DHHS Inspector General, the Chicago region Office of Program Inspections reviewed the implementation of the hospice benefit. On-site interviews were conducted with 77 hospices and 49 representatives of other organizations. In addition, 167 telephone discussions were held with hospice administrators and other interested parties. In a draft of the report, it was estimated that, by April of 1985, only 210 (about 20 percent) of those organizations delivering some type of hospice services would be Medicare-certified. The report cited three areas of "primary disincentives" to certification:

- The cap amount of $6,500 was seen as the greatest barrier to participation. Payment rates, particularly the routine home care rate, were perceived as too low. It was feared the core services requirement and the new record-keeping procedures would raise the cost of care for all patients, not just Medicare beneficiaries.
- Some hospices were concerned that certification would force them to make decisions conflicting between the palliative needs of the patient and the economic needs of the hospice program.
- The role of the hospice medical director was seen by some as in conflict with that of the attending physician. Home care hospices anticipated difficulties in contracting with hospitals for inpatient care in which the hospice would retain professional management responsibility.[22]

The report concluded that the payout under the benefit would be less than originally estimated: under $22 million in FY 1984 and $104 million in 1985.[F] It was recommended that the benefit be considered "as a demonstration program in a market setting," that fraud and quality abuse be monitored, and that the hospice option be actively publicized by DHHS.

The National Hospice Organization took exception to the Inspector General's findings. A June letter asserted that a better classification of disincentives was reimbursement, core services, and misunderstandings.[G] The main problem was the rates. Hospices were prepared to make the changes necessary to be certified, said NHO, if they could be assured of adequate reimbursement.

In September 1984, the Senate Finance Committee's Subcommittee on Health, concerned about the limited participation of hospices, held a hearing to review the implementation of the Medicare hospice benefit. Representatives of NHO and others testified that the primary barrier to program participation was the inadequacy of the home care rate. The witnesses also pointed out that HCFA had failed to begin the collection of hospice cost data HCFA Administrator Carolyne Davis countered that low participation was more a result of restrictive conditions of participation than of payment rates.

Once again Congress sent a message to hospices and to HCFA that it intended for the hospice benefit to succeed. On October 11, the Panetta/Gradison bill (H.R. 5386) was passed. As a result of this legislation, noted the NHO in a

"Hospice Bulletin" on October 12, "hospice providers will be better able to meet their actual costs." Perhaps more important than the rate increase was another provision that mandated an annual review of the rates by HCFA. Previously, there was no requirement for a rate review at any point in time. The bill was signed by the President on November 9. The rate increase went into effect on October 1, 1984.

The other hospice issue receiving legislative attention was core services. Small rural hospices complained it would be difficult for them to hire their own nurses. They preferred to contract for this service with existing agencies. NHO responded by drafting a "rural waiver" bill, which was passed by the Congress in June. It allows DHHS to permit a nonurban hospice to contract for nurses if the hospice was in existence prior to January 1, 1983, and made a good faith effort to hire nurses directly.

A fact of overriding importance for hospice providers in the debate over the merits of the benefit is the sunset provision by which Hospice reimbursement under Medicare is scheduled to end on November 30, 1986, unless renewed by legislation. This has several implications. Hospices should decide if the changes necessary to participate in Medicare can be modified if the benefit is not renewed. HCFA must report on the effectiveness of the benefit and Congress will consider whether to let the benefit expire, change, or continue in present form. But perhaps most important, hospice providers must demonstrate, through expert management and excellence of patient care, that the benefit is truly a cost-effective and humane approach to the care of the terminally ill.

PROVISIONS OF THE MEDICARE HOSPICE BENEFIT

Many of the administrative adjustments from prior operating procedure that need to be made by a participating hospice are the result of the philosophical premise of the legislation. The benefit centers on beneficiary needs rather than on those of the provider. Central fiscal and professional management responsibilities were included to protect the interests of the patient and the taxpayer and are the key to an understanding of how the hospice benefit functions.

The hospice is the direct recipient of all payments for care related to the terminal illness of patients under the benefit, with the exception of reimbursement to the patient's personal physician. This precludes the brokerage of services to other providers in which billing would bypass the hospice. The hospice controls revenue and must be prudent in negotiating fees it will pay contract providers.

Professional management requirements were designed primarily to ensure that patients could look to one organization to be responsible for the quality of all service components. It also gives the hospice an opportunity to control costs by limiting contract services to items appropriate for hospice care and authorized by the hospice.

Coverage

The following discussion is not intended to replace the hospice administrator's careful study of the published regulations. However, it is useful to review the coverage and to itemize those items, services, and protocols that are new and unique to the hospice benefit. Rather than a collection of existing coverage under a new name or the fragmented extension of provider services, these benefits are provided in a centralized package intended to fully meet the care needs of the patient/family.

Medicare will cover these services when provided by a qualified hospice program:

- Nursing care
- Physician's services
- Medical social services
- Counseling
- Chaplaincy
- Home health aides and homemakers
- Physical therapy, occupational therapy, and speech-language pathology
- Medical supplies and equipment
- Drugs and biologicals used for pain and symptom control
- Short-term inpatient care for pain control or acute or chronic symptom management
- Short-term inpatient care to provide respite for family or others caring for the patient at home

Many items and services are covered (or required) under hospice that are *not* covered through any other provider:

- Drugs and biologicals for home use
- Service coverage regardless of whether or not the patient is homebound
- Inpatient respite care
- Continuous care at home during periods of crisis
- Counseling services at home for both the patient and the family
- Homemaker services
- Bereavement counseling
- Copayments limited to 5 percent of outpatient medications and inpatient respite care
- Volunteers must be available

- Care must be continued if benefits run out
- Personal comfort items
- Inpatient unit must have homelike decor

Eligibility

As in the section on coverage, this brief summary of eligibility and those on conditions of participation and reimbursement should not substitute for a thorough review of the regulations.

In order to be eligible to elect hospice care under the benefit, an individual must (1) be entitled to Medicare Part A and (2) be certified by the attending physician and a hospice physician as being terminally ill with a life expectancy not exceeding six months. An eligible patient becomes entitled to the benefit by signing an ''election'' statement provided by the hospice. A significant other may sign on behalf of an incompetent patient as permitted by state law. This indicates an understanding of the palliative, rather than curative, nature of hospice care and the knowledge that certain other Medicare benefits will be waived.

This election has been controversial among hospices. Some have never required that patients be ready to forgo concurrent curative therapy in order to receive hospice care. Others perceive the election and waiver process as difficult to administer and confusing to the patient/family.[H]

As indicated, the beneficiary must waive his or her right to have payments made for comparable or other services related to the terminal illness rendered by all other providers, with the exception of the personal physician. However, should the beneficiary require services not related to the terminal illness, regular Part A or Part B benefits continue to be available. Although not all examples of this are as clear-cut as the patient who needs trauma care following an automobile accident, a body of experience will develop, as it has in other provider categories of Medicare coverage, to address inevitable gray areas. At the outset, nonhospice providers should be circumspect with regard to care rendered to beneficiaries who have a hospice election in place.

The election process was designed to promote the development of hospice as a comprehensive alternative form of care and to ensure a substitution, rather than add-on, reimbursement effect for the Medicare program. Without a demonstrable substitution of hospice care for more expensive traditional care, it is unlikely the benefit would have been enacted and equally unlikely it will be renewed.

Hospice services are covered for 210 days, broken into three benefit periods of 90, 90, and 30 days (in that order). The patient can opt out of the benefit once in each period and once again be eligible for regular Medicare coverage. Reelection is permitted and begins the first day of the next benefit period. Concern about the potential abandonment of patients once their hospice coverage days are exhausted led to a prohibition against the discharge of, or service diminution to, such patients based solely on the ability to pay for services rendered. This does not imply that the hospice may not charge those who have adequate financial resources or that a hospice must admit all patients regardless of ability to pay. Rather, it is intended to protect the terminally ill patient from exploitation by hospices that might place financial considerations above their patient care commitments.

Conditions of Participation

The prospective hospice in the Medicare program must be a public or private organization or subdivision engaged primarily in the delivery of care to the terminally ill, including bereavement counseling for survivors. The hospice must be surveyed against standards established by HCFA. The Medicare-certified hospice must offer the assurance of continuity of care through a comprehensive, interdisciplinary approach in home, outpatient, and inpatient settings. At least nursing care, physician services, and drugs/biologicals must be available on a 24-hour basis.

The law and regulations distinguish between "core" and "non-core" services. Designed to promote both continuity and accountability, the four core services— nursing, physicians, medical social work, and counseling—may not be provided under arrangements, that is, by contracting with another organization. They must be provided directly except when there are above-average caseloads, significant staff absences, or other extraordinary circumstances. All other services, including inpatient care, are considered non-core. In spite of full congressional debate on this provision, it remains one of the most controversial of all the conditions of participation.

Objections, now that the rural waiver has been passed, come primarily from coalition model hospices. Directors of these programs fear disruption of established service patterns and/or wish to remain primarily volunteer organizations delivering psychosocial support without responsibility for medical services. Hospital-based programs with no experience in home care have also had problems with this requirement.

On closer inspection, however, the issue is not core services but the central financial position of the hospice. Under the prospective reimbursement system, hospices cannot afford the luxury of routine delivery of nursing services by contract. Such arrangements invariably will require paying the contractor fees that include the contractor's administrative overhead in addition to the nurse's salary and benefits. This would be imprudent for the hospice that has its own overhead and fixed per diem reimbursement. For the same reason, non-core service contracts must be evaluated closely by the hospice administrator and compared with the cost of directly employed staff. One suspects that the contract option would be rarely utilized if it were available for core services. This could be tested by a review of contracts for high-volume, non-core services such as home health aides.

When non-core services are provided under arrangements, the hospice must maintain professional management responsibility. The contracts must be in writing and legally binding. The hospice interdisciplinary team must develop a care plan for all settings and ensure its execution. Medical records must be centrally maintained by the hospice and a quality assurance process be in place for both direct services and those delivered under arrangements.

The method of contracting, especially for inpatient care, presents the hospice with both opportunities and challenges. Liability, appropriate sites, and reasonable costs are issues for planners and managers to consider. (These issues are discussed in detail in Chapter 10.) Creative contracts promoting the hospice concept and giving the program sufficient control to effectively manage inpatient care are possible.[23] A hospice might, for example, contract only for selected services offered by the host institution, delivering others directly. Contracts have been made that call for the lease or purchase of physical space, equipment, furnishings, and various ancillary services while the hospice provides nursing, social services, and counseling.

For programs purchasing care rather than space in which to provide care, the key is to purchase *hospice* care in place of the typical care offered by the contract institution. A hospice must not permit a hospital or nursing home to treat the program as simply a shift in third-party payers. There must be a clear understanding that the services are provided to the hospice so that the hospice can meet the client inpatient needs. In the absence of a fixed per diem rate contract, the inappropriate utilization of inpatient services might result in charges to the hospice that exceed its Medicare payment rate.

Requirements for a designated minimum level of volunteer services grew out of congressional concern for continued commitment to the use of volunteers. The law provides that hospices demonstrate a continuing level of volunteer participation. HCFA decided to implement this through a condition of participation that requires volunteer services to equal at least 5 percent of the total hours of patient care activities performed by paid staff.

A paid or volunteer medical director must be employed by the hospice. The Inspector General's report indicated some programs felt this individual would interfere with the relationship between the patient and the attending physician. Other hospices objected to the reimbursement scheme in which the medical director would be precluded from billing professional services directly to Medicare Part B. Instead, payments flow from Part A to the hospice program and these amounts are included against the hospice reimbursement cap.

It is unlikely that these problems will actually present serious obstacles to participation. The medical director serves primarily as a consultant on specialized matters of pain and symptom control. His or her status as a member of the hospice interdisciplinary team and as a resource in care plan development does not imply negative consequences for the patient-physician relationship. The role of the consultant physician is well established and the concepts of peer review and regulatory impact are facts of modern medical practice. From the hospice's perspective, the payment system compels the close monitoring of resource consumption. Without a medical director to intervene and educate physicians on hospice philosophy and protocols, a possibility exists for overutilizing expensive care modalities.

Physician service reimbursement to the hospice becomes problematic only as total average charges for the various care levels reach the cap amount. Up to that point, Medicare payments for physicians' professional services represent important revenue to supplement existing, perhaps inadequate, income from the per diem rates.

Reimbursement

Participating programs, regardless of auspices, are required to have a hospice provider agreement with DHHS. This is in addition to provider agreements in other categories held by the organization. Payments will come to the hospice in five streams: the four level-of-care per diem rates and the professional component of hospice physician services. The per diem rates are set prospectively by HCFA and the physician payments are 100 percent of reasonable charges. Per diem rates apply regardless of the amount of services, if any, provided daily. Only one level of care may be billed per day. The rates are applied by Metropolitan Statistical Area using an adjusted wage component and a nonwage component that is not adjusted.

The continuous home care rate is the only one that may vary according to the length of service. There is a base amount for the first eight hours and an hourly increment thereafter. This care is authorized only in periods of crisis when the patient is maintained at home. It must consist primarily (at least 51 percent) of services rendered by a nurse. The prudent hospice should, subject to patient/ family need, commence continuous care so that the minimum eight-hour qualification in each of the 24-hour periods (midnight to midnight) is met.

As a condition of participation, total inpatient days for Medicare patients under the benefit must not exceed 20 percent of all days. HCFA, through regulation, has expanded this to a reimbursement limitation as well. If, at the end of each cap period, the total is less than 20 percent, no adjustment is necessary. If it is more, a complex calculation is required. First, the ratio of allowable inpatient days to actual inpatient days is applied to total payments for inpatient days. Then the number of excessive days is multiplied by the routine home care rate. The two products are added together and this sum is compared with total payments for inpatient days. The difference must be refunded by the hospice.

While the cap amount will be adjusted annually by the medical care component of the Consumer Price Index, the rates are not subject to automatic indexing. Rates are to be revised using cost data gathered from participating hospices.

Certification: Yes or No?

In late November of 1983, DHHS Chief of Staff George Sigular met with NHO representatives, congressional committee staff, and Representative Willis Gradison to discuss the proposed routine home care rate. He told the group that it might be difficult to operate a hospice with less than "30 units of production." The reference was not to widgets, but to terminally ill hospice patients. Despite Sigular's insensitivity, it is clear that the prospective payment system in general and the established rates in particular mandate careful analysis prior to seeking certification. The hospice administrator must determine if there will be a sufficient number of patient days over which to spread the fixed costs of the program so that the total cost of care stays within the Medicare rate structure. It is not essential that the cost of each individual day category be under its respective rate. If, for example, the cost of routine home care is above the rate, this might be compensated by other rates and/or additional revenue generated by hospice physician services.

Planning for certification is best accomplished through the use of budgetary models. Revenue and expense should be projected at various attainable levels of patient service volume.[1] If patient care revenue does not exceed total expenses, the hospice must consider reducing costs or increasing income. Costs might be lowered by greater reliance on volunteers and donated goods or services. The cost of contract services should be examined to determine if direct employment is more economical. Conversely, consideration should be given to utilization of contracts for low-volume, non-core services. Income might be increased by higher charges to non-Medicare patients or, in nonprofit hospices, by more aggressive fund raising. Of course, these approaches to income have the result of either shifting costs onto private payers (a much-used strategy in hospitals) or subsidizing the cost of Medicare services with funds originally intended for indigent care.

While smaller hospices may be more disadvantaged by inadequate rates, they can often obtain a higher proportion of their budget items through volunteer services and in-kind donations.

Beyond purely financial considerations, a hospice program must examine its mission. Medicare certification imposes certain organizational standards the government considers necessary to ensure safety and quality care for Medicare beneficiaries. Coverage provisions of the benefit are comprehensive, including various care settings and both medical and psychosocial services. Hospices considering their mission as limited to one setting, such as a hospital-based program, may want to forgo certification. Hospices that deliver only psychosocial support services, such as counseling and friendly visiting, may not want the responsibility for professional medical services required by the Medicare conditions of participation.

Thus, a decision on Medicare participation depends on various factors. Because misunderstandings exist about certification requirements and reimbursement policy, the hospice should ensure that its deliberations result in a fully informed decision. The Medicare hospice benefit can be of great value to the patient/family and it is likely that other third-party payers will be influenced by its example.

THIRD-PARTY REIMBURSEMENT BY PAYERS OTHER THAN MEDICARE

One of the earliest serious discussions of third-party payment for hospice care was a paper prepared by staff at the Blue Cross Association in February of 1978. Noting that "while many issues remain unresolved, initial evidence indicates great promise for both major quality improvements and cost containment effects in the hospice concept," the authors concluded that "an opportunity exists for the Blue Cross organization to become involved in this potentially valuable innovation."[24]

This initial enthusiasm was followed, however, by a tepid official statement by Blue Cross and Blue Shield. Approved by their boards in November 1978, the statement took a less sanguine view of any cost-saving potential. "There is not sufficient evidence or experience," the statement read, "to be able to state conclusively whether hospice care is more or less costly than alternative modes of health care."[25] While supporting the basic ideas, concept, and philosophy of hospice, the Associations were reluctant to take the reimbursement plunge. They suggested to local BCBS plans that payment be limited to a small demonstration project and that any other reimbursement be made under existing benefit provisions.

A cost-containment survey conducted by BCBS in the spring of 1979[26] reflected the existing benefit/pilot project approach. Of 59 plans that responded to hospice-related questions, only eight were currently covering hospice care, none under a separate benefit, and only three had an active hospice pilot project. But 37 more were considering hospice coverage and 12 were either planning a pilot or otherwise formally studying the issue.

In 1983, a new survey was taken.[27] Fueled by previously conducted cost studies, the passage of Medicare hospice coverage, increasing demand from subscribers, and their own payment experience, 13 Blue Cross plans offered a separate hospice benefit. Further, 30 provided coverage as an expansion of hospital, home health, or nursing home benefits. (Eight of these offered both the defined and expansion options.) In addition, 12 pilots were underway.

While the local plans have been moving ahead, the BCBS Association declined to propose hospice benefits in its 1985 contract with the U.S. Office of Personnel Management for coverage of government workers. (BCBSA is the largest health insurer in the federal employees benefit program.) Despite studies demonstrating hospice cost savings, some from Blue Cross plans themselves, the BCBSA took the position that the hospice benefit would substantially increase the cost of coverage.

The Frank B. Hall Consulting Company has conducted annual surveys of hospice coverage in the insurance industry since 1981. That first survey of 11 major carriers indicated "only nominal support . . . for comprehensive hospice services."[28] In 1982, many of the companies were actively developing a hospice "product." And, in 1983, all 11 were offering some form of coverage, mostly under a defined hospice benefit. None had linked hospice coverage with an increase in premiums, although participation (and therefore cost experience) has not been uniformly substantial.

When the NHO study on the delivery and payment of hospice services was published in 1979, there were few instances of reimbursement to report, but many questions about how such payment should be structured. Several of these issues are resolved, while consensus on others remains elusive.

Benefits

There appears to be general agreement that benefits should cover a comprehensive range of home, outpatient, and inpatient services to both the patient and the family. Increasingly, it is understood that a hospice must have broad latitude in planning service that reduces costs by substituting palliative strategies for medically inappropriate hospitalization. Many of these strategies are designed to maintain the patient in the home setting. Third-party payers recognize this can be best accomplished under a defined hospice benefit rather than an expansion of existing coverage categories.

Standards

Another problem in 1979 was the qualification of hospices. Payers lacked a mechanism to measure programs against quality standards so as to preclude payment to providers unable to demonstrate adequate levels of safety, service capability, and clinical expertise. Today there are several useful approaches. A number of states have licensure for hospices, usually accompanied by regulatory standards. Medicare's conditions of participation comprise another test payers can apply. Carriers wishing to qualify hospices through perhaps the most rigorous appraisal may rely on accreditation conducted by the Joint Commission on Accreditation of Hospitals.

Reimbursement

From the preceding discussion of the Medicare benefit, it may be inferred that the issues of appropriate payment mechanisms and levels have not achieved similar resolution. Few of the nongovernmental third-party payers have adopted a per diem approach to reimbursement. Instead, they rely on a charge-based system with a wide variety of deductibles, coinsurance, and payment limits. Typically, payments are made only for specific services rendered. Aside from tracking the differences between carriers, hospices face the more fundamental accounting problem of reconciling this "per item" system with Medicare's per diem method. Hospice managers must know their per-day costs to determine margin on Medicare rates, in addition to costs by the visit, the session, or the procedure in order to set appropriate charge levels.

The promotion of a model hospice insurance benefit and a unified payment mechanism by the National Hospice Organization may help to further standardize third-party reimbursement. Legislation to require health insurance carriers to offer a hospice benefit is another method that has been introduced in several states, including Maryland, Michigan, Colorado, New York, and West Virginia.

A potential source of hospice reimbursement receiving less attention is the Medicaid program. State programs participated in payments under the National Hospice Study and some states, such as New York and Florida, have expressed interest in continuing participation in hospice coverage. One approach is for the state to include the home care element of hospice in a program of home or community-based services approved under the waiver provisions of Section 1915 (c) of the Social Security Act. This permits states to include, in their Medicaid plan, services (other than room and board) necessary to keep patients in the community and preclude a nursing home admission, as long as the average per capita expenditure for the care of patients under the waiver does not exceed expenditures otherwise required.

The problem with this path is that it does not enable the state to offer a comprehensive hospice benefit. It is more practical to have a hospice benefit under Section 1905 (a) (18). This paragraph permits payment for medical or remedial services, not specifically listed elsewhere, which are recognized under state law and approved by the Secretary of DHHS. State and federal cooperation to effect this approach could extend the hospice benefit to those who need this care but can least afford to pay for it.

STATE LICENSURE OF HOSPICE PROGRAMS

The drive for licensure of hospices centers on one or both of two factors: "truth in advertising" and legality. The first stems from the perception that organizations that hold themselves out to the public as hospices or as offering hospice services should conform to certain minimum standards of quality and provide a specified array of services. These requirements could be applied regardless of the size or reimbursement status of the hospice.[J]

The second is prompted by the fact that many hospices grew out of community-based organizations unaffiliated with traditional providers of medical services. When these programs began to provide nursing care and other professional services, they discovered no rubric under which to operate legally. Hospice licensure provides this, as well as a potential basis for third-party payers to qualify provider hospices.

Utilizing existing hospital licensing laws as a statutory base, Connecticut promulgated hospice regulations for inpatient care in 1978. The rules were styled specifically to the needs of the Connecticut Hospice, which was planning an inpatient building.

Florida became the first state to enact specific state laws establishing hospice as a medical-legal alternative within the recognized and licensed health care system. The legality of hospice care in Florida was under challenge from the state's home health industry, which viewed hospice competitively in a state already overcrowded with home health providers.

In response to the home health challenge, Hugh Westbrook conceived the idea of special hospice licensing and certificate-of-need legislation. Don Gaetz, at the time an official of Methodist Hospital in Jacksonville, joined with Westbrook to establish the first state hospice organization with the goal of passing a hospice law.

Despite intense opposition lobbying from the Florida Association of Home Health Agencies, the Florida legislature passed the "Florida Hospice Act" without a single dissenting vote in early 1979. The Medicare hospice benefit passed by Congress in 1982 includes many of the features of the Florida law.

Nationally, the home health industry rallied behind the Florida Association of Home Health Agencies with court challenges to the implementation of the Florida Hospice Act. The Florida State Hospice Organization, Methodist Hospital, several hundred terminally ill patients, and their families joined the State of Florida in defending the law. Ultimately, the state's Supreme Court threw out the home health industry's challenge and the law went into effect in 1980.

Methodist Hospital Hospice in Jacksonville became the first hospice licensed under the first state hospice law in the nation.

According to a survey conducted in June 1984 by the National Hospice Organization, 15 states and the District of Columbia have enacted some form of hospice licensure and 13 others have legislation pending or under development.[29]

A related concern on the state level is the place of hospice within the health planning system. About the same number of states that have licensure laws have hospice included in their certificate of need (CON) process. (The lists are not identical.) Many of these, however, require a CON only when inpatient facilities are involved or when an existing institution adds hospice to its services. Depending on one's perspective, CON functions for hospice, as it does for other provider categories, as either a useful restraint on unnecessary and undesirable proliferation or a regulatory intrusion on the competitive marketplace. Given its nascence as a reimbursed service and limited community need, it may be wise to include hospice in the health planning process at least until the effects of third-party payment, particularly Medicare, and community education efforts can be assessed.

NHO, which in the past has taken a limited role in the development of state licensure law, appears ready to draft a model bill and make a more forceful case for the value of this type of legislation. Coupled with the increased attention of third-party payers, this may lead to a significant increase in state hospice licensure.

FINAL THOUGHTS

An instructive parallel may be drawn between the current polymorphism of the hospice movement and the sectarian character of the medical profession in late nineteenth-century America. That period, according to Paul Starr, was one of "feuds and divisions," which weakened any collective effort to improve the status of physicians. This grew partly out of a democratic impulse in the country that held that professional licensure and other standards were merely an attempt by doctors to "establish exclusive privileges" and to perpetuate a "machinery of mystification and concealment." Starr says the "issue was defined by the regular physicians as science versus quackery; by the irregulars, as free competition versus monopoly." What destroyed early attempts at licensure "was the suspicion that it was an expression of favor rather than competence." William James argued in 1898 that "licensing would interfere with freedom of research in medicine."[30]

There are clear echoes of all this in today's hospices, many of which assert, according to the DHHS Inspector General's report, that standards such as those imposed by the Medicare hospice benefit present " 'one right hospice' model [which] at the very least implies that some kinds of hospices are more 'correct' than others and ultimately could bureaucratize and institutionalize what heretofore has been a pluralistic, community-based movement."[31]

For those who agree with Santayana that "those who cannot remember the past are condemned to repeat it," a further quote from Paul Starr is worth reviewing.

> A profession . . . differs from other occupations in part by its ability to set its own rules and standards. But it cannot do so unless its members agree, first, on criteria for belonging to the profession and, second, on what its rules and standards ought to be. . . . Perhaps the foremost obstacle to the collective authority of the medical profession in mid-nineteenth-century America arose from within its own ranks. Mutual hostility among practitioners, intense competition, differences in economic interest, and sectarian antagonisms held the medical profession in check. Internally divided, it was incapable of mobilizing its members for collective action or of winning over public opinion.[32]

Despite the recent emergence of hospice into the health care consciousness of the American public, the movement has accomplished a great deal through the force of its commitment and dedication. Hospice has struck a responsive chord in the desire of Americans for a more humane approach to the care of the terminally ill. But, as in all innovative efforts, there comes a time when a movement must be integrated into the mainstream or face a withering of purpose and energy. Thus, the twin realities of reimbursement and regulation were an inevitable development. It is up to hospice leaders, planners, and administrators to cope with these challenges intelligently, responsibly, and with unity of purpose.

TEXTUAL NOTES

A. A comprehensive review of everything which has been written on the subject of hospice costs is beyond the scope of this chapter. There have been a number of "review of the literature" articles published that summarize any of the several dozen treatments of this subject. For an example, see Charles H. Brooks' "The Potential Cost Savings of Hospice Care: A Review of the Literature," which appears in Charles H. Brooks and Kathleen Smyth-Staruch, *Cost Savings of Hospice Care to Third-Party Insurers* (Cleveland: The Hospice Council for Northern Ohio and others, 1983).

B. Recognizing, however, that the potential patient load would only be achieved over time, HPA reviewed surveys conducted by GAO, NHO, JCAH, and the University of Arizona to come up with an estimate of 12,000 Medicare beneficiaries actually receiving comprehensive hospice services in 1981. Using the 20 percent medium estimate of potential use, HPA then recalculated the potential participation estimates beginning with the 12,000 1981 base. This yielded a rate of build-up to potential of 35,000 in 1985, 45,000 in 1990, 53,000 in 1995, and 60,000 in the year 2000.

C. Actually, given the election feature of the Medicare hospice benefit, which precludes the concurrent use of hospice and most nonhospice services for the treatment/palliation of the terminal illness, all the users would be "new." Beneficiaries who, in the past, had utilized existing coverage to pay for elements of hospice care would not "add on" the new benefit. This implies that the savings estimates should have been considerably higher.

D. The exemption was to the cap amount, the limitation on the frequency and number of respite care days, and the aggregate limit on the number of days of inpatient care. It applied only to the Connecticut Hospice. A later exemption, part of the Technical Corrections Act of 1982, signed into law in January 1983, extended the National Hospice Study demonstration project until September 30, 1986, for hospices not providing care directly but acting as a channeling agency for hospice care. This applied only to the Genesee Region Home Care Association in Rochester, New York.

E. Among the HCFA officials were Robert Streimer, Director of the Office of Coverage Policy in the Bureau of Eligibility, Reimbursement and Coverage, and Tom Hoyer, Chief of the Bureau's Institutional Services Branch, both of whom would be deeply involved in the regulatory process.

F. It was projected that less than 23 percent of Medicare patients receiving hospice services in FY 1985 would have payment made on their behalf under the new benefit.

G. One important misunderstanding was, once again, the idea that the cap applies on a per-patient basis. One hospice asked, "What if one patient required prolonged, expensive care or a costly inpatient stay? The bill might be $30,000 and the reimbursement $6,500, which could easily bankrupt a smaller program." In reality, losses sustained as a result of the cap would occur only when the average of all Medicare bills per case exceeded $6,500.

H. For a detailed discussion of the hospice election, see Chapter 9 on legal issues and Chapter 12 on ethics.

I. Various formulas are included in Chapter 2.

J. At least one state, Florida, has provided exemptions for all-volunteer hospices that do not charge for services.

NOTES

1. General Accounting Office. "Hospice Care—A Growing Concept in the United States," Publication No. HRO-79-50.

2. Ibid.

3. National Hospice Organization et al., *Delivery and Payment of Hospice Services: Investigative Study* (Vienna, Va.: National Hospice Organization, September 1979).

4. Joint Commission on the Accreditation of Hospitals survey on hospices, 1982.

5. Health Policy Alternatives, Inc. "Summary and Statement of Conclusions of Analysis of Proposed National Hospice Reimbursement Bill to be Introduced by Congressman Leon Panetta et al. First Session of Congress," November 1981.

6. U.S. Congress. Congressional Budget Office. *Cost Estimate [of H.R. 5180]*, June 25, 1982.

7. Charles H. Brooks and Kathleen Smyth-Staruch, *Cost Savings of Hospice Home Care to Third-Party Insurers* (Cleveland, Ohio: The Hospice Council for Northern Ohio and others, 1983).

8. David S. Greer et al. *National Hospice Study Preliminary Final Report*, Health Care Financing Administration, January 1984.

9. James Lubitz and Ronald Prihoda, "Use and Costs of Medicare Services in the Last Years of Life " (Draft), Health Care Financing Administration, June 29, 1982.

10. ———, "Use and Costs of Medicare Services in the Last Years of Life," *Health, United States, 1983*, DHHS Pub. No. (PHS) 84-1232 (Washington, D.C.: U.S. Government Printing Office, December 1983).

11. James O. Gibbs and John F. Newman, *Study of Health Services Used and Costs Incurred During the Last Six Months of a Terminal Illness*, Research and Development Department, Blue Cross and Blue Shield Association. Prepared for the Department of Health and Human Services, November 1982.

12. *Congressional Record*, July 2, 1980. Referenced under Leon Panetta.

13. Dennis Rezendes, Written testimony submitted for a hearing before the Subcommittee on Health of the Committee on Ways and Means, House of Representatives, 97th Congress, 2nd Session on HR 5180, to provide hospice care under the Medicare Program. March 25, 1982.

14. Ibid.

15. Donald J. Gaetz, Speech to the 5th Annual Meeting of the National Hospice Organization, November 1982.

16. Leon Panetta, Testimony at a hearing before the Select Committee on Aging, House of Representatives, 98th Congress, 1st Session, May 25, 1983.

17. Donald J. Gaetz et al. Letter to Members of Congress. A discussion of cuts to the Medicare benefit proposed by the Office of Management and Budget, November 15, 1983.

18. National Hospice Organization, *Hospice Bulletin*, December 12, 1983.

19. "Medicare Program; Hospice Care; Final Rule." *Federal Register*, December 16, 1983.

20. David Greer, Letter to Hugh Westbrook of the National Hospice Organization. November 16, 1983.

21. Ibid.

22. U.S. Department of Health and Human Services, Inspector General. "A Program Inspection on Hospice Care" (Draft), June 1984.

23. Stephen H. Bandeian, *The National Hospice Reimbursement Act, How a Hospice and a Hospital Can Structure an Agreement to Provide Inpatient Hospice Services*. Arlington, Va.: National Hospice Organization, 1984.

24. Blue Cross Association, "Hospices, Status and Issues." Staff discussion paper, February 24, 1978.

25. Blue Cross and Blue Shield Associations, *Initial Statement on Hospice Care and Payment for Hospice Services*, November 8, 1978..

26. National Hospice Organization et al., *Delivery and Payment of Hospice Services*.

27. Blue Cross and Blue Shield Associations. *Hospice Care Benefit Coverage: Results from a Survey of Blue Cross and Blue Shield Plans*, May 1983.

28. Frank B. Hall Consulting Co., *1983 Hospice Reimbursement Survey*, October 24, 1983.

29. National Hospice Organization, "State Legislative/Regulatory Activity." Survey conducted by staff, Licensure and Reimbursement Committee, June 1984.

30. Paul Starr, *The Social Transformation of American Medicine* (New York: Basic Books, 1982).

31. U.S. Department of Health and Human Services, Inspector General, "A Program Inspection on Hospice Care."

32. Starr, *The Social Transformation of American Medicine*, p. 80.

BIBLIOGRAPHY

Gaetz, Donald J., et al. Letter to Margaret Heckler, Secretary of the U.S. Department of Health and Human Services. A discussion of hospice cost projections being relied on by the Office of Management and Budget, July 21, 1983.

————. Letter to Margaret Heckler, Secretary of the U.S. Department of Health and Human Services. A listing of alternatives to the proposals to cut the Medicare hospice benefit attributed to the Director of the Office of Management and Budget, July 22, 1983.

National Hospice Education Project. *The Grassroots Report*, August 1982.

National Hospice Organization. *Leadership Report*, April 1983.

————. *NHO Report*, June 1983.

————. *Hospice Bulletin*, December 16, 1983.

————. *Hospice 84: Financial Planning and Budgeting for Hospice Survival*. Syllabus for regional training conferences, Spring 1984.

————. *Hospice News*, July 1984.

Pryga, Ellen A., and Bachofer, Henry J. *Hospice Care Under Medicare*. American Hospital Association, Office of Public Policy Analysis, June 24, 1983.

Rosen, Michael P. *An Analysis of Proposed Federal Legislation Relating to Home Health, Hospice and Long Term Care*. Florida State Hospice Organization white paper, September 1980.

————. *Issues in the Development of Medicare Hospice Regulations*. National Hospice Organization, December 1982.

U.S. *Congressional Record*. Vol. 129, No. 161, November 18, 1983.

U.S. Department of Health and Human Services, Health Care Financing Administration. Unpublished discussion paper on strategic choices in the implementation of the Medicare hospice benefit. Undated, but first distributed in November 1982.

————. "Notice of Proposed Rulemaking—Hospice Care—Medicare Program" (Draft), December 1982.

————. "Notice of Proposed Rulemaking—Hospice Care—Medicare Program" (Draft), April 1983.

————. "Medicare Program; Hospice Care; Proposed Rule." *Federal Register*, August 22, 1983.

————. "Hospice Cost and Data Report" (Draft), May 15, 1984.

Chapter 9

Legal Issues Facing Hospice Programs

John D. Blum

In recent years health administrators have experienced a growing awareness and concern about the impact of the law on the delivery of health care services. While it is hardly a flattering commentary that there is little escape in any enterprise from legal issues, we are at a point in the health field where the pervasive influence of the law must be taken as a given fact. Legal considerations will most certainly influence hospices as they have affected other provider organizations. Although the law acts not only as a sword but also as a shield that can protect a program, this realization may be of little comfort to hospice administrators who see their programs threatened by legal jeopardies.

The impacts of the law on hospice are difficult to assess for two primary reasons. First, because the hospice concept is new and largely untested, legal analyses in an area without case law are, for the most part, a matter of speculation. Second, hospice is hardly a unitary concept with defined protocol. It remains loosely defined in order to address individual patient needs. Nevertheless, regardless of the difficulties in developing a comprehensive legal assessment, treatment of the terminally ill through palliative therapy, in a nontraditional program, gives rise to legal issues that can be ascertained in case and statutory law.

This chapter provides hospice managers, program planners, and administrators with an overview of key legal areas they are likely to encounter in program operations. It is not intended to be a detailed discussion of legal theory. And it should be noted that legal issues, while significant, should never be viewed as a barrier to development and innovation in the hospice movement.

MAJOR IMPACT AREAS

There are a range of vantage points from which to assess the impacts of the law on a hospice program. Every major legal subject area may, in some fashion,

229

be related to hospice development and operation. Issues could be explored concerning business law problems that a hospice provider may encounter regarding tax status, corporate structure, personnel policies, employee relations, property issues, and the broad area of contracts.

Another major area of legal inquiry centers around regulatory issues. The advent of Medicare certification in 1983 created extensive requirements to which hospice programs must comply to be eligible for federal reimbursement.[1] In other sectors of the health industry both Medicare and Medicaid reimbursement have spawned extensive legal controversies waged in administrative and judicial forums; there is no reason to feel that the federal law and regulations concerning the hospice benefit will be an exception.

Aside from federal regulatory activity there are important developments in state hospice regulations. State regulation is the first line of regulatory concern for affected programs. Without appropriate state approval a hospice will most likely be unable to function.

NEGLIGENCE, WRONGFUL DEATH, AND SURVIVAL ACTIONS

While the areas mentioned above are of great importance to hospice managers, this chapter focuses on negligence issues arising in the delivery of services to hospice patients and families. General negligence is loosely defined as an act or omission on the part of an individual (or group of individuals) that violates acceptable standards of behavior. Furthermore, this act causes injury and may require the perpetrator to provide restitution for damages.[2] Broadly speaking, negligence as it relates to hospice can be split into two areas: individual negligence and organizational or corporate negligence.

The discussion in this chapter rests more with malpractice than with general negligence. However, it is important to recognize the potential problems hospices can face in the area of general negligence. For example, if a family member visits a hospice patient in an inpatient hospice unit, slips, falls, and injures himself or herself because a waxed floor wasn't cordoned off, this constitutes negligence and could result in a liability suit.

Some managers, unexposed to the legal system, may question why a hospice program should be concerned about patient negligence claims. The patient is dying and the likelihood of that individual filing a liability suit seems remote. Most administrators, however, realize that a legal cause of action is not terminated by death, but can be pursued by the claimant's heirs or personal representatives. Under state law, *wrongful death* and *survival actions* for negligence continue for a number of years after a patient's death.[3]

A *wrongful death* action is one filed to recover for negligent occurrence causing death. For example, if a hospice patient was improperly medicated and that error resulted in death, a lawsuit is possible under a state wrongful death statute. Where the tortious action (a civil action) does not result in death but causes a measurable injury, a suit brought on behalf of the deceased is a *survival action*. To succeed in either case the party bringing the suit must demonstrate that the alleged negligence caused an injury. In the case of a terminal patient who suffered multiple complications, it is difficult to show that the alleged negligence directly caused death or injury.

MALPRACTICE: DEFINITION AND SPECULATION

There is no professional group associated with hospice, clergy included, that does not face a potential malpractice threat. *Malpractice is the failure of one rendering professional services to deliver those services in an acceptable manner.* In malpractice cases, individuals are judged on the basis of how other members of the same profession would behave in a similar situation.[4] The issue of professional negligence or malpractice is pervasive and troublesome in the broad area of health services delivery. While the focal point of legal discussion concerning malpractice rests on physician's liability, all caregivers are affected by increased malpractice litigation.

Because hospices offer a broad range of professional services, it is difficult to envisage all potential liability areas providers face. For example, a malpractice suit could be brought against a hospice medical director or participating physician who makes an improper diagnosis and recommends palliative care when a curative approach may have been beneficial. In another situation, a hospice physician or nurse could improperly administer medication or administer the wrong medication. Failure by a staff member to follow a patient's plan of care, or to prepare an adequate plan of care, could result in malpractice claims. Bereavement counseling improperly conducted could cause a family member unnecessary emotional distress and may serve as the basis for a liability action. Errors in treatment as well as administrative matters may give rise to professional negligence. This includes failure to document treatment, failure to supervise employees adequately, and so on.

Scenarios of individual hospice professional liability can be easily expanded by the active administrative imagination. Yet any type of professional error does not automatically lead to liability. To have a successful malpractice claim it is necessary to demonstrate that the alleged negligent party's conduct caused a particular injury and that such conduct violated a professional practice standard. The structure of a malpractice case varies by state. However, there are four commonly recognized elements in all cases: duty, breach, causation, and damages. These elements are examined in detail.[5]

DUTY AND PROFESSIONAL STANDARDS

Duty involves a twofold inquiry: (1) whether a professional-patient relationship exists and (2) whether the professional is determined to be responsible for his or her actions. For hospice, duty addresses a staff member's responsibility to patient and family members.

Is a hospice legally responsible to provide such items as bereavement counseling to all family members? While this question is up to a court, it is conceivable that a duty to provide counseling and other support can be viewed broadly to encompass all family members in the geographical area who desire such services.

Demonstrating breach of duty by a caregiver rests upon both establishing a professional standard and obtaining adequate evidence to show that the standard was violated. Generally, standards are established by comparing appropriate courses of action in similar situations. At one time, the standards of medical practice were based upon an assessment of acceptable community practices. This so-called "locality rule" was abolished in most states and replaced by national or regional standards.[6] Medical practice standards are hardly exact. While there are areas of general agreement, there are many illnesses that allow for a wide range of clinical practices.

New professional categories or alternative modes of therapy present problems in identifying applicable standards. Although the law allows for variations in treatment, the basis for assessing clinical acceptability of such variations rests largely with physicians. When other health providers develop standards seen as conflicting with those established by physicians, the former are likely to face difficulty in having standards legally upheld. For example, it has taken years for non-MD (non-allopathic) practitioners such as podiatrists and chiropractors to have their own practice standards legally recognized and reimbursed. Today, problems continue if those standards deviate significantly from medical or osteopathic schools of practice.

It is unclear whether the law will recognize unique standards for hospice. There are differences of approach to the treatment of the dying patient in a hospice program. However, differences stem from use of palliative therapy and not from the model in question. Within the framework of palliation, an acceptable range of practices can be identified and will undoubtedly be more focused as hospice care evolves. Peer identification of acceptable professional behavior in the field, as well as in programs and organizations, will mold practice standards for hospice professionals. The court's role is limited to recognizing appropriate hospice standards as a basis of evaluation. This is generally established through testimony of experts in the field.

Hospice professionals will likely be held to a range of standards including acceptable palliative care practices, as well as recognized curative therapies. While a curative approach is not pursued in hospice, that does not absolve the practitioner from being aware of all accepted modes of therapy and their rami-fications. For example, an attending hospice physician who is a general prac-titioner may not be judged by the same standards as an oncologist, but that general practitioner should have a detailed knowledge base in the cancer field, far beyond palliative care. It is reasonable to assume that any health professional working in a hospice has a high degree of expertise and broad knowledge in his or her area as it relates to terminal illness. Conceivably, the scope of knowledge requirements for hospice professionals may be dictated by some type of specialty certification.

While there are currently no widely recognized hospice-specific standards, guidance for certain professionals in the area can be ascertained from regulation and individual program policies. Federal and state regulations and JCAH ac-creditation standards serve as valuable guideposts for determining the scope of responsibility of individual practitioners.

For example, federal and state regulations establish responsibilities of a hospice medical director. At the federal level, regulations charge that the medical director assume overall responsibilities for medical aspects of a hospice program.[7] Al-though the federal standard provides little detail, it identifies the broad scope of a medical director's clinical activity. Under many state laws, detailed descriptions of the medical director position exist. In Florida nine specific areas of respon-sibility are delineated.[8]

Aside from regulatory guidelines, the scope of responsibilities of hospice staff can be found in individual program bylaws, job descriptions, policy statements, and contracts. Although the factors above may not be legally binding, they provide the courts with a range of hospice practitioner activities. Determining the appropriate activities of professionals addresses only part of the standards issue. The more difficult issues concerning a caregiver's performance are not answered and will be evaluated on the basis of expert opinion and field expe-rience.

CAUSATION AND DAMAGES

The third element in building a malpractice case requires a *showing of caus-ation*. It must be demonstrated that (1) the act or omission caused the injury that precipitated the lawsuit and (2) the event is recognized as negligence. *Causation requires a demonstration of two factors: cause in law and cause in fact.*

Cause in law, often referred to as proximate cause, is difficult to explain because it involves an extensive test dictated by state law. For purposes of this chapter, intricacies of legal causation are not critical. What is important is that proximate cause concerns whether the law will recognize certain conduct as negligence and allow damages to be assessed against a person or agency.[9] Proximate cause is most difficult in cases where the alleged negligent conduct has never been subject to litigation. In most situations, legal causation is not evaluated by totally new analyses but through precedent.

Factual causation requires adequate proof to illustrate that the defendant's action resulted in a particular injury. Traditionally, factual causation was proven by the so-called "but for rule." "But for" the defendant's actions the plaintiff would not have been injured. The "but for" factual causation test has been replaced by requiring proof that the defendant was a substantial factor in causing the alleged injury.[10]

Conceptually, the factual element of causation is not difficult to illustrate. However, it presents highly problematic issues in cases where multiple causes contribute to an injury. In the case of hospice, a patient malpractice claim may involve a dying person suffering from a host of complex medical conditions. To have a successful malpractice action, the negligent occurrence must be established and a connection must exist between the negligence and the patient's injury.

For patients suffering from a host of medical problems, it may be difficult to isolate a negligent occurrence as a primary cause of an injury. A negligent event will not lead to liability if it is demonstrated that the negative outcome would have occurred regardless of the event. As a practical matter, a case involving hospice professional malpractice would most likely be a wrongful death-survival action. In this instance an autopsy may be required.

The fourth factor in a malpractice case concerns the issue of damages. If there are no measurable damages, there is little incentive to pursue a lawsuit. Generally, legal damages in malpractice fall into the following categories: (1) actual compensation for the past/future medical costs, (2) past/future loss of income, (3) physical pain, and (4) mental anguish. The other two damage categories are punitive, for willful or malicious conduct, and nominal, for proven claims where exact damage amounts cannot be established.

A major component of damages for seriously injured patients falls into the area of future income loss. For a dying patient, where the action is not for wrongful death, projections of future earnings would be minimal. Some states have established a minimum floor for damages in cases involving patient negligence in long-term care.[11] At this point, state regulations concerning nursing home liability damage requirements have not been extended into the hospice field.

Two damage areas of particular interest to hospice providers are damages for emotional distress and loss of consortium. As a general rule, it is very difficult to recover damages for an emotional injury where there is no accompanying physical injury. Under traditional legal doctrine, if a family member of a hospice patient witnesses an act of negligence that causes the patient pain and suffering, and even death, it is generally not possible for the family member to claim damages for psychic injury without some type of physical involvement. The law, however, in this area is undergoing change as requirements to show neg- ligently induced emotional trauma as well as physical injury are no longer nec- essary.[12]

As awareness and knowledge of psychic injury expands, courts may abolish restrictive policies against recognizing independent emotional trauma. The New York case of *Lafferty v. Manhasset Medical Center Hospital* provides insight into psychic trauma.[13] In the Lafferty case the decedent erroneously received the wrong type blood transfusion and died. The New York court allowed the woman's daughter-in-law, who witnessed the wrongful transfusion and subse- quent suffering and death, to receive damages for emotional trauma. Critical in the court's decision was the fact that the daughter-in-law had witnessed the negligently induced suffering while actively caring for her mother-in-law. A situation may exist in which an individual, while assisting a dying family mem- ber, witnesses negligence perpetrated by a hospice practitioner and sues using the Lafferty rationale for remuneration due to emotional distress.

In a malpractice case involving a hospice patient, damages may be obtained for loss of consortium.[14] Generally speaking, loss of consortium is a broad concept involving recovery for deprivation of society, fellowship, and affec- tionate relations; it is a damage claim that can be made by the patient's spouse, child, or parent. While awards for loss of consortium seem reasonable in the hospice context, they may, as for other damages, be limited because the patient in question was terminally ill prior to the events which constitute malpractice.[15]

CORPORATE LIABILITY: TRADITIONAL DOCTRINE

For managers, considerations of liability issues in the context of a hospice program are much broader than those issues regarding individual professional liability; they include programwide liability. Organizational negligence, or cor- porate liability, attaches to an entire program, holding it accountable as if it were an individual. Corporate liability extends to the board of trustees, the ultimate site of an entity's legal authority. Individual trustees can be held per- sonally accountable for their actions on behalf of the organization. In the field of health care, corporate liability has been expanded as its concepts are applied to a wide range of facilities and programs. There is no reason to feel hospice will be immune to this trend.

Perhaps the most basic program responsibility possessed by a hospice is a custodial one: the duty to maintain premises in a reasonably safe manner. Cus- todial duty is applicable to a program if it owns or leases property, although ownership could heighten legal responsibilities. If a hospice, for example, owns its facility, it is responsible to ensure that individuals accessing that building are not exposed to dangerous conditions. If someone using the hospice's building is injured as a result of the program's failure to maintain the premise, the hospice is liable. At one time, the law conditioned such liability on the status of the injured party (trespasser, guest, invitee), but these distinctions are no longer strictly enforced.[16]

An interesting question related to a hospice's responsibility for custodial care concerns contracting with third parties. If a maintenance company is contracted by a hospice to provide custodial services, does the hospice corporation bear the liability for the service company's negligence? The answer to the question is clearly yes. A well-established rule in corporate law is that a corporation's legal duties are nondelegable.[17] Thus, a manager who feels he or she can insulate the hospice program from liability by contracting responsibilities is mistaken. However, even though the hospice bears ultimate legal responsibility for executing its duties, it can sue the contractor for liability the hospice must bear due to the contractor's actions.

As an outgrowth of custodial liability a health care program has to ensure the safety of patients, employees, and the public. The safety responsibility is particularly acute as it relates to patients. In the context of hospice, a program has a responsibility to ensure that a patient is supervised in order to guarantee physical safety. It is questionable whether the home-based hospice patients are owed the same safety duty as those in inpatient settings. Under a hospice's 24-hour accountability, a program must ensure the safety of all its patients regardless of care site. However, it seems reasonable to argue that the extent of the safety duty may be mitigated in a home setting because a program would not have the same degree of control over the individual as it would in an inpatient setting.

Custodial and safety questions also address liability issues involving defective treatment equipment. While a hospice is clearly not as technologically intensive as other medical treatment programs, use of various technologies is integral to patient care and undergoing rapid change. Two issues often raised related to equipment are: a duty to possess and a duty to maintain. A health provider must possess equipment that adequately provides the type of care being offered. Specific duties concerning what to possess vary among programs. There is no duty to have the latest piece of equipment or technological system. A hospital intensive care unit has a greater legal responsibility to have extensive technologies than a hospice. However, within the context of hospice certain hospice programs, such as freestanding facilities, should possess a higher degree of responsibility with more extensive medical equipment and technologies than home-based programs. Courts will most likely find that the type of equipment a hospice uses has a greater relationship to its philosophy of care than organizational structure.

In the area of equipment maintenance, a hospice program has a duty to maintain equipment in a safe and workable fashion. If a device is overtly defective and that defect injures the user, the program may be liable. If there is a latent defect, one that is not obvious, liability still attaches to the program and possibly also to the manufacturer.[18]

A major source of liability for any health provider stems from the provider's status as an employer. Under the doctrine of *respondeat superior* an employer is vicariously liable for the tortious conduct of employees. If an individual, regardless of profession, is an employee of the hospice, the *respondeat superior* doctrine applies. In a Medicare-certified hospice individuals providing core services, including volunteers, are considered employees and, as such, their liability is attributed to the employer program.[19] The underlying theory is that the employee carries out responsibilities on behalf of the employer. If the individual acts in an improper manner, the consequences attach to the individual and the employer. The *respondeat superior* doctrine exposes the hospice employer to a range of liabilities. However, it does not apply in situations where the employee's activities were outside the boundaries of the individual's job. For example, in the case where a hospice employee drove a patient's relative home and was involved in an accident, the hospice may not be liable under the *respondeat superior* doctrine.

Liability becomes more complicated when the wrongdoer is an independent contractor. Under the independent contractor arrangement (seen most commonly in the hospital sector) the provider corporation is not held liable for the contractor's negligence because the provider has no control over the contractor's activities. In a hospice setting, if services were provided under contract by a health professional, the program bears no liability for the individual contractor's malfeasance. The impact of independent contractor liability on the contracting institution is undergoing change in the hospital field, but this trend has not affected other provider entities.[20]

In addition to independent contractor status, a nonemployee may be an agent of the hospice corporation. An agent, unlike an independent contractor, performs a task. Within the boundaries of that task, the provider corporation, and the principal, bear liability for any negligence.

A home health aide who is not an employee of a hospice but conducts home visits under contract is not an independent contractor, but is an agent of the hospice. If the home health aide is an agent, can other hospice professionals working under contract be similarly classified? Health professionals working under contract in a hospital (with the exception of Medicare certification requirements) are viewed as independent contractors. The reason for this rests in licensure status. It is difficult and legally suspect for these individuals to be corporately controlled in the exercise of their professions. Health providers' organizations are not licensed to practice. Practice decisions by a provider organization would be legally suspect. In the case of hospice, however, contracted professionals have an agency relationship with the employing entity. While the hospice health professional has some latitude in providing care, discretion is restricted by hospice philosophy and practices. The more structured and rigid the hospice's approach to care of the terminally ill, the stronger the argument that professionals providing services are acting in the role of agents, rather than independent contractors. Therefore, their liability in performing professional responsibilities reverts to the hospice.

A significant issue regarding vicarious liability concerns legal culpability of a hospice for the negligence of volunteers. Under the Medicare regulations volunteers are employees. Thus if a court uses these regulations as authority, certified hospice programs would be vicariously liable for volunteer negligence.[21] Aside from the Medicare regulations, strong legal principles exist to apply *respondeat superior* to volunteer negligence.

The historical immunity of charitable organizations from liability for negligent acts by volunteers is largely abolished.[22] Organizational liability for volunteers' negligence is determined by two factors. First, is the volunteer in question acting in the scope of the voluntary activity? And second, what sort of control does the hospice exert over that individual? The more control exercised through special training, supervision, and operational policy requirements, the more difficult it is to argue against application of *respondeat superior*.

The hospice using volunteers is caught in a difficult situation. It may escape vicarious liability if it does not control volunteers, but failure to adequately control and monitor voluntary personnel could serve as a separate basis for negligence. The failure on the part of the hospice to adequately control volunteers' activities would pose more serious problems and may result in corporate liability, as well as licensure, certification, and accreditation difficulties.

The best argument a hospice can make to avoid liability for volunteer mistakes is that the event fell outside of the scope of the volunteer's hospice activity. For example, if a volunteer nurse drives another hospice worker home and causes injury to the passenger in an automobile accident, the negligent driving would likely fall outside the scope of the nurse's hospice responsibility. On the other hand, if the nurse regularly transports other hospice personnel (even if it is not a part of her voluntary function), negligence in so doing could be vicariously attributed to the hospice corporation. Whether a volunteer's action is outside the scope of his or her voluntary function is situational, conditioned by the organization's interpretation of the function and by the individual volunteer.

A hospice may avoid voluntary personnel liability by establishing a separate corporate entity designed to provide voluntary services. If a volunteer is liable in providing services, that liability would vicariously attach to the new entity and not the hospice. The spin-off corporation can be an effective liability check, if it is distanced from the hospice. Distance is created if the new entity also provides voluntary services to nonhospice organizations and formalizes its hospice relationship(s) via contractual arrangements. If volunteers employed by a separate entity are providing core hospice services, the hospice may still bear liability for volunteer negligence. The spin-off corporation, however, acts as a buffer and reduces the hospice program's liability in non-core areas.[23]

INFORMED CONSENT

Informed consent is a difficult issue for hospices, considering the impaired mental competency of many terminally ill patients. Legally, informed consent entails negligence action when there is a failure to adequately disclose information. It is based upon an individual's legal right of self-determination. Historically, informed consent grew out of the law of battery. Today it is an action that rests in negligence law and contains the four elements discussed earlier: duty, breach, causation, and damages.

Broadly speaking, an informed consent statement should include facts concerning the risks of hospice care, the alternatives to hospice care, and the implication of electing no medical treatment. A number of states have passed informed consent statutes that delineate specific requirements. While statutes provide helpful guidance, determining compliance with state informed consent laws is still a matter of considerable discretion.

To the lawyer the legal doctrine underlying the concept of informed consent is a fascinating one subject to much debate. For administrators, however, an immediate and practical policy in the area is necessary. This is particularly important because both state law and Medicare certification require hospice programs to obtain informed consent.[24]

Hospice programs tend to provide information in general terms, often as a result of philosophical convictions. While it is laudable on the part of a hospice to avoid upsetting patients and families, sufficient details must be provided to all concerned parties to make informed decisions. Essential information includes facts that the hospice is for dying patients, the overall philosophy of care, the regime of palliative care and how it differs from curative approaches, the basic treatment routines and administrative procedures, the nature of family involvement, and, very important, policies concerning resuscitation and feeding tubes.

There is no standard required list of information. As a general policy, program managers should provide patients and family members with all material facts needed to make decisions about electing and continuing hospice treatment. Informed consent should be used as a mechanism for avoiding uncertainties and controversies with patient/family about the nature of hospice services. Information disclosure should be viewed as an ongoing dialogue among all the interested parties.

Legally, informed consent must be documented through appropriate consent forms. A useful consent form provides a basic set of information and allows space for specific commentary tailored to the parties in question. The more standardized the informed consent document, the less effective it is. In addition to a particular form, it is important to document conversations between patient/

family and hospice provider to indicate ongoing information disclosure and to cover areas not originally discussed and documented.

The issue of patient competency makes informed consent in the context of hospice difficult. Whether a patient is competent to make decisions about his or her care is judgmental and generally addressed by the assessment of health professionals.[25] As long as a patient has lucid periods, the chances are good that the individual can provide a valid consent. If the patient is unable to consent, a family member or legal guardian should provide consent. Competency aside, a hospice should identify a family member or other trusted surrogate to assist in making treatment decisions for the terminal patient. This individual should review and cosign any hospice consent form. If there is a disagreement between patient and surrogate, disputes should be resolved in the patient's favor.

QUALITY OF CARE AND CORPORATE NEGLIGENCE

The area of health care institutional and programmatic liability is significantly expanded by evolving doctrines of corporate negligence and theories of *respondeat superior*. With the landmark Illinois decision of *Darling v. Charlestown Community Hospital* in 1965, the traditional distinction between administrative responsibility and medical practice is subject to ongoing erosion.[26]

In *Darling*, a high school football player's broken leg was negligently set in the local hospital emergency room by an attending physician with little experience in orthopedics. The care provided the boy while in the hospital by the same physician was negligent, so that the patient had to be transferred to another hospital, where his leg was amputated. Both physician and hospital were sued, but the former settled out of court. In the case against the hospital it was alleged that the institution allowed an unqualified physician to practice orthopedics, failed to review physician qualifications and privileges, and ignored the nurse's notes that the boy's condition was deteriorating. The hospital argued that it should not bear liability for the boy's injuries because it was not licensed to practice medicine and, as such, could not interfere in treatment decisions. In deciding this case the court judged the hospital's conduct by use of the state licensing act, the institution's own bylaws, and JCAH accreditation standards. On the basis of the criteria used it was clear that the facility breached its duty to monitor the treatment provided and uphold acceptable standards of care.

While a modern health facility is not licensed to practice medicine, it has a duty to uphold the interests of patients and ensure that they receive medical care of optimal quality. This legal responsibility in the patient care arena, stemming from *Darling*, is a broad-based duty for health care providers. It covers all aspects of a patient's care and supervision in a particular program or facility, ranging from admissions to discharge planning.

As a medical program, hospice provides health services directly. Thus, a hospice needs to address the scope of patient care liability. Administrators, attempting to understand the scope of a hospice's corporate legal duty, should consider legislation, regulation, accreditation standards, program bylaws and statements, and customs and practices of other hospices and health care providers.

A Medicare-certified hospice provider falls under an extensive set of regulations that constitute legal obligations and provide specific direction concerning a program's duty. For example, Medicare requires certified hospices to provide care to enrolled patients after their benefits expire, without regard to the ability to pay.[27] If a certified hospice provider excludes enrolled patients for financial reasons, that constitutes a breach of legal obligation. Further, failure to adhere to state regulations mandating certain programmatic behavior is also viewed as a breach of corporate duty that would result in organizational liability.

Program managers should be aware of the fact that in addition to regulation, hospices voluntarily seeking JCAH accreditation are judged by the standards of that organization. Thus, an accredited hospice may be held to higher corporate duty than a nonaccredited program. Courts may also use JCAH standards for assessing any hospice provider's obligations, even if the program in question is not accredited.

A hospice can also create legal obligations through statements included in its bylaws and policy manuals. A bylaw, and to a lesser extent, a policy statement can be interpreted as creating a contractual obligation. While a hospice may not be obligated to adopt a particular bylaw or policy, once it does it has a responsibility to live up to such a provision. If, for example, a hospice program's bylaws state that if space is available it must admit all terminal patients with six months or less to live, the program is legally obligated to do so. It is imperative that a hospice, prior to adopting bylaws or other official policies, consider whether it can meet potentially binding obligations.

Where no guidelines exist or those available prove inadequate, a court may assess a hospice's corporate responsibilities on the basis of custom and practice. Just as any individual health professional is judged by a comparative standard derived from other professionals' experiences, so too could a court judge a hospice program by comparisons with other reputable programs. It seems unlikely that a court, in determining corporate duty, would apply a locality rule. Rather, it would be influenced by comparisons with similar programs, regardless of location.

Because hospices operate in a given way does not mean their operations set a standard. In turn, the failure of a hospice to follow the norm does not necessarily render a particular practice unacceptable. The benefit of comparing programs is that it affords some evidence as to how the practices at issue are generally handled. Over time, if consensus develops concerning certain program policies or behaviors, it may be hard for a hospice to argue for alternatives without strong justification.

Unquestionably, legal precedent offers key sources for assessing the scope of responsibility of a hospice program. At this time judicial precedent involving hospice liability is nonexistent. Once legal opinions are drafted concerning hospices, those initial decisions will be highly influential in all jurisdictions. Until a body of precedent dealing with hospice is developed, courts will consider various types of cases for guidance in the area. If a hospice is a component of another provider, for example, a hospital, a skilled nursing facility, or a home health agency, a court would use cases involving the parent organization as precedent. If a hospice is not part of another provider organization, it is likely that courts would use judicially recognized standards involving other health care providers for guidance, especially those regarding hospitals and skilled nursing facilities.

Beyond issues of determining how the law will frame the duty of a hospice program are very real concerns of hospice administrators about the likely areas of program vulnerability that could result in corporate liability. Just as it is impossible to predict what liabilities individual hospice practitioners will face in providing care for patients, it is equally as difficult to make predictions concerning specific areas of programmatic liability.

There are certain areas that can be highlighted as being potential ones for hospice corporate liability. As discussed, the hospice can be held negligent for the conduct of its employees. In addition a hospice can be held liable for hiring unqualified staff. The fact that a hospice hires a licensed provider does not make the employee qualified if he or she has no experience in dealing with terminally ill patients. Furthermore, hospices have a clear duty to train, monitor, and supervise staff members. In the area of recordkeeping, questions of access and confidentiality could create liability problems. Admission standards could generate legal difficulties. While a hospice, as other providers, is not obligated to admit a patient, the soundness of its admitting criteria may become an issue. A program must guard against charges of being arbitrary and discriminatory. In turn, a program that improperly discharges a patient without making adequate arrangements for his or her care could be held liable for abandonment.

INDEMNITY CLAUSES

One important question managers often raise concerns issues of liability in the context of contractual arrangement between hospices and other providers. It is not uncommon for a hospice to contract with an inpatient facility for bed space. The issue of liability in such contractual arrangements concerns who should bear the legal responsibility for injuries in the contracted space. Suppose, for example, a hospice contracts for bed space in a skilled nursing facility and all services to hospice patients therein are provided by the hospice. If patient negligence occurs, the caregiving hospice, and not the skilled nursing facility, would bear liability. However, there is a strong legal bias to attribute negligence to a facility if it occurs in that facility's four walls, regardless of the perpetrator.

In order to deal with the assignment of legal responsibility between contracting parties, hospice administrators should be sure that contracts contain indemnity clauses (often referred to as hold harmless clauses). These clauses indicate who shall bear liability for injuries in leased space. Contracts often state the lessee (the hospice) should bear the liability for negligence resulting from its services in the physical area in question. The hospice program should be cautious of contracts (allowed in some states) that transfer all liability to the lessee for negligent occurrences in the leased space, even those caused by the lessor institution.[28] For purposes of insurance coverage, liability between two organizations must be carefully delineated.

LIABILITY FOR NONTREATMENT

One challenge to hospice providers concerns a program's perceived legal obligations to sustain life and its posture toward upholding the wishes of patient, family, or guardians concerning a decision to forego life-sustaining treatment. By selecting a hospice program, patients and family members reject a curative, life-saving approach. Because a family enters the hospice with this perception, the program may erroneously assume that its responsibility for providing heroic treatment is reduced. This may not be the case. To waive responsibility, a hospice must obtain a family's signatures on specific informed consent documents indicating that at the time of death, a hospice patient will not be subjected to any extraordinary life-saving measures. The consent should conform to relevant state laws concerning nontreatment to be sure that failure to treat is not viewed as a form of active euthanasia.[29] In formulating policy in this area, the hospice may confront ambiguous state laws. The program should develop a nontreatment policy carefully detailing all elements of procedure, and where there is no relevant state law, those policies should be reflective of national trends.

A specific problem area involving nontreatment deals with removal of a respirator or feeding tubes from a hospice patient. Some hospices will not admit a patient whose life needs to be sustained via a respirator or feeding tubes. With technological changes, portable respirators and other high technology life supports in home settings are now feasible. Carefully developed policies concerning the removal of a respirator or feeding tubes are essential. If a state requires appointment of a guardian and court proceedings prior to removing life support, the hospice needs to follow the prescribed policy. While court action in this area may be an unreasonable intervention, if mandated, the hospice manager puts a program at considerable risk for doing otherwise.[30]

Another issue concerning nontreatment involves the impact of a state natural death act, or living will, on hospice policy. In states with living wills, patients are allowed to make an advance   directive to avoid extraordinary life-saving treatment in the event of incompetence. Where the living wills are legislated, difficulties arise in interpreting such statutes and in assuring compliance. Some state living will statutes tend to be procedurally cumbersome and have a number of restrictions placed on their application.[31]

In a state that has no living will statute, a patient-family may still present such a document to the hospice provider. In this case, the existence of the living will and its contents should be noted in the patient's record (as would be done in hospices where a statute exists). Until the effect of a living will without statutory basis is assessed, a hospice should try to comply with the request. However, this should not be done at the risk of violating state law concerning nontreatment. Regardless of the existence of special statutes, hospice policies concerning living wills need to be carefully delineated with patients and families.

SAFEGUARDS

Discussions of individual programmatic liability often convey the impression that legal problems are inevitable. While this is not always the case, the successful hospice administrator should understand safeguards that can minimize liability exposure.

It may sound overly simplistic, but a general awareness of law and legal jeopardies represents a first step in liability avoidance. Believing that because a hospice program performs a valuable, humanistic function it will not be subject to legal challenges is naive. Hospice personnel do not need to be lawyers, but they should understand situations that could lead to liability and know when to seek legal consultation.

A more formalized approach to reducing exposure to liabilities, and one that is mandated by law and JCAH accreditation, involves implementation of a quality assurance program.[32] While quality assurance is not just a program geared to minimize liability, there is no question that utilization review and medical audit serve as valuable tools to address potential patient liability problems.

As an adjunct to quality assurance, a hospice may establish a risk management program. Risk management is a formal process designed to reduce liability exposures and to foster awareness of legal liability. A risk management program needs to be tailored to a particular hospice and to contain certain elements. Basic elements of risk management include:

- continuing review of insurance to determine adequacy of coverage
- ongoing review of the physical premises and equipment to discover and correct defects
- ongoing personnel performance appraisal review and revision of hospice policies so that those policies reflect adequate quality of care measures

- maintenance of systems for investigating adverse incidents to prepare a defense and to develop procedures for avoiding future occurrences
- support of patient-family grievance procedures to handle complaints, solve problems, and prevent litigation [33]

Hospices interested in creating a risk management program should look to hospitals and long-term care institutions for guidance. These institutions widely use risk management techniques. Finally, considerations of how a hospice program deals with liability must include insurance coverage. Although insurance is no hedge against liability, it is a necessary operational cost and acts as an incentive to decrease liability occurrences so that claims can be reduced and premium costs kept down. Hospice administrators must determine the amount and type of insurance coverage needed.

Although the hospice's model, location, contractual arrangements, scope of services, etc., all condition insurance needs, there are certain kinds of insurance all programs should carry. Included in the list of necessary insurance is general liability for bodily injury and property damage recovery, contractual liability coverage, and tenant's liability. Hospices should have property coverage to protect the physical space used by the program and the space's contents, as well as professional liability insurance to protect the program from negligence claims against hospice employees or contractors. The hospice may also want to request its health professional staff to carry malpractice insurance and purchase coverage protecting directors and officers from losses and expenses resulting from claims brought against a program.

The purchase of other types of insurance, such as automobile insurance, ERISA, liability coverage, accounts receivable coverage, and employee dishonesty, depend upon individual program needs. In contract arrangements with other facilities, special insurance may be purchased covering occurrences in that provider's facility for which the hospice is contractually liable. Insurance, as any product, is subject to wide variation in price and quality. Administrators should be demanding in negotiating with insurance brokers, being careful to purchase policies tailored to individual program need. And those needs should be well understood prior to any purchase negotiations.

SUMMARY

The scope of legal issues potentially related to hospice programs is very broad. Each of the areas discussed, such as malpractice, corporate liability, and informed consent, should be evaluated with reference to an individual program. Although there are general principles that govern our legal system, for every rule of law there are numerous exceptions. This makes the law both frustrating and challenging.

From this chapter, administrators, program planners, and providers should get some sense about how legal principles might be applied to particular hospice programs. With no cases in the area, applying law to hospice is speculative, but that situation will change with increased hospice development. The legal problems discussed warrant expert assistance. The administrator who fails to obtain needed legal assistance places the hospice operation in considerable jeopardy.

While caution in dealing with hospice legal issues is essential, the law should not be viewed as a paralyzing force, blocking innovation and development. In planning and operations, the hospice administrator who considers legal effects will find that there are ways of running a progressive operation within legal boundaries. The critical factor is that the hospice program leaders are aware of legal issues and confront those issues in a timely manner.

NOTES

1. *Federal Register*, 48, "Medicare Program-Hospice Care: Final Rule." December 16, 1983, 56036.

2. William L. Prosser, *The Law of Torts* (St. Paul, Minn.: West Publishing, 1971), Sec. 30.

3. Ibid., Sec. 126, 127.

4. Angela Holder, *Medical Malpractice Law* (New York: Wiley, 1974), 40–43.

5. Ibid.

6. David M. Harney, *Medical Malpractice* (Indianapolis, Ind.: Allen Smith, 1973).

7. *Federal Register*, 48, "Conditions of Participation-Medical Directa." December 16, 1983, Sec. 418.54, 56028.

8. Florida Administrative Code, Sec. 10A-12.14.

9. Prosser, *The Law of Torts*, Sec. 42.

10. Ibid, Sec. 41.

11. N.Y. State Public Health Law, Sec. 2801-d.

12. 77 ALR 3d 447, see also *Molien v. Kaiser*, 167 Cal. Rpt. 831 (1980).

13. *Lafferty v. Manhasset Medical Center Hospital*, 425 N.Y.S.2d 244 (1980).

14. Holder, *Medical Malpractice Law*.

15. Ibid.

16. Prosser, *The Law of Torts*, Chapter 10.

17. Arthur Southwick, *The Law of Hospital & Health Care Administration* (Ann Arbor, Mich.: Health Administration Press, 1978), 404.

18. Ibid., 402–409.

19. *Federal Register*, 48, "Care Service." December 16, 1983, Sec. 418.80, 56030.

20. Southwick, *The Law of Hospital & Health Care Administration*, 378.

21. *Federal Register*, 48, "Definitions-Employees." December 16, 1983, Sec. 418.3, 56027.

22. Southwick, *The Law of Hospital & Health Care Administration*, 346.

23. 82 ALR 3d 1213.

24. See Georgia, Rules of Dept. of Human Resources 290-5-43.13(2).

25. President's Commission for the Study of Ethical Problems in Medicine and Biomedical and Behavioral Research, *Deciding to Forego Life-Sustaining Treatment* (Washington, D.C.: U.S. Government Printing Office, 1983), 121–126.

26. 211 N.E. 2d 253 (1965).

27. *Federal Register*, 48, *Continuation of Care*. December 16, 1983, Sec. 418.60, 56029.

28. 49 ALR 3d 321.

29. *In the Matter of Claire Conroy*, 464 A 2d 303 (1983).

30. John Blum, "Withdrawing Life Support: A Legal Assessment and a Possible Response," *The Hospital Medical Staff* 13, no. 4 (April 1984): 17.

31. See Texas Rev. Civ. Stat. Ann. Art. 4590h.

32. See Rhode Island Rules and Regulations for Licensing Hospice Care, Sec. R23-17-HPC,23.

33. Richards, *Medical Risk Management: A Preventive Legal Strategy* (Rockville, Md.: Aspen Systems, 1982).

BIBLIOGRAPHY

Holder, Angela. *Medical Malpractice Law*. New York, N.Y.: Wiley, 1975.

Harney, David M. *Medical Malpractice*. Indianapolis, Ind.: Allen Smith, 1973.

Prosser, William L. *The Law of Torts*. St. Paul, Minn.: West Publishing, 1971.

President's Commission for the Study of Ethical Problems in Medicine and Biomedical and Behavioral Research. *Deciding to Forego Life-Sustaining Treatment*. Washington, D.C.: U.S. Government Printing Office, 1983.

Richards, *Medical Risk Management: A Preventive Legal Strategy*. Rockville, Md.: Aspen Systems, 1982.

Southwick, Arthur. *The Law of Hospital and Health Care Administration*. Ann Arbor, Mich.: Health Administration Press, 1978.

Chapter 10

The Caring Aspect of Hospice: A Study

Nancy Burns and Kim Carney

Hospice care is appealing emotionally, philosophically, and practically. Yet few managers and planners have objective information about what actually occurs in a hospice care program. Who renders hospice services? What types of "care practices" are provided to patients and families? Exactly how does hospice care differ from nursing home and hospital care? Who are the primary hospice providers and what types of services do they provide?

In addition to a lack of information about the caring aspects of hospice, recent studies claim there are really no differences between hospice care and other types of providers.[1] Can this be true? Are the claims made by hospice workers across the country merely slogans? This question will be a difficult one to answer. Not only are the processes of care in both settings poorly defined, but it is difficult in any setting to relate the process of care to outcomes. This chapter, with its emphasis on the process of hospice care, will provide important information to planners and policymakers in answering this question.

In spite of the inability to explain care, there is some consistency in care provided throughout the institutionalized health care system. The philosophy (and the mandated standards of care that have emerged from the philosophy) is consistent enough to direct the care that occurred, ill defined though it was. The definition of quality of care depends upon beliefs and values that emerge from a philosophy of care defining desirable outcomes. Hospice emerges from a distinct philosophy of care that defines quality differently from the traditional system.

Many articles have been written describing hospice care and its philosophy. These articles describe a multidisciplinary team, emphasize patient and family as a unit, discuss intensive efforts to maximize comfort through medical and nursing interventions, and explore the psychosocial and spiritual aspects of care. Open communication is encouraged and there is concern for the patient's and family's continued growth. Families are cared for after the patient's death with the expectation that this care will have long-term effects on levels of mental health and social functioning.[2] However, these discussions may be oriented toward the ideal (what ought to be), rather than the real (what is).

Before determining whether hospices actually provide the care they claim to, and whether that care is actually different from care provided in a hospital or other institutional setting, we must first find ways to measure and describe the hospice care. Measures of hospice care will lead to more thorough examinations of the differences between hospice and hospital care. It will also give us a better way to understand nursing care, regardless of the setting.

STUDYING HOSPICE CARE

We became interested in hospice research at the same time the call for proposals for the national hospice study was released. Because of the National Hospice Study, it was difficult to get funding for other hospice research. Therefore, we confronted the necessity of developing a study that was feasible for us to conduct without outside funding. The joining of an economist and a nurse in studies to examine health care services is unusual but extremely important and gives us insight to make clinical as well as financial decisions. It also provides a unique opportunity to examine interaction between care and economic factors.

The study was conducted in a small, hospital-based hospice located in the Southwest. The hospice serves primarily one county in a large metropolitan area and was developed by a Catholic hospital, which manages it administratively. However, direct management of the hospice and staff were distinct from the hospital and had considerable autonomy. The administrative director of the hospice was a nurse. The staff consisted of two registered nurses, a part-time medical director, a part-time social worker, a licensed vocational nurse, a home health aide, and a secretary. As the hospice developed, a full-time social worker was acquired, a second home health aide was employed, and, more recently, a director of volunteers was hired. The licensed vocational nurse position has been deleted and plans are being made to add a third registered nurse.

Physicians admitting patients to the hospice were not required to have staff privileges at the hospital. The hospice planners wished to ensure that the hospice could indeed serve the entire community. The hospice provided only home care. No inpatient hospice beds were available. If patients needed hospitalization, they were admitted to one of a variety of hospitals in the area. Admission policy for the hospice has now changed because of Medicare requirements. Admitting physicians are given courtesy staff privileges. The hospital has three beds assigned to hospice. If patients prefer another hospital, they must be discharged from hospice care. These changes were made recently.

During the time of our study, hospice staff visited hospitalized patients. However, they were unable, in most cases, to influence the care given and served primarily in a supportive way to the patient/family unit. The nursing staff of the hospice used primary care nursing to provide home care. This means one nurse had the major responsibility for planning and providing nursing care for a particular patient. This increased the stress on hospice nurses but was considered important for quality care.

We chose this hospice because of the unusually comprehensive recordkeeping techniques introduced by the first hospice director. These records included detailed notes of all hospice visits and phone contacts and gave us data previously unavailable for examination. We developed the study to examine three aspects of hospice: demand, care, and cost, a combination other studies lacked.

As we approached the research design, two concerns emerged. First, there was an inadequate theoretical base from which to develop studies. Second, the mechanics of extracting data from hand-written patient care notes seemed overwhelming. We decided that our investigations must be designed to provide a base for developing theories related to hospice care. These theories would serve as bases from which to extract hypotheses for further testing.

Our emerging theory is described in detail in Chapter 11. It incorporates nursing and economic theories, using ideas of Grossman's human capital model and Yura and Walsh's nursing process.[3] Within our theoretical structure, hospice care is defined in terms of services, mix, intensity, order, and rhythm that merge into patterns. Care results from an interactive process between the patient/family unit expressing need, personal preference, and demand for services and the hospice staff offering a supply of services (see Figure 10-1). This interactive process leads to decision making about the care to be provided. The outcome is differing patterns of care. The process is continuous because supply and demand factors continue to influence changing patterns of hospice care.

Figure 10-1 Interactive Process Leading to Care

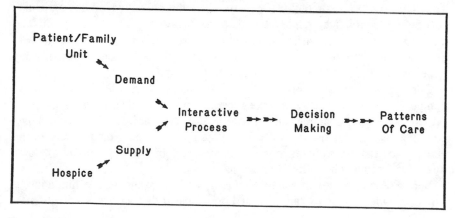

We decided to examine care across time. In this way we could study the care of patients from admission through the time of death. We also examined changes in care occurring as the hospice matured. Given the early developmental stage of hospices in general, it seemed likely that care patterns would change as the hospice grew institutionally. Our approach to the study of hospice care is practical. Rather than imposing a theoretical model upon administrators we use actual practice data to develop a model of care. The use of existing clinical techniques not only makes wise sense, but also provides administrators with specific evaluative data from which to make program and patient care assessments.

Patient Data

Information about the patients and their families was limited to data available from the patient's chart and discussions with hospice personnel. Because of patient confidentiality issues, the study was conducted without direct patient or family contact. We obtained information on varied aspects of the patient including his or her admission date, date of death, place of death, age, gender, race, marital status, religion, source of referral, source of third-party reimbursement, relationship of primary caregiver to patient, sex of primary caregiver, age of primary caregiver, residence of primary caregiver, attending physician, primary medical diagnosis, and identified nursing problems. Nursing problems are classified into nursing diagnoses.

A Tool to Measure Hospice Services

Policymakers and hospice managers have few, if any, means to evaluate care given in their programs. Care as a concept is elusive and poorly defined. The need for an easily assessible and complete measure of care is sorely needed. The tool developed for our research involves the collection of demographic patient and family data. While we realize that many programs are operating on a limited budget and provision of patient care taxes the budget, we nevertheless emphasize the importance of maintaining a data collection system. Not all data collection systems need be cumbersome or expensive.

Our approach to data collection identifies services provided and classifies components of care. The system does more than merely identify the individual providing care (for example, the nurse, social worker, or aide). It examines the patient's chart notes and patient care protocols. Examining data collected on charts also provides staff rendering care an opportunity to explain and explore their own attitudes, behavior, and service patterns.

Before describing our data collection tool, we must point out two limitations. First, only that portion of care recorded on the patient's chart can be identified.

There may have been a tendency to emphasize the recording of those activities most likely to obtain third-party reimbursement. Thus, nonreimbursable activities, such as psychosocial care, may have been less carefully recorded than reimbursable activities, such as skilled nursing visits. It is possible that some care activities are not even recognized by the caregiver but are performed intuitively. For example, providing support nonverbally could occur without the conscious recognition of the caregiver.

Second, the analysis of recorded clinical comments by a data collector requires subjective judgments of how care, described in narrative form, should be categorized. The data collector must avoid "reading into" the written narrative activities that are not described but rather expected to have been performed in a given circumstance. Training a data collector involves comparing results with the performance of previous data collectors on the same patient chart. Our degree of concordance was 85 percent.

There are problems inherent in classifying components of hospice care as discrete services. Hospice care is a very complicated collection of services. Any method used to catalogue services loses something of the wholeness of hospice care. In addition, differing care environments may modify the services. For example, the care provided in one patient's home may differ from the same care provided in another patient's home because of environmental factors.

In spite of these difficulties, we developed a classification system consisting of 66 services. Table 10-1 lists the services identified. These services are categorized by nursing process stage, dividing the intervention stage into care activities and teaching activities. The evaluation phase is merged with the assessment phase since care is examined longitudinally rather than cross-sectionally.

Measuring Care

The strategies used to examine care are useful to hospice managers and they can serve as a guide to developing additional techniques for evaluating hospice services. Our first task was to measure patterns of care by examining site of contact, minutes of care provided, hospice staff providing care, and changes in pattern from admission to patient death. In addition, we examined differences in patterns of care by medical diagnoses and nursing diagnoses.

The focus of hospice is home care. Home death is positively valued and considered desirable in terms of the quality of life and future family mental health. It is also valued because the cost of a home death is considerably less. The mode of death, however, may preclude home death, even though the patient/family unit desires it. Furthermore, not all families are willing to experience a patient's home death. Some patient/family units may decide, prior to hospice

Table 10-1 Activities By Stage of Nursing Process

ASSESSMENT:
1. Assess psychosocial situation
2. Perform social service intake
3. Perform assessment and evaluation
4. Assess patient's condition
5. Assess spiritual situation
6. Inquire about health of family member
7. Inform of patient's death
8. Inform of admission to hospital
9. Inform of patient's condition
10. Evaluate effectiveness of management
11. Assess family's condition
12. Complain

PLANNING:
1. Discuss symptom management
2. Discuss pain management
3. Discuss diet management
4. Discuss physical care management
5. Discuss drug management
6. Participate in discharge planning
7. Inform patient going home
8. Obtain physician order
9. Introduce other hospice personnel
10. Discuss situation with other health professionals
11. Arrange time of visit
12. Refer for hospice care
13. Convey patient or family concerns to physician
14. Convey physician comments to patient or family or hospice
15. Discuss psychosocial management
16. Discuss alternatives for providing care
17. Discuss plans after death
18. Plan care
19. Plan funeral
20. Discuss Medical management

INTERVENTION:
1. Rearrange environment for care
2. Discuss legal concerns or obtain legal assistance
3. Provide physical care
4. Provide spiritual support
5. Allow expression of feelings
6. Counsel and advise
7. Visit at time of death
8. Explore financial concerns
9. Reassure family that they are providing good care
10. Encourage family to take care of themselves

Table 10-1 continued

11. Discuss spiritual situation or request spiritual assistance
12. Obtain needed equipment or supplies
13. Obtain community service
14. Obtain financial assistance or discuss situation
15. Request help or respond
16. Arrange for someone to stay with patient
17. Arrange admission to health facility
18. Provide respite care
19. Provide support
20. Discuss feelings about impending death
21. Provide access to prescription of drugs
22. Public relations
23. Unsuccessful attempts to contact
24. Social interaction
25. Errands
26. Obtain specimen/analysis

TEACHING:
1. Teach physical care
2. Teach treatment technique
3. Teach hospice pain management
4. Explain hospice
5. Teach stages and management of dying symptoms
6. Teach procedure after home death
7. Explain bereavement care
8. Discuss expected physical changes

---

admission, to receive home care as long as possible but to seek hospitalization during final stages of the dying process. Despite these situations, a standard measure of a hospice program's success is the number of patients who died at home. Place of death is a major variable throughout our analysis.

In addition to place of death, two other variables are reviewed that are important because of their relation to reimbursement. Age is examined in detail because reimbursement patterns are significantly different for those over 65 years. Duration is the second major concern for both policymakers and hospice managers. In most studies, the mean duration is 55-60 days. However, the median duration, which is not affected by outliers (those at the extremes of the sample), is 28-32 days. These statistics have remained consistent across studies and also hold true for our sample. Most people live about four weeks after admission to hospice. There is some expectation, however, that with reimbursement, this may change. The care component of our study examines differences in care patterns as duration varies.

FINDINGS

Our research involves a longitudinal case study. Because it is a case study, we cannot say that other hospices are likely to have similar patterns of care to the one described; however, we can provide managers and planners with important insights and with techniques for assessing their own clinical practices. Because this study is largely descriptive, our capacity to explain the causes of our findings is limited. Thus, our discussion about causes is speculative. We ask that managers be cautious in using data and consider the uniqueness of their own program.*

Examining Services

The services examined include the 66 variables listed in Table 10-1. Those were extracted from patient charts. These care activities provide the core for our examination.

Who Provided the Care?

An important question related to hospice care is who provides the care. Table 10-2 indicates the percent of care within each stage of the nursing process provided by various hospice staff. A major portion of care was provided by the registered nurse. Most planning and teaching activities were performed by the RN, who coordinated the care activities of the other hospice staff members. All of the hospice staff, including pastoral care and volunteers, were involved in assessment activities. This is a clear indication of the teamwork involved in hospice care and of the importance placed on continual assessment of the situation.

Primary services provided by the social worker included psychosocial assessment, managing legal concerns, obtaining needed equipment, obtaining financial assistance, obtaining community services, and discussing psychosocial management. The home health aide was involved in providing physical care, rearranging the environment for care, assessing the patient's condition, and assessing the psychosocial situation. Pastoral care activities included assessing the psychosocial situation, assessing the spiritual situation, informing the hospice of the patient's condition, providing spiritual support, allowing expression of feelings, and discussing the spiritual situation with the patient's pastor.

---

*The study is being expanded through funds from the American Cancer Society. This money will allow us to further examine the impact of Medicare reimbursement on hospice care.

Table 10-2 Percent of Care Provided by Stage of Nursing Process by Hospice Staff in Third Year of Hospice Operation

Hospice Staff	% of Assessment	% of Planning	% of Intervention	% of Teaching
RN	74.0	88.8	64.6	96.8
LVN	1.6	1.1	1.1	0.6
Aide	14.1	0.3	12.7	0.2
MSW	5.2	7.2	11.7	0.7
Pastoral Care	0.9	0.1	1.8	1.4
Volunteer	3.4	2.0	6.8	0.3

No activities were provided all the time by one type of hospice staff. Although roles of different staff can be identified, there is some blurring of roles. Staff responded to present patient/family needs by providing multiple dimensions of care. Table 10-3 illustrates the percent of staff time invested in each stage of the nursing process. The RN is involved in all activities but spends the greatest amount of time in planning. The greatest portion of most hospice staff time is spent in providing interventions.

Managers and planners can assist staff in providing less familiar types of care by offering opportunities for mutual sharing of ideas and techniques used by each type of staff, thus strengthening the capacity for multidimensional care. For example, volunteers, aides, and pastoral care personnel may have approaches to care not well understood by traditional health care givers and yet very effective. These activities can be incorporated into the practice of other staff members.

Table 10-3 Percent of Staff's Patient Care Time Invested in Each Stage of the Nursing Process

Hospice Staff	Time in Assessment	Time in Planning	Time in Intervention	Time in Teaching
RN	23.6	43.5	24.6	8.3
LVN	34.5	34.5	27.8	3.2
Aide	47.2	1.6	51.1	0.1
MSW	17.2	36.3	45.9	0.6
Pastoral Care	24.2	3.1	61.5	11.2
Volunteer	23.1	21.6	54.7	0.6

Each type of staff has strengths that are important for administrators to recognize and nurture. The expertise of each staff makes a unique contribution to quality hospice care.

How Did Services Vary with Site of Care?

We identified six sites of care activities: telephone, home visit, hospital, nursing home, the physician's office, and the hospice. A seventh category of "other" was included for infrequent contacts. The majority of contacts were either home visits or telephone contacts.

Because of the large number of encounters occurring by phone, we targeted those services most frequently provided. Table 10-4 lists services rendered during phone conversations more than 50 percent of the time. These activities, provided most often by registered nurses, reflect coordination of care with other health care professionals, community agencies, and the primary caregiver (PCG).

The PCG was seen as a partner in care. Planning of care between the registered nurse and the PCG occurred frequently by phone. With this in mind, it appears that an effective working relationship between the registered nurse and the PCG may facilitate the capacity of the PCG to maintain the patient at home. If this holds true for other hospices, it will be important for hospice managers to provide adequate time for registered nurses to communicate by phone. This allows them to interact therapeutically with patient/family units and coordinate care with other health professionals. This could increase the quality of care, decrease the need for home visits, and raise the number of deaths that occur at home.

Examining Services-Mix-Intensity
How Does Age Influence Services-Mix-Intensity?

To examine this question, care activities for patients over and under age 65 are compared. Our sample included 120 subjects under 65 and 146 who were 65 or over. The proportion of patients 65 and over has increased over time. Differences in services related to age are listed in Table 10-5. Our findings indicate that the PCG working with older patients needed more assistance providing care than those caring for younger patients. In our sample, the PCG was usually the spouse. The increased needs may be due, in part, to an older PCG. The PCG caring for older patients also needed more assistance in dealing with the patient's psychosocial responses to the situation than those caring for younger patients. They were less confident in their ability to perform in the role of PCG and needed encouragement and a great deal of community support. These older patient/family units were passive during interactions with physicians, placing the hospice staff in the role of intermediary.

Table 10-4 Services Provided by Phone More Than 50% of the Time

ACTIVITY	% of Time Activity Occurs		Primary Staff
	Phone	Home	
Obtaining physician orders	93	1	RN
Arranging time of visit	93	6	RN,SW
Informing of admission to institution	93	5	PCG
Arranging for someone to stay with patient	92	7	RN
Informing of patient's condition	90	9	PCG
Requesting help	88	11	PCG
Conveying patient or family concerns	85	11	RN
Arranging admission to health facility	81	7	SW
Discussing situation with other health professional(s)	80	9	RN,SW
Discussing spiritual situation	77	15	PC
Conveying physician comments to patient or hospice	77	18	RN
Obtaining financial assistance	76	14	SW
Informing that patient is going home	74	0	PCG
Providing access to prescription medication	67	19	RN
Informing of patient's death	65	33	PCG
Discussing legal concerns	64	29	RN,SW
Obtaining needed equipment	62	33	RN,SW
Reassuring family that they are providing good care	61	36	RN
Exploring financial concerns	58	38	RN,SW
Inquiring about health of family member	57	40	RN
Counseling and advising	56	42	RN
Discussing physical care management	55	42	RN
Participating in discharge planning	55	3	RN
Discussing pain management	54	43	RN
Discussing psychosocial management	54	39	RN
Discussing alternatives for providing care	51	42	RN

Patient/family units with a relatively younger dying member had greater difficulty dealing with the impending death than did the older patient/family units and needed greater emotional and spiritual support. Younger patients were more actively involved in their care than were older patients. They expressed feelings more openly and sought information about expected physical changes. Although they had more difficulty dealing with the impending death, they tried to maintain

Table 10-5 Care Provided by Age

	Average Number of Services per Patient	
Service	Under 65	Over 65
Providing physical care	6.14	9.00
Inquiring about health of a family member	0.47	0.99
Obtaining community service	0.62	0.83
Arranging for someone to stay with patient	0.41	0.77
Arranging admission to a health facility	0.11	0.31
Conveying patient or family concerns to physician	0.40	0.60
Conveying physician comments to patient/family unit	1.63	1.92
Discussing psychosocial management	6.43	7.99
Providing respite care	0.64	1.12
Performing errands for patient/family unit	0.20	0.36
Discussing legal concerns	0.85	0.47
Providing spiritual support	0.65	0.47
Obtaining financial assistance	1.96	1.19
Planning funeral	0.15	0.09
Allowing expression of feelings	4.75	4.29
Providing access to prescription drugs	1.10	1.34
Exploring financial concerns	1.03	0.85

control over the dying process and sought greater understanding of expected changes. They were also involved in planning the funeral. It could be that younger people in our society are more open to discussions related to death than older people. These younger families had greater difficulties with financial and legal concerns than older families. This may reflect the abrupt and unexpected disruption of an income stream, less protected in our society than that of the older person. It may also be a reflection of differing reimbursement mechanisms for hospice care between the two groups, with the younger group receiving considerably less third-party reimbursement for home care than the older group. Differing needs of various age groups are important to consider in planning hospice care. Directly identifying the needs, and planning ways to meet those needs, decreases the probability that staff will respond impulsively to the age groups based on bias and cultural expectations.

How Does Gender Influence Services-Mix-Intensity?

Our sample included 138 males and 128 females. Unlike the age ratio, the sex ratio remained relatively stable over time. An examination of care in relation to the patient's gender reveals some interesting differences (see Table 10-6). In our study, the PCG was usually the patient's spouse. In the care of females, the patient's PCG was usually her husband. For female patients, psychosocial and spiritual support and counseling activities increased above that provided to male patient/family units. Furthermore, there was an increase in planning activities between the hospice staff and the PCG. Legal concerns also were increased. The PCG providing care for a female patient was more involved in planning life changes after the patient's death than the PCG caring for a male patient.

The male PCG, on the other hand, needed greater reassurance that he was providing good care than did the female PCG. In our society, the female has traditionally had the role of providing needed care to family members. Many of the services listed in Table 10-6, increased for female patients, may involve efforts to provide help to a male PCG who may have less experience in this role.

Many female PCGs who were spouses attempted to work a full-time job and provide care to the spouse the remaining 16 hours. This led to extreme fatigue and associated stress. Other female PCGs had never worked, did not drive, and

Table 10-6 Care Provided by Gender

	Average Number of Services per Patient	
Service	Male	Female
Discussing legal concerns	0.53	0.77
Providing spiritual support	0.34	0.78
Allowing expression of feelings	4.59	4.41
Counseling and advising	3.67	3.83
Reassuring family they are providing good care	0.62	0.84
Participating in discharge planning	0.04	0.22
Receiving communication from family to hospice staff that patient was being discharged	0.16	0.34
Informing of admission to health care facility	0.75	0.98
Assessing family's condition	1.37	1.24
Discussing family's plans after patient's death	0.71	0.49
Inquiring about health of a family member	1.04	0.45
Encouraging family members to take care of themselves	0.41	0.30
Providing respite care	1.22	0.57
Performing errands	0.37	0.20

were not skilled in decision making. The increase of interventions for male patients could be reflective of those two subpopulations. However, the data reflect differences in care primarily related to the more active female PCG. Hospice staff expressed more concern for the female PCG taking care of herself and inquired more frequently about her health than the male PCG. Respite care was also provided more often for female PCGs.

The working female PCG was more likely to be in the under 65 group and the dependent female PCG tended to be in the 65 and over group. Our society has been in the process of changing expectations for the female role. The older female developed the dependent lifestyle earlier in her life when this was an expected behavior. Although the role of PCG is stressful for the more active PCG, the death and subsequent lifestyle readjustments are likely to be more difficult for the more dependent female. In the first year of our study, the under 65 group and the 65 and over group were roughly equivalent. However, as the number of older patients increases we expect that females will function in more active roles, even in the older groups. Hospice managers can encourage consideration of differences in care needs based on sex and an interaction of sex and age when care is being planned. A clearer delineation of differences in care needs of the two sexes would enhance the quality of hospice care.

How Does Race Influence Services-Mix-Intensity?

Our sample contained 216 white patients, 37 black patients, and 7 Chicanos. In our study the number of black patients was proportional to the percent of black population in the community. However, the Chicano community was underrepresented. There has been some claim that hospice is a white, middle-class phenomenon that does not respond to the needs of other races. Need may be related to numbers admitted to the hospice or to the care provided after admission. Because of this expressed concern, differences in care by race were examined (see Table 10-7). Because of the small sample of Chicanos, data on only black and white subjects are presented. The data indicated decreased frequency of psychosocial services for black patient/family units. Providing physical care, obtaining community services, responding to financial concerns, and intervening with the health care system were the only items increased for blacks. These differences may be reflective of economic and cultural differences between the patient/family unit and the hospice staff. However, prejudice may have played a role in modifying the supply of services offered by the hospice staff.

In addition, the way the black community responds to a dying situation may be different from that of the white community. For example, the black community may be more willing to express feelings and deal with psychosocial issues within the family unit than with outsiders. The black family may have a stronger tendency to accept the present situation and deal with the present rather than plan for the future. Black patients may have had lower incomes, needing more

Table 10-7 Care Provided by Race

Service	Average Number of Services per Patient	
	White	Black
Assessing psychosocial situation	7.82	5.30
Teaching stages and management of dying symptoms	1.57	0.89
Discussing physical care management	6.28	3.76
Providing spiritual support	0.58	0.27
Allowing expression of feelings	4.86	2.41
Inquiring about health of family member	0.81	0.49
Encouraging family members to take care of themselves	0.42	0.11
Discussing psychosocial management	8.01	4.32
Discussing alternatives for care	2.29	1.14
Discussing feelings about impending death	1.80	0.89
Assessing family's condition	1.45	0.76
Discussing plans after death	0.69	0.27
Planning funeral	0.13	0.00
Providing physical care	7.55	9.14
Exploring financial concerns	0.90	1.05
Obtaining community service	0.70	1.08
Arranging admission to health facility	0.19	0.43

financial assistance and community services. It is possible that there is a differential demand for hospice services by black patient/family units, with the black patient/family unit desiring a different mix of services. Or black patient/family units may not be able to communicate demands to a white hospice staff. However, since these are speculations, and there are some obvious differences, we recommend that hospice managers examine not only admission patterns but differences in care related to race that may occur in their hospice.

Finding reasonable solutions to these concerns is complex. One obvious suggestion is to hire black hospice personnel. The hospice under study had one black home health aide. Other staff were white. However, if there is a differential demand for a different mix of hospice services, this solution may not alter the care. Another approach would be to seek the advice of representatives of the black community.

Hospice administrators must be sensitive to claims of discrimination if there is a problem in the program. It is important to ask whether similar differences in care occur in other hospices. Are differences due to problems of supply, demand, or an interaction between the two? Are they perceived by the patient/family unit as a problem? If the family is receiving the care they wish, is there a problem simply because the care is different? Should whites impose their behavioral expectations on the black family? In short, managers must clearly ascertain if there is a problem, what it is, and how it can be resolved.

Unlike blacks, the Chicano population was underrepresented in the study hospice. This may be due to differing cultural patterns related to management of the dying family member but it may also be due to an expectation of prejudicial treatment. As with the black community, dialogue with leaders in the Chicano community could provide information on why few Chicanos use hospice and what type of services are needed to draw these individuals. A simple marketing strategy, similar to the one described by Lamb in Chapter 2, which assesses the marketplace, would work well in this case.

How Does Socioeconomic Status Influence Services-Mix-Intensity?

Care was examined by five levels of socioeconomic status: upper, upper middle, middle, lower, and poverty. This categorization was based on an estimation by the nurse coordinator of reported income level, type of home, neighborhood, social behavior, and job or previous job history (see Table 10-8). There were 8 upper-class families, 71 upper-middle-class, 118 middle-class, 56 lower-class, and 11 poverty families.

There seemed to be little difference in the care provided to upper-middle-class, middle-class, and lower-class patients. The average number of services received by the poverty-level patient was lower in every category than those received by other patients. The one exception was in providing access to prescription drugs, which increased for poverty-level patients. Greater social distance was experienced between hospice personnel and those at the extremes of socioeconomic status than between hospice personnel and middle-income groups. This is demonstrated in the data by decreasing psychosocial interventions for both upper-class and poverty groups.

Differing social expectations related to these groups may be involved. For example, upper-income individuals are expected to be more private and independent than other groups. Hospice staff may be reluctant to touch them or to intrude psychologically into their personal space. Poverty-level patient/family units may expect and seek only minimal help from hospice staff and be unskilled in asking for needed help. They may not know what services are available or understand the effect of help on their situation. Their problems are often complex and may seem unsolvable, leading to feelings of helplessness (and avoidance) by hospice staff.

One would also expect differences in health beliefs and socially expected health behavior among groups that influence responses to services offered. Upper-class people may be more oriented to preventive health actions than the poverty-level person. This may be one of the factors involved in a differential demand for hospice care after admission. The difference we found in care may

Table 10-8 Care Provided, by Socioeconomic Status

Service	Average Number of Services per Patient				
	Upper	Upper Middle	Middle	Lower	Poverty
Assessing psychosocial situation	8.13	6.69	7.66	8.68	2.00
Assessing patient's condition	17.25	14.96	14.34	15.68	7.27
Teaching physical care	1.88	1.79	1.76	1.54	0.64
Teaching treatment technique	1.38	1.20	1.39	1.55	0.73
Teaching hospice pain management	1.75	0.93	1.18	1.07	0.73
Explaining hospice	1.13	1.04	1.07	0.96	0.55
Teaching stages and management of dying	2.88	1.66	1.34	1.41	0.36
Teaching procedure after home death	1.25	0.62	0.74	0.52	0.18
Discussing symptom management	5.00	5.89	6.09	6.27	0.73
Discussing pain management	8.25	5.58	6.13	7.32	1.45
Discussing diet management	2.75	3.10	3.31	3.13	0.73
Discussing physical care management	9.75	6.06	5.50	6.55	1.55
Providing physical care	8.88	8.89	7.11	8.55	2.36
Allowing expression of feelings	7.75	4.27	4.58	4.68	2.18
Counseling and advising	3.75	3.21	3.97	4.61	0.82
Discussing drug management	5.75	4.87	4.72	5.89	0.27
Obtaining needed equipment	1.38	2.76	3.14	3.16	0.73
Requesting help	8.63	5.00	4.19	6.18	1.45
Arranging time of visit	11.38	8.69	7.50	7.98	2.82
Informing of patient's condition	12.38	11.07	9.22	11.39	1.18
Discussing psychosocial management	11.75	8.03	5.95	9.73	2.00
Providing support	11.88	9.69	8.97	11.16	1.55
Discussing feelings about impending death	2.00	1.79	1.54	1.91	0.00
Assessing family's condition	1.38	1.27	1.26	1.73	0.09

be due to the low number of poverty individuals in comparison with other groups. However, managers and planners must be aware of the potential of a class-status differential in hospice care provision. This differential may exist throughout the traditional health care system and may be reflected in this micro look at hospice programming.

Provision of adequate care for the poverty-level patient requires careful assessment and planning. Managers should examine possible barriers to the provision of care with the poverty-level person. The difference in care is probably due to an interaction between willingness and ability of the hospice staff to provide care and willingness and ability of the poverty-level patient/family unit to request and accept it.

The hospice staff may need increased awareness and skills to adequately care for the poverty-level person. If so, the hospice manager would be responsible for providing the needed training. Recruitment of volunteers from diverse backgrounds who could comfortably respond to the needs of poverty-level persons may be beneficial. Developing ways to help the poverty-level patient/family unit accept needed care is also important.

The difference in care given to poverty-level people compared with other patient/family units is striking. It is vital that hospices examine the provision of care to the poor. If they find they are providing significantly less care to the poor than to other classes, it is imperative that managers: (1) explain reasons for these differences and (2) determine whether adjustments in the care plans should be made. The poor are less likely to be able to verbalize their needs and make their demand for services explicit than are higher socioeconomic groups. This places an increased responsibility on hospice staff to carefully assess the situation and develop means to provide quality care in complex situations. Providing adequate care to the poor may require increased investment of time, energy, and commitment on the part of hospice managers and staff.

How Does Family Coping Influence Services-Mix-Intensity?

We have found that family coping is closely related to place of death, and place of death is associated with a significant difference in minutes of care and numbers of care activities. Differences in care activities between families classified as coping and families classified as not coping were examined (see Table 10-9). In our sample, 184 families were classified as coping and 74 as not coping. The categorization was made by the nurse coordinator, who made a subjective, forced-choice decision placing each patient/family unit into one of the two categories.

Families considered to be ''coping'' were reassured more frequently that they were providing good care than those classified as not coping. There was an increase in social interaction between coping patient/family units and the hospice staff. However, the frequency of most interactions was equal to or lower than those provided to families categorized as not coping. When the family was not coping, services were increased. It appears that hospice staff recognized the coping difficulties early and invested increased amounts of time in psychosocial interventions to enhance the family's coping. Pain management and physical care management activities are increased in patient/family units classified as not coping. This suggests that the diminished coping could be related to patients

Table 10-9 Care Provided, by Coping

Service	Average Number of Services per Patient	
	Coping	*Not Coping*
Assessing psychosocial situation	6.94	8.97
Discussing pain management	5.80	7.16
Discussing physical care management	5.86	6.17
Allowing expression of feelings	4.07	5.84
Counseling and advising	3.57	4.47
Discussing drug management	4.50	8.05
Obtaining financial assistance or discussing situation	1.21	2.37
Requesting help	4.67	5.56
Discussing situation with other health professional(s)	5.67	8.32
Informing of patient's condition	9.65	11.19
Arranging admission to health facility	0.11	0.49
Discussing psychosocial management	6.90	8.85
Discussing alternatives for providing care	1.81	2.91
Providing support	9.17	11.37

who are experiencing greater amounts of pain and types of physical deterioration that families could not successfully manage.

Use of a coping/noncoping dichotomy can assist staff and administration in determining the level of potentially necessary services. It also provides a forum for discussing differences among patient care programs and may provide insights into the care needed by individual patients and their families.

How Does Place of Death Influence Services-Mix-Intensity?

Because of the seeming importance of place of death, differences in care occurring between those dying at home and those dying in an institution were explored (see Table 10-10). In our sample, 180 died at home and 86 died in an institution. In preparation for a home death, hospice staff invested greater time in teaching activities and establishing an effective supportive framework so that the patient/family unit could manage death at home in the most healthy way possible.

Patients who died in the hospital had an increased tendency to have been hospitalized previously during their hospice care relative to those who died at

Table 10-10 Care Provided, by Place of Death

Service	Average Number of Services per Patient	
	Home	Institution
Assessing patient's condition	13.94	15.69
Teaching physical care	1.84	1.30
Teaching treatment technique	1.47	1.08
Teaching stages and management of dying symptoms	1.76	0.79
Teaching procedure after home death	0.84	0.24
Rearranging environment	1.21	0.29
Discussing symptom management	6.33	4.62
Providing spiritual support	0.32	1.05
Allowing expression of feelings	4.07	5.41
Visiting at time of death	1.07	0.12
Discussing drug management	5.67	3.05
Reassuring family that they are providing good care	0.88	0.38
Participating in discharge planning	0.08	0.22
Informing that patient is going home	0.17	0.42
Obtaining community service	0.88	0.43
Discussing situation with other health professional(s)	5.72	7.55
Informing of admission to institution	0.40	1.84
Arranging admission to health facility	0.03	0.60
Conveying physician comments to patient	1.59	2.21
Discussing psychosocial management	6.70	8.51
Discussing alternatives for providing care	1.68	2.88
Providing respite care	1.14	0.42
Providing support	8.97	10.78
Discussing expected physical changes	2.03	1.09
Discussing feelings about impending death	1.73	1.41
Providing access to prescription drugs	1.37	0.94
Assessing family's condition	1.51	0.88
Discussing plans after death	0.73	0.34

home. This tendency to increased hospitalization was reflected in services such as discharge planning, informing of admission and discharge from the hospital, and efforts of hospice staff to facilitate hospital admission.

When patients died in the hospital, care seemed to focus on interactions with other health care professionals and the PCG. There seemed to be fewer direct hospice interactions with these patients than occurred with those who died at home. Furthermore, patients who died in a hospital received less teaching and actual patient care and increased discussion of alternatives for providing care than those who died at home. This indicates interactive decision making between hospice staff and patient/family units regarding hospitalization of the patient.

Services provided reflect less emotional involvement of hospice personnel with the patient/family unit when the patient died in an institution. Did the patient/family unit choose to be less involved or did hospice staff react to these patient/family units differently? Did the difference in care lead to an increased probability of hospital death or did different patient/family choices or a different physical illness situation lead to differences in care? Why do staff avoid involvement with these families? Could it be that hospital deaths are viewed as a personal failure? Does involvement with some subgroup of patient/family units place the hospice staff at greater emotional risk in some way?

Although the cost of providing hospice care alone is greater for the patient who dies at home, the total cost of care (hospital and hospice) is greater for the patient who dies in the hospital. It is important to identify strategies that facilitate successful home deaths. It is also important to understand how staff respond to institutionalized patients, and whether their involvement discourages the increased use of home care strategies. Managers should consider education for hospice staff as well as early efforts at problem resolution for patient/family units experiencing difficulties.

How Does Medical Diagnosis Influence Services-Mix-Intensity?

We examined each care activity in relation to the patient's medical diagnosis to allow comparisons of care. Our sample consisted of 51 lung cancer patients, 9 with head and neck cancer, 37 with urinary tract cancer, 38 with cancer of the breast, ovary, or uterus, 6 with brain tumors, 20 with soft tissue malignancies, 77 with cancer of the gastrointestinal system, and 4 other types of cancer.

The highest incidence of assessment of psychosocial situation occurs in patients with head and neck cancer. There is a high incidence of teaching treatment technique to patients with urinary tract cancer. Discussing pain management occurs most frequently in patients with head and neck cancer. Patients with urinary tract cancer and breast, ovary, and uterine cancer seem to require the greatest amount of physical care provision by hospice staff. Discussion of psychosocial management occurs most frequently in patients with head and neck cancers and brain tumors. Patients with head and neck cancer had the highest average number of activities for 15 of the services, followed by patients with cancer of the urinary tract who had a high average number of activities in 13 services. Patients with these two types of cancer required the greatest intensity of care. Hospice administrators should review admission diagnoses and consider the potential impacts on staff time. Understanding differential patient needs is useful management information and assists in planning for service availability.

Examining Services-Mix-Intensity-Order
What Is the Order of Care by Week in Relation to Services-Mix-Intensity?

Examining order of care by week provides increased understanding of the care process and aids hospice managers in planning for staffing needs. Presently, we have little understanding (other than intuitive) of changes in services provided after the patient is admitted and moves toward death. With this knowledge, managers can efficiently determine the type of care needed and compare it with the care actually given. In addition, managers can anticipate the level of intensity for patient care and use this information to balance hospice staff patient care loads.

Using the subset of patients who lived at least 28 days, we examined the frequency and average number of each service by week. Since some patients in the subset lived only four weeks and others lived several months, we divided the care by week into the first three weeks and the last four weeks. Services that occurred with greatest frequency the week of admission included performing the admission assessment and evaluation, teaching physical care, teaching treatment technique, teaching hospice strategy toward pain management, explaining hospice, and discussing spiritual needs. The first week's activities seem to revolve around teaching activities and efforts to establish a situation conducive to home care.

Those services occurring most frequently the week of death included assessment of the patient's condition and psychosocial situation, teaching of the stages and management of dying symptoms, teaching the family how to manage the situation after a home death, inquiring about the health of family members, reassuring the family they are providing good care, encouraging the family to take care of themselves, rearranging the care environment, providing physical care, allowing expression of feelings, visiting at time of death, informing of patient's condition, providing support, discussing expected physical changes and feelings about impending death, assessing the family's condition, discussing plans after death, and planning the funeral. These activities indicate an increase in not only the intensity of physical care but also in bereavement activities. This result appears consistent with findings of others regarding service to patients during the final days. Managers can use this information to better plan hospice staffing needs

How Does Duration Influence Services-Mix-Intensity-Order?

In our sample, 40 patients died within seven days after admission, 28 patients had a duration of 8-14 days, 55 had a duration of 15-28 days, and 141 patients lived longer than 28 days. We were interested in those services provided with greatest frequency to the patient/family who died within seven days of admission. We suspected that care would be more intense and thus more costly in relation to length. Further, we were concerned that staff would not have time to address increased patient care demands. In the last week of a patient's life, services to family members increased. Services showing the greatest frequency of occurrence included assessing the patient's condition, discussing pain management, providing physical care, counseling and advising, discussing the situation with other health professionals, informing of the patient's condition, discussing psychosocial management, and providing support. Because of the urgency of care, hospice staff seemed to focus on immediate needs. Staff had less time to perform teaching activities and to address psychosocial concerns when patients lived less than seven days after admission compared with those living longer than seven days. It is usually too late to interact at an emotional level with the patient. Further, staff had little, if any, time to deal in depth with family dynamics and psychological issues.

Services that showed the greatest increase when the patient lived longer than 29 days included assessing the psychosocial situation, assessing the patient's condition, discussing symptom management, discussing pain management, discussing diet management, discussing physical care management, providing physical care, allowing expression of feelings, informing of the patient's condition, evaluating the effectiveness of management, discussing psychosocial management, providing support, discussing expected physical changes and discussing feelings about impending death. With longer-term patient/family units, hospice staff were more likely to focus on changes in symptoms such as pain, eating patterns, and physical care need than with shorter-term patients. Much more time was spent interacting with the patient, discussing feelings, facilitating preparation for death, dealing with family dynamics and communication patterns, and providing support and encouragement to patient and family.

Examining Services-Mix-Intensity-Order-Rhythm

We have compared the incidence of services in patients with the three most frequently occurring cancers: lung, gastrointestinal tract, and breast-ovary-cervix, across 28 days of care (using the suɒset of patients who lived at least 28 days). Our data show differences in rhythm of specific care activities. Teaching activities occurred most frequently at the beginning of hospice care. Psychosocial interventions were maintained at a relatively steady pace across the first three weeks and then intensified the week of death. Physical care activities gradually increased across the period of hospice care and were greatest the week of death. Figure 10-2 illustrates the rhythm of care for providing physical care. Figure 10-3 illustrates the rhythm of care for discussing pain management. Figure 10-4 illustrates the rhythm of care for providing support.

Changes in the frequency and average number of services per patient identify important information about the patterns of hospice care. When a hospice opens, the staff are usually inexperienced in the process of hospice care. Across time, a learning curve occurs, and care is modified. Staff identify problem areas and shift interventions to achieve greater effectiveness. Types of staff available to provide care change. The ratio of patient/family unit to hospice staff may also change. Most services have increased strikingly over time. This indicates an increase in intensity of care as the hospice develops. Because of this, cost estimates based on the first year of care will be very low.

We have examined changes in pattern of care across the three years of the study in relation to week of care and age. Intensity of care was lowest for all patients the year the hospice opened. The second year, average minutes of care increased greatly. The third year, this trend had moderated but remained above

Figure 10-2 Rhythm of Care for Providing Physical Care

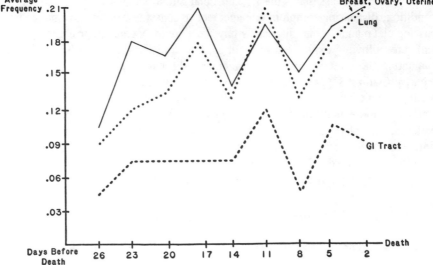

Figure 10-3 Rhythm of Care for Discussing Pain Management

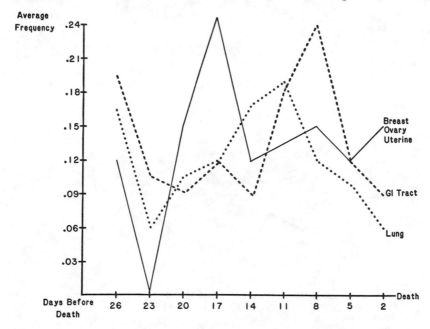

the first year. There was a decrease in intensity of care (as measured in average minutes of care) in patients under 65 whose duration of hospice care was at least 28 days (see Figure 10-5). In this same set, patients who were 65 and over had an increase in intensity of care from the first year (see Figure 10-6). In the first year of hospice care, patients 65 and older received fewer minutes of care each week than younger patients. In the second and third years, minutes of care for older patients increased in intensity considerably beyond the younger set.

Increased intensity of services as the hospice develops was mentioned by Lamb in Chapter 2 and is an important administrative issue. Administrators need to be aware of the increased and rapidly escalating program growth during the first three years. According to Lamb, the curve can be expected to stabilize after the program has been in operation for a period of time.

SUMMARY OF STUDY

We have begun developing a picture of the process of hospice care as it changes over time. Care activities occurring with greatest frequency in specific types of hospice patients are detailed and provide a basis for more clearly un-

Figure 10-4 Rhythm of Care for Providing Support

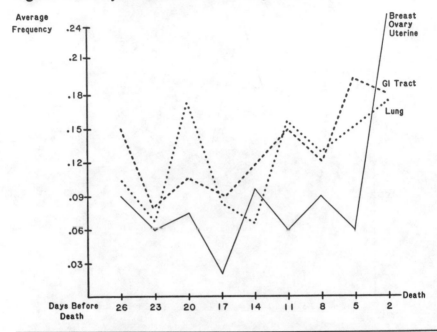

derstanding patterns of care. These patterns can be used to measure a program's performance and facilitate future service planning.

In our study, *there were differences in care provided to the elderly, the black, and the poverty-level patient/family unit.* It is essential that these differences be examined carefully in hospices across the country. The bias may be due, in part, to a lack of knowledge of how to effectively deal with the more complex care situations involved or it may simply be a reflection of larger cultural prejudices. Changes in care patterns do occur as hospice staff learn to manage new situations. For example, the patients over 65 had the lowest level of care the year the hospice opened. By the second year, their care had increased considerably. By the third year, care had moderated to what is probably a more reasonable level. This same pattern may occur in care of blacks and those in poverty.

Our work raises many questions. Like other researchers, we hope these questions will stimulate further investigations. However, some of the answers may be readily obtainable through introspective examination and evaluation by hospice staff. Becoming aware of potential differences in care can lead to modifications. Effective problem resolution can be accomplished through creative strategies to manage complex situations.

At the present time, hospice managers have little specific information, other than verbal explanation by staff, of what is or should be occurring during hospice

Figure 10-5 Average Minutes of Care by Week for Patients Under Age 65

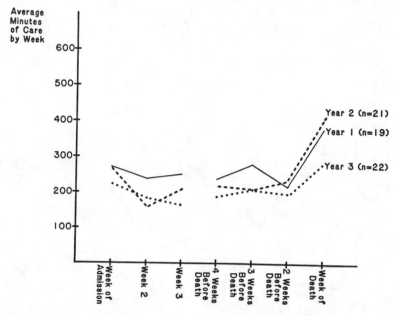

care. Administrative judgments are based on peripheral information such as numbers of visits, length of life, and patient/family satisfaction with care. Standards of care must be developed to evaluate the care that is occurring. This study provides useful insights for administrators developing new hospices or providing staff learning experiences. The awareness of care patterning can improve the quality of patient care and allow management to make better judgments about how staff time can be most effectively utilized.

The process of accreditation is an important issue in hospice circles. These standards attempt to encourage high-quality care without inhibiting the growing process that must occur in the development of hospice care. However, the present JCAH standards are fairly restrictive. Research such as ours provides a valuable tool for assessing existing certification standards, including Medicare. Moreover, it provides hospice decision makers and advocates with valuable, documented insights from which to assess state and national policies.

Decisions related to reimbursement of hospice care by the federal government and private insurers will continue to be made by policy planners for the next few years. Sound policy decisions are made from a firm data base. Hospice investigations provide new knowledge to the field and insights for policy makers and managers.

Figure 10-6 Average Minutes of Care by Week for Patients Age 65 or Over

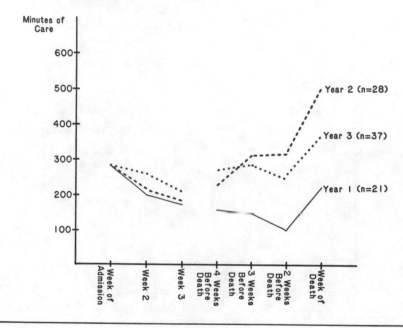

SUGGESTIONS FOR FUTURE RESEARCH

Because of the critical need for more understanding of the process and outcomes of hospice care, it is imperative that those participating in the provision of hospice care become involved in the study of hospice. Insights acquired from practical hospice work need to be utilized in the development of further investigations. Policymakers also participate in the provision of hospice care. Their unique perspective is invaluable as a base for the design of studies that will influence future decisions about hospice care.

Many of those involved in the practice of hospice care are inexperienced in research techniques. These practitioners may feel that the studies are best left to those more experienced. But the insights of the hospice practitioner are critical to the design of meaningful research. Ideally, hospice investigators should involve practitioners, scientists, and policymakers. The practitioner may be the one to initiate a study, because of more immediate concerns related to hospice care. Establishing a research partnership with an experienced researcher can help hospice managers to avoid many pitfalls. One good source of skilled researchers is a nearby university. Faculty should be sought from disciplines that would be interested in the area to be studied. Faculty who are actively involved in research will tend to be more interested and have the experience and knowledge needed to conduct a clinical study. Relationships with local decision makers may lead to funding assistance and provide a base for broad research support.

Research requires a great deal of planning. It is not unreasonable to invest a year in planning before initiating data collection. Planning involves examining previous related research, identifying variables, selecting an appropriate design, searching for effective ways to measure the variables to be studied, determining how and where data can be collected, and, often, going through the procedure to get approval to conduct the study. Sufficient time must be allotted for this process. The success and significance of the study depend on it.

One of the most important sources of data in hospice research is the patient's chart. Hospice managers have a distinct advantage over scientists in this case, because the manager has the power to determine what data will be included in hospice records. Thus, an important first step is to examine hospice forms and consider modifications that can be made to allow for recording of pertinent information. Consideration must be given to the time required by staff to complete the form. Also, if staff do not consider the data important, that section of the form will be left blank. Therefore, it is important to involve staff in planning research-related activities requiring their cooperation.

Staff will consider data important only if it influences decisions related to patient care. They must be helped to realize that data collected for research can have an impact on patient care. Staff in the hospice we have been studying had difficulty understanding the need to determine the age of the PCG. Therefore this information was often left blank and we had inadequate data for that analysis. More recently, we have met with staff to discuss the significance of these data. We pointed out our concern for problems that might be encountered by the older PCG, which could indicate a need for additional hospice services. If we found in our analysis that this was occurring, the hospice could modify care to meet these unique needs. The information is now being provided more frequently.

As noted in Chapter 3, the process of data collection can be frustrating and tedious. When hand-written notes are being used for data, as in our study, care must be taken to ensure that each person collecting data is as consistent as possible in interpreting the meaning within the notes. If questionnaires or scales are employed, they must be administered to each person in as consistent a way as possible. And yet, there is nothing consistent about clinical practice. Even when great care has been taken to ensure consistency, the unexpected will inevitably occur. It is best to view these events philosophically to decide how to best handle the situation that exists, and continue the study. It is important to report these events because they do influence how the findings are interpreted, but any clinical researcher worth his or her salt has had similar experiences.

Many of the studies currently being reported regarding hospice care are case studies. Such studies provide detailed information that is sorely needed. However, what is even more badly needed at this point is research that combines information from several hospices across the country. This can lead to larger samples and greater generalizability. Policymakers need studies that have been repeated five or six times in various parts of the country. In this way, a single researcher, in coordination with a number of hospices, could plan and implement a well-designed study that could have significant impact on the future of hospices. Hospice personnel could contribute by pooling information from patient records and by assisting in the data collection process. Studies need to be designed that can more effectively measure differences in care among hospices and other types of care for the dying. Although these studies will be more costly than the typical descriptive study, they are crucial.

A serious problem in hospice research relates to communicating research findings. Many who have done small studies feel that their study is not "important enough" to report. If so, then it was not important enough to conduct. There is a "rule" in academia that a study is not complete until the results have been published. It is the only effective way we have of sharing our new knowledge with others. The reluctance to report findings is due to two main concerns. One is the risk of revealing one's work to others. We tend to fear the criticism we may receive. We are all afraid of not being "good enough." It is much safer to keep the information to oneself. But then it is of little use.

The other concern is related to writing skills. In the first place, we do not feel we write well enough to get something published. In the second place, we tend to fall in love with whatever we write and think it is the most wonderful thing ever written. Then we are afraid to submit it, because someone might criticize it. Again we are taking a risk by revealing something about ourselves. Editors almost always send papers back with suggested revisions. A majority of writers never return the revised paper, assuming and fearing rejection. Resubmitting a paper is the best way to begin to improve writing skills. However, before a paper is submitted, it is very helpful to seek out someone who is skilled in writing to give feedback. It has been said repeatedly that the good writer is not one who can write well but one who is skilled in rewriting.

We have much work left to develop a clear picture of hospice care and to document how hospice differs from other forms of care. This is no small effort and must involve use of time, energy, and money from many within the hospice arena. As a consequence of our joint endeavors, however, we may serve as a hallmark to those studying other facets of health care.

NOTES

1. D. S. Greer et al., *National Hospice Study Preliminary Final Report Extended Executive Summary*. National Hospice Evaluation Study, Health Care Financing Administration (Grant #99-P-97793/1-0), Robert Wood Johnson Foundation, and John A. Hartford Foundation. Brown University,

1983; R. L. Kane et al., "A Randomised Controlled Trial of Hospice Care," *The Lancet* 1 (1983): 890-894.

2. C. Gotay, "Models of terminal care: a review of the research literature." *Clinical & Investigative Medicine*, 6(3) (1983): 131-141.

3. M. Grossman. *The Demand for Health: A Theoretical and Empirical Investigation* (New York: Columbia University Press, 1972); H. Yura and M. B. Walsh. *The Nursing Process: Assessing, Planning, Implementing, Evaluating* (New York: Appleton-Century-Crofts, 1978).

Chapter 11

Hospice Care: Some Insights on Nature, Demand, and Cost

Kim Carney and Nancy Burns

Hospices in America have developed at a rapid pace. Although this pace reflects a responsiveness to widespread concern about care for the dying, it also means hospices are in early stages of development. Because of this newness, there has been limited time for research on numerous issues pertaining to hospice care. In addition, a scant eight years after the opening of the first American hospice, legislation was passed making hospice care a reimbursable service under Medicare. Although the financial resources resulting from the legislation were welcomed, there was a concern that making hospice care a reimbursable service would, in some manner, change the nature of hospice care. Reflecting both of these, i.e., the early stage of hospice development and the possible impact of reimbursement on the nature of hospice care, the legislation includes a sunset provision. Under this provision reimbursement is adopted only temporarily. Congress will be required to assess the impact of reimbursement before extending the legislation.

This chapter provides an economic and nursing framework from which hospice policymakers and planners can analyze hospice care. In addition, findings from a three-year case study of a hospice supplement the analytic framework. With the analytic framework and the empirical data, we examine (1) the nature of hospice care, (2) some determinants of demand for hospice care, and (3) factors influencing the cost of hospice care.

ANALYSIS

Cost Concepts

Cost is frequently discussed with respect to hospice care. Because cost of care is related to other concepts, namely price and expenditure, it is useful to define these items individually. In economic terminology, the *price of a good or service is the amount paid by the consumer or purchaser.* Price is determined by the interaction of demand (representing the behavior of the consumer) and supply (representing the behavior of the producer or supplier). *Cost, on the other hand, refers to the cost of producing the good or service.* The supply curve embodies cost information.

In common usage, the distinction between price and cost is rarely maintained. After all, the price of bread is perceived as a cost by the purchaser. Nevertheless, the distinction is important and will be maintained throughout the chapter. The economic concept of cost differs from the accounting concept in that the former includes "opportunity costs." *Opportunity costs are those costs necessary to keep the producer in business in addition to the normal costs of production.* In a competitive model, price and economic cost approach one another. When equilibrium occurs, the two are equal.

In contrast to price and cost, both of which refer to the individual unit of good or service, expenditure reflects both price and quantity. Total expenditure is the total spent for a particular good or service and is, therefore, the sum of all the prices involved. Expenditures can, as a result, rise when either prices or quantities or both increase.

A consideration of cost, price, and expenditure of hospice care is complex because hospice care, like other forms of health care, differs from most goods and services subject to economic analysis, for example, a bushel of wheat or a haircut. In contrast to these items, hospice care is (1) comprised of a collection of services and (2) delivered over a period of time.

In policy discussions on the cost of health care, two problems emerge. First, prices in the health sector have risen considerably more rapidly than other prices in the economy. Second, the total quantity consumed has expanded more than expected based on factors such as prices, income, and population. Total expenditures for health services, in other words, have risen. As noted in Chapter 1, the share of Gross National Product comprised of health services has significantly increased. Thus, discussions of new health services, or more particularly, financing of new health services, is appropriately concerned with both price and expenditure.

The debate about hospice reimbursement under Medicare was largely focused on the broad issue of the cost of care for dying patients. Supporters of the legislation were committed to the notion that hospice care would be less costly than traditional care. As a result, there is no attempt in the legislation to limit the number of patients seeking hospice care. The legislation is, however, concerned with limiting the total amount spent per hospice patient.

Just as the interaction between demand and supply determines price, that interaction also determines the quantity consumed. Thus, any discussion of either price or expenditure must also consider demand and supply. And, since demand and supply always relate to a particular good or service, it is necessary to explore the complex good in question, i.e., hospice care.

The Law of Demand

Demand is a basic economic concept referring to the quantity of a good or service consumers are willing to purchase. While a variety of factors determine demand, the "law of demand" refers to the inverse relationship between the price of the good and quantity demanded when all other variables are held constant. According to this law, the higher the price of the good, the smaller the amount that will be demanded. The other variables that must be considered are the income of the consumer, the size of the population, the "taste" for the good in question, and the price of goods and services that are either substitutes or complements for the good in question.

Since demand defines quantities of a good or service consumers are willing to purchase at various prices, it is an important concept for planners and managers to understand. *Demand differs from need, a concept generally defined by providers*. (See Lamb's treatment of need in Chapter 2.) Need generally implies a situation where some benefit is expected as a result of an intervention. Demand specifies the price the consumer is willing to pay for a perceived or expected benefit. Need is usually larger than demand.

Demand in the Health Sector

Early attempts to examine demand for health services faced two difficulties. One related to the difficulty of defining services. For example, the demand for hospital services is usually defined in terms of days of hospital care, regardless of the intensity of care provided. The second difficulty concerns the price of services. The relevant price for demand analysis is the price paid by the consumer; in the health sector it is the amount paid out of pocket by the patient. The existence of third-party payers drastically reduces out-of-pocket payments; the actual out-of-pocket cost may be known to the consumer only after the service has been provided. Researchers may be unable to determine the out-of-pocket price.

Initially, policymakers suspected that economic demand analysis was inappropriate for the health sector on the grounds that demand did not respond to price changes. Demand was assumed to be unresponsive, or in the economist's terminology, "inelastic," to changes in price. Demand would not change when price changed. However, it became apparent, as third-party coverage increased, that demand was surprisingly elastic, or responsive to changes in price. Demand changed when price changed.

A recent development in economic theory proposes that consumers' demand for health sector goods and services is indirect. For example, families produce a commodity that is unavailable in the market, such as recreation. To produce recreation, the family combines time with various market goods and services such as skis, other ski equipment, an airline ticket, and lodging accommodations.

Grossman has adapted this approach to the health sector.[1] He suggests that the family produces health using time and medical and nonmedical inputs. He proposes that the family desires health for investment reasons (to protect an income stream) and for consumption reasons (to enjoy feeling well). The educational level of the family, particularly that of the wife and mother, influences family efficiency in the production process.

The Grossman approach, thus, begins with a production function—a mathematical statement defining the relationship between the inputs, which are also the independent variables—time, medical goods and services, and nonmedical inputs—and the output or dependent variable—health. From this function a demand function for medical services generally, or for a particular medical service, is derived. The dependent variable of the demand function is the quantity of services. The explanatory variables include the prices of relevant medical and nonmedical goods and services, family income, the time cost of obtaining the various inputs, and the educational level of the family

Demand for Hospice Care

Grossman's model has been extended to hospice care.[2] For patients, hospice care is strictly a consumption good. Hospice enrollment indicates that the patient is no longer seeking to protect an income stream. However, family members may perceive hospice care as an investment good since it is known that family members are at a higher risk of illness than usual during and following the terminal illness of a family member. Unique to hospice care is the high time cost, not only for the patient, but for the person serving as primary caregiver (PCG). Presumably, the lower the income-earning capacity of the potential PCG, the greater the willingness to assume the role. However, in somewhat of a contradiction to this, it seems that the ability to fulfill the demanding role of the PCG rises with education. Thus, the higher the educational level of this individual, the greater the possibility of being an effective PCG.

Defining demand for hospice care is complex. There are three components to demand: (1) the decision to seek hospice care in contrast to care in the traditional setting, (2) the decision concerning the illness stage at which hospice care is sought, and (3) following the decision to enter a hospice, decisions concerning which hospice services to seek. Although the demand for hospice care is a demand for a combination of services, that combination is not firmly defined. The determination of the services is carried out by the patient/family (demand for services) and the hospice staff (supply of services). A phone call from PCG to the hospice reflects a demand for services; and that phone call may result in a (previously unplanned) visit to the patient or family.

We suspect that the responsiveness to price changes, or the elasticity of demand, varies with the three elements of demand we identified. The decision whether to enter a hospice may not be highly elastic. The patient and/or family may have a strong philosophic preference for hospice care over traditional care, for example. However, the decision about when, in the stage of a patient's illness, to enroll is probably more elastic. The family may have a concern that admission be postponed until it is reasonably certain that third-party benefits will not be exhausted prior to the patient's death. And the third element, the demand for services once hospice enrollment has occurred, may be very elastic. *All three elements of demand—whether to enter a hospice, when to enter, and how many services to seek—influence the quantity of hospice services provided.* And the quantity provided is a crucial factor in determining total expenditures for hospice care.

In demand theory the price paid by a consumer for a good or service is usually the most important determinant of the amount of the good or service consumed. Determining the role of price in the demand for health services is difficult because of the importance of third-party payers. Third-party coverage has typically paid a larger proportion of the cost of hospitalization than of outpatient care.

Prior to Medicare coverage for hospice care, reimbursement for hospice care, most of which was outpatient care, was lower than reimbursement for care in the traditional setting. Thus, although the cost of hospital care is perceived to be considerably higher than the cost of hospice care, patients may have paid more out of pocket for hospice care than hospital care because of limited third-party coverage. However, it has been the policy of many hospices to provide care at little or no payment by the patient and family. In such cases, the difference between the price charged either to third parties or patients has been met by philanthropy. Philanthropy is a type of third-party payer, although considerably less important today for the health sector than the major third-party payers: private insurance and government. Philanthropy is also considerably less important for other portions of the health sector than for hospices. Philanthropy entails either monetary contributions or volunteer services.

Supply of Hospice Care and Determination of Prices

The typical economic supply curve is one in which the quantity supplied is directly related to price. The higher the price of the good, the larger the quantity that suppliers are willing to supply. The supply curve is derived from the production function and the cost function. These are discussed more fully later. Now we will note that the cost function is normally U-shaped. This implies that in the short run when at least one input, such as the physical plant, is of a fixed size, there is an optimum level of output associated with the existing plant size. If either more or less than the optimum is produced, unit costs rise.

Other factors in addition to price affect the supply curve or are determinants of supply. For example, changes in technology are likely to affect supply, as are external factors such as weather and work stoppages.

It is useful to examine the demand and supply concepts graphically in order to see how the two interact to determine price and quantity. Since the variables employed in graphing are price and quantity, the assumption is implicit that all other variables are held constant. It is also understood that a particular period of time, perhaps a given year, is being examined. It is possible to consider various market sizes. For example, we can explore supply and demand for hospice care in a particular community or we can consider aggregate supply and demand for hospice care in the entire country. The good or service being considered must be well defined. For example, the results will be very different when we consider supply and demand for the following: food, meat, tenderloin steak. Thus, if we want to consider supply and demand for hospice care it is necessary to specify clearly what is being examined.

Some possible relationships between supply and demand are shown in Figure 11-1. For example, in Figure 11-1A supply and demand curves are brought together. The equilibrium price (that price which market forces will tend to produce) is p(e), and the equilibrium quantity will be q(e).

A change in taste might cause the demand curve to shift out. In the case of hospice care, the shift might reflect the growing interest in and awareness of hospice care on the part of the public. If the demand curve shifted from D(1) to D(2) as shown in Figure 11-1B, and no change in supply occurred, the price would then rise from p(e) to p(e)' and the quantity would increase from q(e) to q(e)'.

If, however, supply also responded, as has surely been the case with regard to the supply of hospice care, the price might increase, decrease, or remain the same. One of these outcomes, namely unchanged price, is shown in Figure 11-1C.

It is also possible that a supply curve might be horizontal, as shown in Figure 11-1D. In this case suppliers are willling to supply any amount at a given price, indicated by the curve. In this situation increases in demand will not induce increases in price.

Hospice Care as a Product

Defining and measuring hospice care, a seemingly simple task, has been difficult. The first reason is that the nature of hospice care is complex. The second reason for the difficulty is the differences in the orientation of the two disciplines, economics and nursing. Both disciplines can provide important insights from which to expand our understanding of the nature of care.

Figure 11-1 Price and Quantity Determination by Supply and Demand, Selected Situations

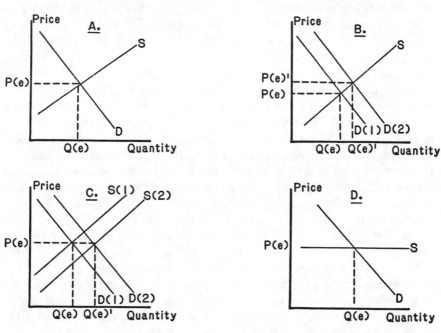

As a starting point, hospice care is defined as a collection of services, which may differ considerably among patients and over time. There are a number of services from which to select. Differing quantities of the services may be used as well as different proportions among them. Since services are provided over time, they can be ordered in different ways. Further, the rhythm or tempo in which services are provided may vary greatly from those provided at regular intervals to those clustered irregularly. Thus, in order to examine hospice care, it is necessary to consider the following five elements:

1. Services
2. Mix or proportion of services
3. Intensity of services
4. Order of services
5. Rhythm of services

The term "pattern of services" is used to refer to all five of these individual elements.

A Nursing Perspective

From a nursing perspective, care is an abstract holistic process that cannot be completely captured in quantitative, measurable terms. The nursing process is the application of nursing knowledge through analytical reasoning to achieve the goal of health. According to Yura and Walsh,[3] during actual nursing practice, the nursing process is indivisible. However, for purposes of analysis, they have identified four phases: assessing, planning, implementing, and evaluating.

In nursing, care is seen as an interactive process between the nurse and the patient/family unit. Therefore, characteristics of both the patient/family unit and the nurse would influence the nature of care. Thus, variables such as family skill in the production of health, coping abilities, income, and education influence the nature of care. In addition, care is also influenced by the characteristics of the nurse, including nursing philosophy, education, motivation, experience, and institutional support (psychological and financial). In this sense, nature of care depends on the willingness and ability of the patient/family to receive care, on the nurse to provide care, and on both to plan jointly, coordinate, and implement care activities. Diminished willingness or ability on the part of any of these individuals will negatively affect the elements of hospital care.

Because nursing care is oriented to the production of health and medical care to the curing of illness, hospice care generally functions within a nursing model. Two ways in which the nursing approach is evident are the emphasis on the family unit and the importance of the interactive process.

An Economical Perspective

Hospice care, from an economic perspective, is an output. Therefore, a logical starting point for discussing the nature of care is the production function. Typically, an economic production function defines the relationship between inputs in terms of the production process, such as capital (physical equipment) and labor. The function shows the level of output for a given level of inputs and the varying proportions in which inputs may be combined. Interest in the production process is predicated on the assumption that there is some degree of substitutability of one input for another or that the mix of inputs may vary. The production function presupposes technical efficiency, i.e., the function defines the maximum level of output achievable for each combination of inputs. The choice between an optimal and suboptimal level of output for each combination of inputs is understood to be a technological question and is of little interest to economists. Economists are concerned with the choice of input combination from among the set of all combinations producing a given level of output. It is assumed that the least costly combination will be chosen. This decision may be described in either of two ways, i.e., maximizing output for a given expenditure or budget constraint or minimizing costs for a given output level. In general terms, the problem is maximization given a constraint.

The production function approach may be readily extended to hospice care in either of two ways. The first is to define output as an individual hospice service. In this instance, there is a production function for each hospice service. As before, the factors of production, labor, and capital are the inputs. Labor may, of course, be further broken down according to the provider of care, such as the RN, LVN, MSW, etc. In the case of a hospice providing only home care, it might be appropriate to eliminate the capital and only consider labor inputs.

The second approach is to examine the production of hospice care with a production function when output is defined in terms of patient and family care and inputs are the individual hospice services. To use this approach, managers must define the amount of care needed for an individual patient and family. If that definition is fully specified by both amount of care and the provider of care, the production function approach has little interest. But if the definition is more general, perhaps specified in terms of the number of contacts per week or the length of time to be spent, then the production function analysis is of interest to administrators and to policymakers. Alternatively, it would be possible to start from a budgeted amount allotted per family and determine, using the production function, what combination of services in what amounts could be provided with the allotment.

It may be the case that the hospice production function differs considerably among hospice programs. This suggests that the technologically efficient production function for hospice care is still in the developmental stage. If restrictions are placed on the process of producing hospice care, such restrictions will serve to constrain the production function. For example, the function will be modified or constrained if standards require that certain types of services are rendered only by particular provider groups such as RNs.

The two proposed production function approaches are of interest to managers since they focus on cost. In the first approach, the effort is to minimize the cost of producing an individual hospice service. In the second approach, the emphasis is on combining services economically. For either to be useful there must be some flexibility in the provision of services available to the hospice manager.

The production function itself must define both the type and number of appropriate services. Technological efficiency is also assumed. The proportions of inputs are then determined using the production function and information about relative costs. Now that our model has been discussed, let's look at a practical application.

APPLYING AN ECONOMIC ANALYSIS

The scene of the investigation is an urban hospice affiliated with a hospital but without assigned inpatient beds. The results are based on data from the first three years of the study, which were also the first three years in the life of the hospice. Information was obtained from existing records. The data base is an unusually rich one and cooperation from hospice staff has been extensive.

The sample studied consists of patients who died in hospice care. During the years under examination 266 patients died in hospice care. Two types of data were generated on each of these patients. The first consisted of demographic data, facts about the illness, hospice admission, etc. Dating of events such as admission on the hospice and day of death was handled by numbering days consecutively throughout the years from 1 to 1,095. Thus, a file might show that a patient was admitted on day 37 and died on day 72, indicating a period of hospice enrollment, referred to as duration, of 35 days.

The second type of data pertained to patient encounters and services provided. Encounter is defined as any contact, by phone or face-to-face, between a member of the hospice staff or a hospice volunteer with the patient, family, or another person for the purposes of consulting about the case. Consultation of this sort was most frequently with physicians; however, there were also consultations with pastors, social workers from outside agencies, and others. Because the number of encounters varied depending on the intensity of care and how long the patient survived after hospice enrollment, there was great variation among patients on the size of their individual encounter file. From the individual's file information regarding the encounter data, length in minutes, site, persons involved, etc., was obtained. Information on phone calls was included in the file along with home visits. In addition, the hospice providers (professionals as well as volunteers) recorded what transpired during each encounter. We created a tool for the classification and collection of this information, which is described more fully in Chapter 10.

Demand, Supply, and Nature of Care

Care actually delivered by a hospice reflects the interaction of supply and demand. A study of a single hospice cannot separate these effects. With regard to demand it has been noted that there are three elements: whether to enter hospice, when to enter a hospice, and what services to seek. A study of a single hospice tells little about the decision whether to enter a hospice. However, the timing of hospice entry and the seeking of services can be explored and is discussed below. The research data presented include comments of interest to hospice planners and decision makers.

We designate the hospice as SW since it is located in the Southwestern region of the United States. The racial composition of the 266 patients who died during the study period was: 82 percent white, 14 percent black, 3 percent Chicano, and 1 percent other. Although SW is affiliated with a Catholic hospital, the hospice enrollees are overwhelmingly (84 percent) Protestant. Seventy percent of hospice enrollees were married at the time of enrollment. The average age of patients at the time of admission was 64.7. For the most part, hospice enrollees appeared to match the population with terminal cancer and the composition of the community. Two exceptions may be noticed: (1) the hospice enrollees are slightly younger than the population with terminal cancer and (2) the Chicano population is underrepresented. There is great similarity among hospice patients across hospices.

When to Enroll in Hospice

The duration of hospice enrollment, that is, the number of days between hospice enrollment and death, varies greatly. If we assume, as seems reasonable, that the impact of hospice enrollment on duration is neutral, or the same across age, socioeconomic, and ethnic groups, the variations in duration reflect the decision of when in the course of the patient's illness to enroll in hospice care. This is the second component of demand identified earlier in this chapter.

During our three-year study period, the range of duration (death day less admission day) was from 0 to 430 days, with an average duration of 54 days and a median duration of 32 days.

Age appears to be a factor, with persons 65 and over surviving 8.5 days longer than younger persons. Place of death (although the direction of causation is questionable in this case) is related to duration. Persons dying in a hospital or nursing home survived 69.6 days after hospice enrollment, whereas those dying at home survived only 46.5 days. White persons survived 54.4 days, whereas those from other racial backgrounds survived only 47.0 days. Marital status is also related to survival. Married persons, who may have been able to cope with their illness longer before enrollment, survived 48.6 days, whereas others, not currently married, survived 66.3 days.

It appears that there is considerable variation in the decision about when to enroll in a hospice according to demographic factors. It may be possible for a hospice manager, using this understanding of demand, to forecast staff requirements based on the demographic characteristics of the hospice patient population. This approach will be more helpful for managers of large hospices than of small hospices since in the latter case the existence of a few patients far from the mean will have a large effect on the hospice needs.

Services Provided

During the first three years of the hospice, the total number of encounters was 15,457. Of these, 10,035 or 65 percent of all encounters were phone contacts. From these data, it appears that many problems encountered by patients and families can be managed through access to expert guidance by telephone, reducing the number of required home visits. The presence of a phone in the home of the PCG or the ready availability of one at all hours of the day or night might well be perceived as a necessity for hospice care.

It was previously noted that services provided reflect a combination of supply and demand factors. The supply influence appears, in part, through staffing patterns. For example, an LVN was not employed for several months after the hospice opened. The social worker, primarily employed by the hospital, was available for hospice work only ten hours per week. Pastoral care was provided by a nun who also had heavy hospital responsibilities. The volunteer program was not begun until well into the first year of the program's existence.

The number of encounters is influenced by the length of hospice stay. The average number of telephone contacts was 38, with a range of 1 to 163. Phone calls averaged 6 minutes in length; home visits averaged 81 minutes, not including transportation time. The longest visits were made by volunteers, followed in length by those of home health aides. RNs made the largest number of visits and a majority of the phone calls.

Place of Death

Because of the positive value placed by many hospice personnel on dying at home, factors related to the place of death were identified. Results show that the higher the income the more likely the patient is to die at home. Age also appears to be a contributing factor. As age increases, the possibility of dying at home decreases. Five subjective variables, related to the ability of a patient and family to respond positively to hospice care were also identified. These are (1) the patient's ability to cope, (2) the family's ability to cope, (3) the acceptance of hospice philosophy, (4) acceptance of death, and (5) classification of the family as "not difficult." Comparing home and hospital death on these factors, the inability of the family to cope is associated with a hospital death.

These relationships raise more questions than they provide answers. Does the family cope poorly because the dying period is protracted? Or does a family that cannot cope seek hospice care at an earlier stage of illness than a family that can? Is the age of the patient an issue by itself? Or does the patient's age relate to the age of the primary caregiver (PCG)? Are older PCGs less likely to be able to manage a death at home? Is income itself the relevant factor? Or are high-income families more cognizant of their ability to cope than low-income families? If this is the case, high-income families choosing hospice care may be a self-selecting group of "copers."

Care Over the Course of Enrollment

The pattern of hospice care was examined by considering hospice enrollees who survived a minimum of four weeks after hospice enrollment. Then care over the last four weeks of life was examined. Patients were selected who lived at least 29 days. By defining the set in terms of survivors of at least 29 days and subsequently examining the last 28 days, the day of admission, determined to be the day on which the formal assessment was made when care was probably unusually heavy, was uniformly omitted from this examination. Of the 266 patients who died during the hospice existence, 148 lived the requisite 29 days. The pattern of their care was examined using data on encounters. Both the number of encounters and the length of encounters, measured in minutes, were used.

Although the intensity of care was expected to increase as death approached, nothing was assumed about the nature of that increase. Conceivably, there would be a gradual increase in care over the entire period of hospice enrollment as the patient's condition deteriorated. However, care is provided both by hospice personnel and by the PCG. And, we anticipated that the skills of the PCG and others caring for the patient would also increase as a result of education provided by the hospice team and as a result of experience. Thus, services provided by the hospice staff would likely increase as the patient approached death and would likely decrease as the PCG and other caregivers became more skilled.

We found that the amount of care provided by the hospice staff during the last four weeks of life increased unevenly over that time. Consistently more care was provided in the second than in the first of the four weeks. However, care in the third week generally declined, only to rise in the final week to its highest level. Figure 11-2 illustrates the pattern of care over the last four weeks of life.

Because we expected that care provided during the final week of life to patients who died in the hospital or nursing home would be considerably less than that provided to patients who died at home, the sample was subdivided into two sets: those dying at home and those dying in a hospital or nursing home. Among the patients who lived at least 29 days, there were 92 who died at home and 56 who died in a hospital or nursing home. As expected, the rate of increase in the quantity of care in the fourth or last week of life was considerably lower for those patients dying in a hospital or nursing home than for those dying at home. In some cases those dying in a hospital received less care in the fourth week than in the previous three weeks. This occurred despite the fact that encounters of the social worker and pastoral care worker increased when the patient died in the hospital. These staff persons, already functioning in the hospital setting, had increased contact with hospitalized patients while contact with other hospice personnel decreased.

Figure 11-2 Minutes of Encounters per Patient by Week During the Last Four Weeks of Life, All Patients, and by Place of Death

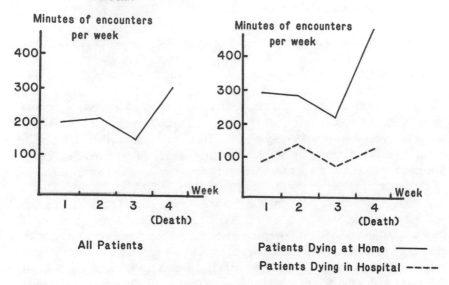

All Patients

Patients Dying at Home ——————
Patients Dying in Hospital ————

Further, patients who died in a hospital or nursing home received considerably less care during all four weeks than those who died at home. A larger sample is required to provide confidence in the results; nevertheless, the differences between the two sets is striking, and the results worth reporting. For example, during the first of the four weeks, patients who died at home received an average of 103 minutes of visits, whereas those who died in the hospital received less than 92 minutes of visits.

The explanation of the variations in intensity of care is not clear. While patients dying in the hospital were probably more likely to have been hospitalized during their illness than the other set, this is insufficient information to explain the large difference found. For example, periods of hospitalization will doubtless reduce the number of visits, but it is not clear that they explain shorter visits. Again a number of questions arise. Did less contact with the hospice personnel influence the decision of families regarding the place of death? Did fewer contacts reflect lower demand, i.e., were these families less committed to hospice philosophy from the time of admission? Or is the issue one of supply—do hospice personnel visit "difficult" patients and families less frequently than other families?

An important question for hospice managers will be whether or not it is possible for them to increase the proportion of home deaths, particularly among that set of patients likely to opt for a hospital death. Will an increase in care early in hospice enrollment increase the proportion choosing a home death? For example, is it possible that some of the study patients who died in the hospital might have chosen a home death if more care had been provided in the early days of their enrollment? If such patients can be identified, it might be less costly to provide more care than these patients seem to be demanding in the early weeks of hospice care than to have them choose a hospital death. Alternatively, it may over time be possible to define a minimum level of care for all patients. This could encourage a high proportion of patients to select home death while the cost of the level of care remains within the reimbursable limits.

Cost of Care

While total spending by hospice SW during a year is fairly easy to determine, it is much more difficult to determine the ''cost'' of care or of particular hospice services. For example, during the first year of existence, hospice expenditures were approximately $125,000. This figure, however, does not include either office space or utilities, which were provided at no cost to the hospice by the hospital. The value of space and utilities has been estimated by the hospice at $8,400, bringing the total to $133,400. The hospice received other benefits that are not reflected in the adjusted figure. For example, no value has been imputed for either volunteer time or transportation; some supplies were also donated. Thus the figure of $133,400 understates total costs of care by SW.

If this amount is divided among 80 patients who died during the first year, the average cost per patient was $1,667. This figure, however, is an overstatement of cost since the count of 80 includes only patients who died during the year. There were others who received services during the first year in addition to the 80 who died. These include patients admitted during the first year who died during the second year, and a small number of patients who were discharged because they moved, their disease went into remission, or they decided to terminate their relationship with the hospice.

With an average duration of 49.4 days, the 80 patients were in hospice care for 3,952 days. (Duration is death day minus admission day or one less than the number of days that the hospice had contact with one patient.) Thus, there are some grounds for using 4,032 days, that is, counting BOTH admission and death day. Using these two day counts, the average daily cost was either $33.76 or $33.09. Again, both figures are overstatements since other patients were served during the year.

An interesting way to consider cost (as well as nature of care) is to use a regression equation explaining or predicting the minutes of care provided. Combining an estimate of the cost per minute of care with predicted minutes produced an estimate of costs under various circumstances.

The dependent variable is minutes of care. The most important explanatory variable is surely the length of hospice enrollment. The result is:

$$TM = 564.9 + 23.2 \text{ DURATION} \qquad R(SQ) = .48$$
$$(123.5) \quad (1.99)$$

where the variables have the following meaning:

TM = total minutes of encounters
DURATION = days of hospice enrollment (death day less assessment of entry day)

Standard errors are shown in parentheses. In this model the constant term represents start-up costs, which are about 9 1/2 hours, and the coefficient represents the length of care per day, which is about 23 minutes. Start-up costs are the costs at the beginning of hospice enrollment that affect every patient and family; initial assessment and training of the PCG would be included. Both the constant and coefficient are statistically significant.

When a dummy variable to account for the place of death is added, the explanatory power of the model increases. The relevant dummy is one affecting the slope rather than the intercept. This is so because there is no reason to assume that place of death affects the start-up costs; instead, it is expected to affect the amount of daily care. The result when this type of dummy variable is employed is:

$$TM = 500 + 18.9 \text{ DURATION} + 9.4 \text{ DURDUM}$$
$$(121) \quad (1.8) \qquad\qquad (2.2) \quad R(SQ) = .51$$

DURDUM is a dummy variable multiplied by DURATION. The dummy is zero when death occurred in a hospital or nursing home and one when death occurred at home. Both DURATION and DURDUM are highly significant.

The addition of the dummy variable clearly improved the results. The implication of this model is that start-up time, indicated by the intercept, is slightly over eight hours. For patients dying in the hospital or nursing home (when DURDUM is zero), an average of 19 minutes per day of encounter time was provided. For patients dying at home (when DURDUM equals DURATION), an average of 28 minutes of encounters was provided. Thus a considerable difference in the quantity of care demanded/supplied is associated with the place of death.

With the regression model it is straightforward to predict the number of minutes of care provided to a patient if duration and place of death are known. If a cost per minute of care is also known, the cost can be estimated under various circumstances.

If the figure of $133,400 is used, it is apparent that the cost per minute of care provided is $1.06. As costs change, it would be possible to substitute a new figure in the regression equation. It should be observed that these figures are for hospice costs and do not include costs of care received in addition to hospice care. In particular, total costs for persons dying in the hospital or nursing home would be considerably higher than the figures shown here. At the average duration of 54 days found at SW, the cost for the care of a patient dying in the hospital or nursing home would be $1,673 and for a patient dying at home $2,231. Table 11-1 lists minutes of care and costs for selected durations, based on place of death.

Table 11-1 Estimated Cost of Hospice Care by Duration of Enrollment and Place of Death*

| | Death Place | | | |
| | Hospital | | Home | |
Duration	Minutes	Cost	Minutes	Cost
1	518.9	$ 550	528.3	$ 560
5	594.5	630	641.5	680
10	689.0	730	783.0	830
15	783.5	831	924.5	980
20	878.0	941	1066.0	1130
25	972.5	1031	1207.5	1280
30	1067.0	1131	1349.0	1430
35	1161.5	1231	1490.5	1580
40	1256.0	1331	1632.0	1730
45	1350.5	1432	1773.5	1880
50	1445.0	1532	1915.0	2030
55	1539.5	1632	2056.5	2180
60	1634.0	1732	2198.0	2330
65	1728.5	1832	2339.5	2480
70	1823.0	1932	2481.0	2630
75	1917.5	2033	2622.5	2780
80	2012.0	2133	2764.0	2930
85	2106.5	2232	2905.5	3080
90	2201.0	2333	3047.0	3230
95	2295.5	2433	3188.5	3380
100	2390.0	2533	3330.0	3530

*Estimates based on regression equation developed in text. Cost per minute employed in estimation is $1.06.

IMPLICATIONS

The implications of the previous discussion, including both the analytic and empirical discussion, fall into three distinct, but not independent, areas. These are (1) the market for hospice care, (2) the distribution of hospice services, and (3) the containment of costs for the delivery of hospice care.

Understanding the Market for Hospice Care

The previous discussion of demand, particularly the first two components of demand—the decision to choose hospice care and the decision pertaining to when in the course of the patient's illness to enroll in a hospice (given that hospice care has been chosen)—provides the necessary background for understanding the market. The hospice manager is able to use this framework along with information from a number of hospices to estimate demand for hospice care in the community. With a general understanding of demand the manager is better able to assess whether or not an apparent increase in demand is temporary or more permanent.The manager can hire permanent staff to meet increased demand or contract for additional services.

Precise estimation of demand for hospice enrollment is likely to prove difficult because of the dynamic nature of demand. Nevertheless, a general understanding of market forces is useful to managers and planners. Similarly, the recognition that patients enroll at different stages of their illness may assist the manager to develop a profile of early enrollers that will aid the hospice staff in handling applications for admission.

Marketing of health services has increased enormously in recent years. With the current expansion of hospice care, managers may find that marketing can put them in an advantageous position.

Equity

The issue of equity in the distribution of health services is a complex one since individual needs differ greatly, as pointed out in Chapter 12. Nevertheless, it is possible to group individuals by categories and examine the provision of care to different groups. For example, the new awareness of inequities of the distribution of health care that developed in the sixties was instrumental in designing divergent types of health programs. At this time it became well known that low-income people received substantially fewer health services than high-income people, despite the fact that low income was typically associated with a higher level of health problems than was high income.

It appears throughout the literature that hospice personnel are idealistic and have a strong commitment to their work. Considering this fact, it is inconsistent to engage knowingly in an inequitable distribution of services. Therefore, it is probably desirable for a hospice to monitor services with the equity question in mind.

One reason that the distribution of services may become skewed is that the demand for services (the third component of demand previously discussed) varies across families. It is important to understand this and to understand that some PCGs, perhaps the more articulate ones, are able to communicate needs to hospice staff clearly and strongly. Any assumption that a family desires less care than usual should be carefully explored. If monitoring of the distribution of services indicates problems, the staff will need to develop strategies to deal with the problem.

The question of equity has been discussed thus far only in the context of its importance for hospice providers. However, it is also likely that federal review of care provided to Medicare recipients receiving hospice care will be concerned with the equity issue. Thus, on both grounds—importance to providers and federal authorities—hospice managers must be sensitive to the question of equity.

Cost Containment

The issue of cost containment will remain an important one for the foreseeable future. Chapter 8 makes this point clear. However, the manager of a hospice—whether nonprofit or for-profit—must also be concerned with costs of providing care for non-Medicare recipients. These patients' care may be financed by private insurance, out-of-pocket payment, philanthropy, or a combination of these. The issue is essentially the same for all types of financing, namely, minimizing the total cost of care—inpatient and outpatient—for dying patients.

Two issues have been raised, in particular, by the previous discussion that are important from the cost-containment perspective. These are the issue of demand for hospice services by the patient and family that have enrolled for hospice care and the relationship between the amount of care provided and the place of death. In a real sense, these two point in the opposite direction. The demand issue suggests that costs may rise for patients and families that are able to demand a large quantity of services. In contrast, the second issue suggests that the provision of too few services may result in death in the hospital rather than at home, with a hospital death obviously associated with high costs.

The present discussion does not provide definitive answers but it does point to the importance of a hospice manager's sensitivity to the issues. Managers and planners must understand the range within which hospice costs can be most effectively allocated to buy the maximum amount of care and the highest quality. This is certainly the challenge for the coming decade.

NOTES

1. Michael Grossman, *The Demand for Health: A Theoretical and Empirical Investigation* (New York: Columbia University Press, 1972); Michael Grossman, "On the Concept of Health Capital and the Demand for Health," *Journal of Political Economy* 80, no.2 (March/April 1972).

2. Kim Carney, "An Economic Perspective on Hospices," *Socioeconomic Issues in Health: 1982*, ed. Robert A. Musacchio and Douglas Hough (Chicago: American Medical Association, 1981).

3. Helen Yura and Mary B. Walsh, *The Nursing Process: Assessing, Planning, Implementing, Evaluating* (New York: Merideth,1973).

Part IV

Major Policy Issues in Hospice Care

Chapter 12

Ethics in Hospice Care

Joanne Lynn

Modern hospice in this country and elsewhere is marked by a striking blend of altruism, effectiveness, generosity, and dedicated providers. Historically, hospice programs and providers have been seen as a marked contrast with the standard care for dying patients provided by the traditional health care system, often perceived as alienating, death denying, ineffective, unconcerned about symptom control, and hopelessly fragmented.[1] Since the stereotypes were largely true, hospice has enjoyed broad public acceptance and an almost unquestioned welcome on the part of patients and public officials.

Over time, hospice and the medical care system changed. Hospice is now a health care program, not primarily an inspired volunteer activity. Potential problems, once presumed to have been averted by good intentions and sterling character, have reappeared as programs grew large enough to have policies, regulations, and paid employees.[2] Some of these problems are common elsewhere in health care: the persistent trouble hospitals have concerning nonresuscitation orders, the long-term-care conundrum of guaranteeing adequate care with inadequate funds and public skepticism, and the home care industry's concern with regulating a cottage industry that accepts certain kinds of death as good outcomes. Hospices must now define the services they will provide, their complicity in suicide, their responsibility for conservation and allocation of resources, and their responsibilities for the care of those who do not qualify for hospice care.

In order to identify and discuss ethical issues that arise for hospice providers, this chapter begins by presenting a framework for analyzing values and issues in health care, including the problems of defining terminal illness and determining who can have access to hospice care. Following a general overview, the ethical problems hospice providers face are delineated.

VALUES AT STAKE IN HEALTH CARE

Three major values are at stake in health care: well-being, self-determination, and equity.[3] *Well-being* applies differently to patients, individuals associated with the patient such as family members and close friends, and society as a whole. *Self-determination* is principally related to the patient, while *equity* is more relevant to the society as a whole. Ideally, a health care system should honor and advance all of these goals. Problems arise both in understanding what advancing each value entails and in resolving conflicts among values when pursuit of one compromises the pursuit of another.

The Well-Being of the Patient

Usually, health care is justified primarily by the expectation that it will improve the patient's health and well-being over what the patient would otherwise face. The patient is given the authority, indeed the social role obligation, to pursue well-being and the physician is held accountable as a fiduciary in this endeavor.[4] The traditions of medicine and nursing demand that all other professional goals are subsidiary to patient well-being.

It can be discerned, in most cases, whether a patient's well-being is being pursued. For example, quality assurance programs measure the adequacy of outcomes for various conditions. Sometimes, however, the definitions of well-being are quite diverse and related to religiously held beliefs or individual preferences. In the case of Jehovah's Witnesses, for example, refusing transfusion is thought to improve chances for life everlasting, while the physician's hope is to give the transfusion to improve the patient's chances in the present life. A woman with breast cancer who refuses a mastectomy may be preserving peace of mind and self-image while risking recurrence.

Self-Determination by the Patient

Well-being can be defined by either professional or lay consensus according to scientific or objective criteria, or it can be decided individually by more subjective criteria. An individual's conceptualization of well-being varies and is influenced by religious, political, economic, and social attitudes held by patients, their families, and health care providers. Respect for the ambiguity and diversity of values and attitudes among patients, providers, and family members requires accepting that there is no clear-cut standard of well-being that applies to all patients in all situations. It is from this respect for others, as well as from an ideal vision that each person can and should shape his or her own life, that the value of self-determination arises.

As ill health becomes more commonly chronic and as increasing medical capabilities are more likely to bring results that are at least partially successful (instead of futile), people have demanded a role in making decisions affecting their own health care. Instead of allowing physicians to make major decisions, patients seek the responsibility, and their claims are legally enforced, most notably with the legal requirement of "informed consent." Competent patients can legally refuse all treatment and may choose from among all reasonable and available medical treatments, even though the choice is not, in the physician's view, optimal for the patient's health.[5] Surrogates deciding for incompetent patients can also choose medically suboptimal treatments if the patient would clearly have so chosen.[6]

The Well-Being of Family and Friends

Except for unusual situations, such as that of a newborn, pursuing the patient's well-being is assumed to also ensure the well-being of the patient's loved one. Thus, conventional health care rarely focuses on the distinct needs of families and friends. In fact, if pursuing the well-being of the patient conflicts with helping friends and family, only two resolutions seem acceptable: (1) if the patient is competent, he or she may consider the interests of loved ones to whatever extent desired; (2) if the patient is incompetent, the surrogate decisionmaker must, in almost all instances, pursue the patient's well-being irrespective of the effects upon others.

Hospice has tried to create a framework in which the family, as a whole, is the "unit of care." The ramifications of this approach are uncertain. As long as the needs of the family do not conflict with the needs of the patient, this care focus is uncontroversial and useful. However, a primary commitment to family care becomes controversial and problematic when meeting the needs of the patient would be compromised by meeting those of the family, for example, when the patient wants to travel away to receive an experimental treatment and family members would be exhausted and impoverished by the effort.

The meaning of the "well-being" of a group of interrelated persons is uncertain. Although events can result in distress to group members, it is difficult to predict whether, over the long term, such care strategies are beneficial or detrimental. Even enhancing the closeness, interdependence, and "smooth running" of a family group may prove harmful for the "well-being" of the group. As hospices proceed beyond platitudes to serving dying patients' families as units of care, an analysis of the degree to which patients' interests can be compromised in order to serve the family and a definition of familial well-being are needed.

Well-Being of the Society

American health care focuses both on general levels of health and well-being of the populace and individual patient outcomes. In practice, this concern is assumed to be met by maximally helping each patient. Only for those endeavors seen as "for the public good," such as immunizations, sanitation, and health education, is the primary measure of success population-based instead of patient-based. In most cases, the underlying assumption regarding the pursuit of public good is reminiscent of Adam Smith's "invisible hand" in economics: by everyone pursuing self-interest, the public well-being is achieved.

In times of economic wealth, conflicts do not generally arise over pursuit of individual versus societal interest. However, in times of economic hardship, resources used for individual health benefits might be used in other social programs.

Maximal pursuit of each patient's interests often means that others, whose well-being could have been more substantially advanced with the same efforts and resources, are not helped. For example societal interests might be substantially advanced by utilizing current health resources in nonhealth arenas such as transportation, agriculture, housing, or defense.

In addition, measuring long-term societal "well-being" has the same kinds of uncertainties that plague measurements of outcomes for families and patients. Something harmful to individual health may well be beneficial to overall social welfare. Consider the complexities of evaluating the effect on societal well-being of a new, cheap remedy that would add ten years to the life span but guarantee recipients severe dependency during those years. In another example, the eradication of smallpox has allowed the immunity to it to lapse in the populace, thereby creating a powerful biological weapon for those nations that retain the virus in culture.

Equitable Allocation of Health Care Benefits and Burdens

In an equitable health care system, benefits and burdens are distributed fairly across the population. Even if the aggregate well-being were the same in two systems, one in which all persons shared in the benefits and burdens should be preferred over one in which only some persons benefited, especially if others, denied benefits, must bear the burdens. Traditionally, ensuring adequate equity in the allocation of health care benefits has been the responsibility of governments and charities, and not of individual health care providers.

Various meanings of equitable allocation, sometimes termed social justice, are possible. For example, each person's benefits and burdens could be justified by individual need, merit, past achievements, or future potential. Ambulance services are usually provided to all in need; Veterans Administration hospitals to those who served in the armed forces; maternal and child health care is targeted for impoverished recipients. Persons could be expected to bear the burdens of the system to the degree that they need the benefits, contribute by voluntary actions to the need for benefits, or are able to contribute without undue burden. Much of health care is financed either by experience-rated group insurance, reflecting at least the aggregate historical need of groups, or by somewhat progressive taxation, reflecting payment by ability to pay. Because examples of a large number of justifications for distribution of the benefits and burdens of health care exist in this country's health care system, the meaning and success of the pursuit for equity is unclear. However, any health care program that aims to serve a select population or to offer limited benefits must offer persuasive justification for the distribution of its benefits and burdens.

HOSPICE AS A PROGRAM OF HEALTH CARE

Chapters 1 and 2 outline the philosophy of hospice care and the divergent organizational structures. Hospice is often described as a "philosophy of care"[7] that accepts death's inevitability and that aims to support the person dying and his or her family and friends by coordinated and effective symptom control, spiritual counseling, and emotional support. Hospice thereby affirms widely accepted values, such as: avoiding suffering is preferable to enduring it; and the suffering of dying persons commonly involves spiritual, emotional, and interpersonal concerns as much as physical pain. Moreover, dying is not primarily a medical problem, but rather a significant personal and community event.

As a philosophy, hospice is fairly straightforward. However, problems arise when these commitments are translated into a program of care. Hospices serve a specific patient population, and if they receive third-party reimbursement, they must justify the population served, which consists entirely of patients with six months or less to live. Further, hospices are required to provide specific services at a cost that is much lower than the traditional system. This latter requirement exists even though hospices are expected to provide numerous nonreimbursable services such as respite care and bereavement counseling. Satisfying these requisites has proved difficult for some programs and has led to multiple problems, some of which are discussed below.

Categorizing and Defining Terminal Illness, Palliative Care, and Related Terms

Hospice programs of care are required to determine a group of "terminally ill" patients for whom it is appropriate to shift care "from curative care to palliative care."[8]

Many assume it is easy to determine when a patient becomes "terminally ill." The Medicare statute, for example, states that a "terminally ill" individual "has a medical prognosis that his or her life expectancy is 6 months or less."[9] This assumes that physicians can prognosticate death with reasonable accuracy, relying principally upon objective signs of disease. This assumption is probably wrong in most cases. Little empirical data exist to guide physicians in making an estimate so close to the end of life. Further, existing data suggest that random events regarding the disease, in addition to factors influencing a patient's will to live, substantially affect life span.[10] In fact, the attention given by the hospice to the patient's comfort and spiritual well-being may prove to be life-sustaining, further confounding the prognostication. Overall, physicians seem to have little reliability in assessing the likely time of death, even in cancer patients.[11]

A further complication with the definition of terminality is that neither the statutory definition nor the hospice literature confronts such simple statistical definitional essentials as whether "prognosis" is the midpoint of the mortality curve, the point of 95 percent or 99 percent confidence of accuracy in predicting death, or some other point. Under the Medicare program, hospices are rewarded for defining the hospice population in a very conservative way, taking little risk that a patient will outlive the 210 days for which Medicare provides benefits. Thus, not only is the reliability of the prediction important, but also the magnitude of any "error" in underestimating long-term survivors. Hospice programs will want to avoid patients with extensive but slowly progressive disease who are dying rapidly because of depression, isolation, or abandonment. These are patients whom hospice would be expected to maximally benefit but, in doing so, will have substantially extended their lives and the cost of care, especially the reimbursed costs.

The central contention that patients with relatively brief life expectancies can reasonably be categorized on that basis is itself a proposition requiring justification.[12] In what ways are terminally ill individuals different from those who are ill but expected to survive for longer periods? Certainly, the care needs of the two groups overlap, as does the likelihood of benefit from care. The prevalence of spiritual and existential concerns might increase as death seems close, but the increase is probably gradual and slight. A close proximity to death generally makes it more appropriate to decline burdensome treatments or other endeavors, but the appropriateness of such treatment does not suddenly vanish at some point prior to death. It is the decreasing expectation of offsetting benefits that ordinarily makes burdensome interventions less desirable as life expectancies shorten.

These observations point up a central problem with the category "terminal illness"—it is defined in arbitrary or procedural ways. While it may sound trite, it is nonetheless true that life itself is a terminal illness. The importance of proximity to death is a very personal matter. One person may live a long life in the shadow of death, with constant concerns about dying. Another may not focus on the impact of dying until the final moments of life.

The term "palliative care" encounters much the same difficulties, especially when seen as the treatment option when cure is no longer possible. Separating "palliation" from curative endeavors requires that the services involved are fairly distinct and that patients are suited only for one or the other set. Neither contention reflects a coherent view, or a practical possibility. The central concerns of palliative care, such as pain control, are appropriate for quality medical care at any time. Moreover, it is lack of effective curative interventions and not their inappropriateness that makes them unavailable to dying persons. If a person nearing death develops a condition that compromises the remaining life and that is curable, such as a urinary tract infection, acute glaucoma, or a drug reaction, those conditions are often quite appropriately treated through curative measures. Patients do not simply pass from being appropriate for curative interventions to being appropriate for palliation. Palliative care has always been part of good care and remains as the potential for curative interventions dims.

Definitions of palliative care and terminal illness often include such terms as "extraordinary care" or "imminent death," which do not define clear and useful categories. Many people use "extraordinary" to mean vigorous, unusual, or artificial treatments, which are not morally relevant considerations in deciding upon the care that must be extended to a patient.[13] Likewise, "imminent" has no statutory or broadly understood meaning. Even among physicians, "imminently" has been shown to imply anything from dying immediately to dying within five years.[14]

Policy and Imperfect Categories

Policies and program are easiest to establish when they reflect real, relevant, and justifiable categories. For example, individuals with permanent kidney failure are the only appropriate targets for a kidney transplant program. Sometimes, however, substantial ambiguity is justified solely on the basis of expected benefits and a lack of countervailing harms. For example, historical disadvantages faced by some minorities in this country are used to justify preferential hiring and educational training practices, even though some receiving the advantages have not suffered from previous policies. Further, there may well be individuals who have not been targeted for preferential hiring and training benefits but who are deserving on the same historical basis.

Whenever possible, public policies are more readily established and managed when the affected population matches the justification well. Whether hospice programs and the public policies that support their development are well enough justified despite the substantial problems encountered in defining categories will be a continuing concern in the ensuing sections, which examine the impact of hospice care programs on the central values in health care described above.

HOSPICE AND INDIVIDUAL WELL-BEING

All of health care is obliged to try to improve the patient's health and well-being. Caregivers must seek to make options available that might be seen as beneficial, to minimize harms, and to establish modes of self-evaluation and improvement. A hospice faces some perplexing problems in pursuing these goals. Most notably, the way hospice programs are organized can restrict the range of patient choice, induce dependency, reduce patient control over dying, and engender difficulties with the development of standards and quality assurance.

Restriction of Treatment Options

The existence of hospice as a treatment option often enhances a patient's range of treatment choices by providing a comfortable setting for living because of adequate symptom control. However, hospice is generally not well integrated into the traditional health care system. This fact is further exacerbated by the Medicare reimbursement. With hospice services kept distinct from conventional care, patients may find access to some options restricted.

Hospices are often unwilling to accept a patient unless all "indicated" conventional curative treatment has been exhausted.[15] This requirement may help protect hospices from having to resolve some thorny issues concerning suicide, but it also limits a patient's authority to control treatment decisions and to use hospice services as he or she desires. A patient might be served best by not seeking a cure rather than by trying all curative options. Such a patient might be averse to suffering, have little for which to live, be concerned about the status of the surviving family's finances, or be devoutly trusting in God. In these instances, it is not beneficial to insist that all "reasonable" and potentially curative treatments be exhausted before a patient can be admitted to a hospice program.

However, hospice policymakers must avoid designing a care system that makes hospice so emotionally or financially attractive that patients are induced to forego aggressive and curative treatment options. For patients who have been emotionally alienated by conventional care, or who have exhausted Medicare benefits, or for whom other modes of care would bankrupt survivors, hospice may be very attractive. This may be the case even if conventional care offers hope for substantial improvement in health or prolongation of meaningful life.

On the other hand, hospice program design can make conventional care more difficult to obtain for hospice patients. If hospice care is providing emotionally supportive care, effective symptom control, and/or reduction of financial anxieties, a patient may be reluctant to lose these concrete benefits for what is likely to seem an uncertain gain in health. This barrier may vanish if hospice caregivers can also attend the patient while he or she is undergoing conventional care, but the Medicare benefit makes this less likely.

Under Medicare, hospice programs will have substantial disincentives against returning a patient to conventional care settings. Hospice care providers are likely to be skeptical that hospital-based or invasive procedures will prove helpful and therefore may not raise the issue with a patient. Furthermore, under such payment schemes as Medicare, the hospice is put at risk for the full costs of an enrolled patient's care, even if the care is given in a conventional care setting. Since the costs of care in conventional settings are likely to be substantially higher than those incurred in hospice care, the hospice program suffers financially for such a choice. Thus, it may be less likely that costly interventions will be offered to hospice patients by program providers.

Furthermore, the Medicare benefit provides hospice professionals with a strong and troubling incentive to act against the patient's interests when there are interventions that might considerably extend the patient's life. Medicare, as well as some state laws, requires hospices to continue care for patients who outlive the duration of the benefit. The program bears the full expense if the patient cannot pay. Therefore, hospice programs are financially benefited by not offering treatments that might greatly prolong life. The thought of actually acting upon this incentive is abhorrent; however, many situations are ambiguous and the outcomes uncertain. The presence of an incentive of this sort could tip the balance. Consider, for example, a patient who, while depressed, turned down an especially onerous (but effective) curative cancer therapy. After some hospice care, the patient's emotional reserves may well be replenished and he or she might be able to reconsider whether to try to delay death by utilizing the once-scorned intervention. The hospice provider may feel that what is best for the patient is quite uncertain. The hospice provider with strong financial constraints might be less likely to offer the intervention. This conflict might not occur if the patient's choice had no impact upon financial status of the hospice. A hospice program could also be financially disadvantaged by employing physicians who emphasize their expertise in curative care modalities, if, as would be expected, that skill utilizes costly interventions rather than curative approaches.[16]

Induction of Dependency

Hospices are very good at their craft. Patients and families often find it hard to believe that anyone less expert could similarly satisfy the patient's needs or that the patient could do much about his or her situation alone.[17] Hospice providers feel that people do better and feel better about themselves if they actively participate in their own care. In fact, reclaiming dying as a human endeavor best experienced among family and community was an early cornerstone of the hospice concept.[18] Obviously, the establishment of professional experts may risk undermining patient and family control over dying. When professional care is more readily reimbursed and less time-consuming than patient or family training and care, experts have strong pressures to accept displacing those directly involved. Hospice planners, caregivers, and managers should recognize that careful attention to the magnitude and likelihood of negative long-term effects can cause professionals to restrain themselves from encouraging dependency and make the dying process one that must be managed by professionals.

Quality Assurance

Developing ways to ensure that the patient's interests are well-served in hospice and home care is difficult. Problems arise both in setting and meeting standards.[19] The outcomes to be desired are quite varied. For example, a patient might well be appropriate for cardiopulmonary resuscitation today and inappropriate even for a feeding tube next week. A patient who died yesterday may have been appropriately treated, may have had a significant treatment erroneously omitted, or may have had dying cruelly prolonged by erroneous administration of a medical intervention. Deciphering which scenario occurred may be impossible, and there may not be a right or wrong answer. In hospice care, as in general medical care, treatment decisions reflect judgment calls and are largely dependent on the expertise of the provider and requests of the patient. Ordinarily, quality control can rely upon independent and concurrent peer judgment and review. In hospice home care, the caregiver present gathers the information, creates expectations, and writes the reports without any real opportunity for evaluation by outsiders.

When death becomes an acceptable care outcome, it must often be seen as an improvement in well-being over continued physical deterioration and pain. However, premature death is always a serious error. Thus, one must develop ways of assessing the relative degree of ''well-being'' gained or lost for each patient at each time that the patient might die. Obviously, such an assessment can depend upon an evaluator's personal values and perspectives more than reliable and verifiable facts regarding the patient's life experience.

Evaluations of outcomes are difficult. Even something as simple and generally well done as pain control yields no easy assessment. One might propose that patients be surveyed as to the degree of pain, and the effectiveness of pain relief, with the goal of eradicating all disturbing pain. However, some patients find meaning in their suffering and are not best served by its eradication. Others have substantial side effects from pain management and are best served by accepting some annoyance from pain so as to retain better mental function or respiratory drive.

Yet, hospices have social, moral, and other obligations to assure patients and others that their services are the best that can be offered. Over the next few years, assessment standards and procedures will have to be developed that are sensitive to the variations among patients and the appropriateness of services in light of patients' diverse and idiosyncratic versions of well-being.

HOSPICE AND PATIENT SELF-DETERMINATION

Hospice, more than almost any other form of health care, has been committed to encouraging the patient to determine the course of his or her life. Perhaps when life is expected to be brief, health care providers, as well as the general public, have felt it important to have patients lead in defining and pursuing goals. Also, in the early days of establishing hospice, relying upon the consent of the patient helped to thwart criticism of the programs by those who felt that aggressive care was always appropriate.

However, many hospice practices actually may limit patient self-determination. Care providers are penalized by offering some valuable treatment options, including transfer to another mode of treatment. To the extent that patients are encouraged to yield important decisions to others, their ability to take charge of the course of their lives is compromised.

Consent and Information

Hospice programs often request a formal consent to admission, as required by Medicare.[20] As noted in Chapter 9, to ask consent for a program of care is somewhat novel, requiring full discussion of included and excluded services in addition to potential financial, physical, and emotional impacts. Hospice patients and surrogate decisionmakers may find it difficult to focus on the range of services and interventions that are unlikely to be made available after hospice admission. And after admission patients may not be able to recognize or to resist behaviors that lead to narrowing the range of choice.

In hospice care, adequately informing patients also requires patients to recognize that physicians feel their life expectancy is limited and that the condition is not likely to be improved by any "curative" care. The effectiveness and the impact of this consent process are uncertain. There are no reports of major ill effects on patients, but there is also little understanding or research regarding the degree to which patients comprehend the information in advance of experiencing the care.

Some kinds of information may prove especially difficult to convey. For example, the financial benefits and risks a patient undertakes in electing hospice under Medicare are substantial and necessitate disclosure. However, such information is complex, requiring that patients envision undesirable future circumstances and deal with risks of potentially devastating events. The usual sick patient confronting financial issues of treatment might find it useless information. There is no published evidence regarding whether patients adequately understand ramifications of their chosen course of treatment. This is particularly problematic in the hospice area where patients have a complex set of criteria from which to draw benefits. The criteria are both insurer- and hospice-program-specific and require that patients understand the implications of withdrawing from the hospice benefit program in order to obtain other third-party benefits.

Limitations to Voluntariness

Not only must patients be well informed to make their own choices but also they must be substantially free of coercion and manipulation. In some circumstances, pressures upon patients to "choose" hospice may actually amount to coercion. Consider an elderly and dying patient with a dependent but younger wife. Imagine that the patient has used up all of the hospitalization days to which he is entitled under Medicare. Caring for such a patient as he dies is likely to be expensive, requiring "spend-down" to poverty before public programs will help and thus assuring that his wife will be left impoverished. Even if the patient wants to continue some potentially beneficial treatments, he may well have to "choose" the hospice benefit to avoid the severely adverse effects upon his wife.

People differ on whether this incident should count as truly coercive, since the patient is made no worse off by the availability of the hospice option than he would have been without it. However, that explanation depends upon a historical accident as to which benefit came first. The more substantial question is whether public policy should regularly put people in the position of accepting an earlier death so as to avoid impoverishment or other related hardships for themselves and their loved ones.

Self-Determination through Surrogate Decision Making

Self-determination for patients who are incapable of making their own choices presents a number of problems, in hospice and in health care generally. Largely unsettled are questions of who should serve as a surrogate decisionmaker, who should decide among potential surrogates, how severe must the patient's decision-making disability become before someone else must make decisions, and what standard should guide the choice. Some major strides have been taken in providing guidelines in this area, especially in affirming that the decision should reflect, to the greatest extent possible, what the patient would have wanted if competent and that the surrogate decisionmaker should be the person best situated to make such a determination.[21]

Hospice programs have often been reticent to accept patients who cannot speak for themselves, though actually many patients have some periods of incoherence when they realistically cannot be directly involved in decisionmaking. Such patients are often more dependent, costly, and emotionally draining to the hospice provider program. Yet, they are often especially benefited by coordinated and competent care. To exclude these persons from hospice is difficult to justify. Still, many hospices accept only coherent patients, claiming that patients must be able to "experience" hospice care, to work through problems with their families, and make choices regarding varied palliative care approaches. These programs have been criticized by established health care providers as "skimming" off the cream of the crop by taking the best patients, that is, those needing the least amount of expensive care.

Hospice, under Medicare, poses additional problems. The final regulations require that consent to admission by given by "someone other than the patient . . . when authorized in accordance with state law" if the patient is incapable of giving his or her own consent.[22] If this is interpreted strictly, patients will have to have been adjudicated incompetent and to have had a guardian appointed before election to hospice care can be undertaken. This creates a substantial barrier to hospice care, as these processes are often expensive and time-consuming. Solutions to these problems will require creative collaboration with traditional care providers and with legislators and lawyers and are likely to be imperfect for some time to come.

THE WELL-BEING OF FAMILIES AND OF SOCIETY IN GENERAL

Determining how to advance the well-being of a patient's family and of society is difficult. As we have noted, achieving benefits for others might compromise the pursuit of the patient's well-being or self-determination. Should a patient's interests ever be compromised and, if so, by how much and for how significant a gain for others? No simple and satisfactory solution to this conflict between individual and societal interest has emerged. However, some general guidelines are helpful. The considerations take on rather different characteristics when the asserted societal interest in the preservation of life itself is at stake and expressed through homicide and suicide statutes.

Balancing Patients' Interests with the Welfare of Others

Concerns about the well-being of others are often part of the concerns expressed by patients themselves. If a patient wants (or would want if capable of formulating and communicating a preference) to compromise his or her own self-interest to benefit others, it is important to respect that decision as a justifiable aspect of patient self-determination. Since there is a risk that patients could be induced to be altruistic in inauthentic ways, caregivers should maintain some skepticism about a patient's desire to be disadvantaged for the benefit of others. This skepticism should ordinarily be muted for the patient who is speaking on his or her own behalf but it should be especially strong when the claim is made by a potential beneficiary on behalf of society.

The appropriateness of compromising the patient's well-being depends largely upon (1) the magnitude of the projected disadvantage to the patient and the projected benefits to the others affected, (2) the personal interdependency of the patient and others who would be advantaged by the patient's disadvantage, and (3) the patient's entitlement to benefits in question by virtue of contract, past merit, or status.

The weighing of these considerations should be accomplished by developing general rules and guidelines rather than by asking those involved in particular instances to develop priorities and definitions *ad hoc*. Thus, if it were decided that patients with life expectancies with treatment of less than a year will not be started upon maintenance hemodialysis because society decides to utilize resources in other ways, then those caring for such patients are restricted by public decision. Likewise, if society decides that people with severe and irreversible dementia prefer to be kept comfortable and to leave loved ones their material goods without depletion by costly vigorous death-delaying interventions, then caregivers and family can apply that generalization in their particular case. If caregivers in such situations were both to apply and to create the rules, these "rules" are likely to be variable, inconsistent, and idiosyncratic. Furthermore, the process of creating them is likely to induce serious conflicts of interest.

Responsible choices regarding this balancing of interests require reliable data about the efficacy and effectiveness of various interventions, including hospice care, relative to the costs and burdens imposed by the interventions. Research must not only ascertain that hospice is effective and well received but it must also establish that its effects are worth the costs and resources displaced. Some care extended to families, such as bereavement counseling, does not directly affect the interests of the patient. While care that does not affect the patient may need less careful scrutiny, it still must prove to be worthwhile relative to other possible expenditures.

When interventions are made primarily for the benefit of someone other than the patient, stringent safeguards are needed. If the intervention is part of research, requiring adequate consent is essential for patient protection. If such an intervention is needed to maintain institutional functioning (as when a patient is restrained or treated to maintain peace and orderliness) then consent, consultation, careful internal review, and possibly court approval may be needed to prevent abuse of the patient.

Balancing a patient's interests with those of the family and the larger society is difficult. Hospice administrators must discuss these issues with staff, volunteers, and board members. A review of the activities of other programs as well as discussions with an attorney or chaplain are useful for identifying the ethical issues. Chapter 9 on legal issues in hospice care contains numerous suggestions.

The Societal Interest in Preventing Suicide and Homicide

In order to protect the lives of all people, society has developed and enforced laws making it a serious crime to cause the death of another or to assist in another's suicide. Nevertheless, most of medical practice, and hospice in particular, considers relief from suffering, even at the risk of a shortened life, preferable to constant pain. Obviously, there will be times when the two concepts both apply—(1) when the action contemplated is likely to result in death earlier than otherwise would happen and (2) when the action still seems to be justifiable because it is essential to easing the patient's suffering. In these instances, are caregivers acting correctly in providing palliative treatment even if it is relatively certain that treatment will result in earlier death? This question arises, for example, with patients having persistent pain requiring narcotics that also predispose them to pneumonia or depressed breathing.

Patients in hospice care rarely seek to die. The compassion, respect, symptom control, and comprehensive attention that mark hospice are effective in diminishing the hopelessness that afflicts many patients not receiving hospice care. However, some patients may not find these modalities sufficient to offset the discouragement or powerlessness or unpleasantness that often attend being sick enough to die. If such a patient seeks to reduce his or her "allotted time," what sorts of actions by the caregivers might count as assisting suicide? Any complicity, including a tolerant attitude, may be construed as actually assisting the patient. However, respect for the patient requires that some self-destructive choices be accepted.

Identifying the differences between treatments aimed to control symptoms and those properly construed as murder or assisting in suicide is surprisingly difficult. If a physician were to cause a patient's death by shooting or cyanide poisoning, even if to relieve pain, the physician would be held guilty of murder. The fact that the patient consented, or that the physician's motives were pure, might mitigate the seriousness of the punishment but it would not exculpate the act.[23]

How is vigorous symptom control using medical interventions to be differentiated from murder if not by motive, consent, and intent?[24] Usually, vigorous symptom control is not as certain to cause death as those steps that are conventionally seen as murder, though sometimes an accelerated death is virtually certain even in good symptom control. Connections between the act and the death are less direct in medical actions than in ordinary murders, but that construction of events rests upon a convention rather than a real difference in whether the act caused death.[25] The only real difference between murder and compassionate medical treatment in such extreme cases is that certain medical professionals have effectively (though somewhat informally) been granted the authority to risk life—and sometimes to cause death—in medical treatment, even though the same actions are considered criminal if committed by others. This is an uncertain protection. The distinction between murder (or assisting in suicide) and symptom control in ambiguous and borderline cases is common. Two especially illustrative examples are the patient dying with respiratory insufficiency and the patient dying with malnutrition or dehydration.

When a patient dies in severe respiratory insufficiency, all senses are overwhelmed in the struggle against suffocation. If there are no reversible causes, the patient may be doomed to struggle until exhausted, with all of his or her last hours being given over to terror. The only readily available treatment is sedation, preferably with narcotics, until the brain is made less responsive to the anoxia and hypercarbia. Doing this almost certainly leads to death, and probably a few hours earlier than would otherwise have happened. The patient slips into a self-perpetuating coma prior to death and dies peacefully, though without awareness. Providing morphine in such cases is recommended in some hospice literature.[26] It does seem to be the only course that offers the patient any benefit. However, the situation is so close to direct killing that it deserves careful consideration, careful explication of why this should be tolerated while poisoning is not, and deliberate examination of alternatives and motives by those involved. If providing morphine in such a case were done unreflectively, inattentively, or by persons not trained and sanctioned to make life-risking decisions, it is likely the actions would be seen as murder.

Many patients have some malnutrition and dehydration at the time of death and most would if no interventions were taken to mitigate these abnormalities. For some, the lack of nutrition and water is a major cause of an early death. Such a patient presents an uncomfortable situation for the caregiver. In most circumstances, providing food and water is a basic obligation. At first glance, failing to do so seems not merely erroneous but outrageous. However, some patients are probably harmed by the medical provision of food and water.[27] Patients may die more comfortably without "normal" hydration and without the discomfort and limitation of mobility occasioned by feeding tubes. Hospice caregivers have found that patients who continue to communicate throughout terminal illness rarely want artificial feeding, even though intake may drop to virtually nothing.

However, a patient who is receiving wholly inadequate food and water cannot live for long. To fail to intervene may be best for the patient, but why is it not murder? The analysis is parallel to that for respiratory insufficiency, depending, most heavily, upon whether the caregivers exercised accurate and reflective risk-taking and thereby were effectively exempted from criminal prosecution.

Vigorous public and professional discussion of these borderline cases between good practice and criminal activity would help clarify and define acceptable standards of practice. Once these are clarified, hospice should be in the forefront of ensuring that substandard practices are eliminated or prosecuted and that defensible ones are not a source of undue anxiety.

EQUITY IN HOSPICE SERVICE DISTRIBUTION

Ideally, society should be arranged so there are adequate justifications for the differences among people in the benefits they receive from societal endeavors and in the burdens they bear when such endeavors are limited or absent. There should be clear, persuasive, and relevant reasons for excluding some and including others in a social benefit. For many reasons, hospice programs in this country have had admission criteria that largely limited their services to a small segment of the population consisting largely of adult, middle-class patients who are dying of cancer and who have a supportive family. Is this a justifiable target category, especially if hospice is to be largely a publicly funded benefit under Medicare? Should only certain classes of patients receive the benefits of community-supported hospice care?

No one consideration adequately defines equity in regard to the allocation of health care resources. Some aspects of health care are allocated on the basis of the need for care, the likelihood of benefit, and the proportionality between the benefits offered and the burdens caused. Health care is an important social good, as well as an individual benefit. Good health and emotional well-being ensures that persons have a range of opportunities in which to invest their lives. These are characteristics that justify efforts to ensure that health care is distributed more fairly than might happen under marketplace economics alone. A recent President's Commission recommended that "all citizens [should] be able to secure an adequate level of care without excessive burdens."[28] If this standard is generally correct, should hospice care be considered a component of an adequate level of care or is it an amenity whose allocation is not a public concern?

Hospice offers some patients benefits that are commonly unavailable elsewhere. However, these benefits are not of the magnitude that compels society to make them widely available. Such endeavors as childhood immunizations and emergency transportation for trauma victims are more obviously effective, cost-effective, and opportunity-enhancing. Hospice programs present a borderline case where social importance can be decided politically. Had hospice not been the subject of major legislation, it might have remained an interesting and instructive oddity in the health care system, if indeed one could count it as part of the health care system. However, Congress decided that, in the short run, the care hospice provides is valuable enough to include in the adequate minimum society will ensure for a select group of citizens.[29] As we have seen, this decision is subject to reconsideration in a few years under a sunset clause. Other third-party payers have followed suit. Thus, the American culture views hospice as a legitimate and appropriate aspect of an adequate level of health care.

Once the question of social importance has been answered, others appear. For managers and policymakers alike, translating a mandate to provide hospice to the population into the programs necessary requires (1) a definition of the population to receive hospice benefits, (2) an identification of the scope of those benefits, and (3) an assessment of potential burdens associated with providing hospice benefits, including whether hospice care is likely to cost some resources above those that would otherwise have been used.[30]

In defining target populations, hospice encounters major ethical problems. Often for very worthy reasons, hospices in this country have utilized multiple admission criteria. Medicare has perpetuated many of these criteria, making them more onerous in some cases.[31] Under Medicare, patients must have a medical prognosis of less than six months; must be likely to be able to be cared for at home, thus must have both a home and a caregiver (usually unpaid) available for most or all of the day; and must have no curative therapy indicated. The requirement that the program continue to provide care even after the 210 days of Medicare benefits provides an incentive to be cautious in prognostication and to also try to enroll patients who can pay for care after Medicare benefits are exhausted.

Who, then, are hospices likely to serve? As we see in Chapter 10, the overwhelming majority of hospice patients are now, and are likely to be white, middle or low income (but not poor), under some type of insurance plan, and dying of progressive cancer. This latter characteristic is true because cancer is one of the few lethal illnesses physicians feel they can prognosticate reliably (though there is little data even in this area). Virtually all hospice patients are going to have homes and reasonably intact families. Furthermore, they will have enough wealth or a feasible employment situation so that a competent caregiver can be at home and not gainfully employed for a rather indeterminate time. In sum, hospices are likely to serve cancer patients who have families with sufficient physical, emotional, and financial resources to allow the patient to die comfortably at home.

In addition, the Medicare program creates an incentive to serve principally those whose care needs can be predicted to remain low throughout their final stages of illness. This incentive arises because Medicare reimburses hospice programs at a fixed daily rate for each of four categories of intensity of care: basic home care, continuous nursing care (which has subcategories of rates), respite inpatient care, and hospital-type inpatient care.[32] Hospices will benefit to the extent that they can select patients whose care needs are low for each category, especially in basic home care, where potential differences between costs and reimbursement can be greatest. If a hospice can serve patients who require one skilled visit each week and emergency telephone access as needed, their balance sheets will look good. If, however, a hospice accepts patients and families with marginal coping skills or more extensive nursing needs, it will be more difficult to pay the bills from the same income. Therefore, in addition to the limits all hospices now have, Medicare hospice programs are likely to show a preference for patients whose care needs are relatively modest.

Is the population targeted for hospice services limited justifiably? Are there other patients for whom hospice-type services would be similarly advantageous? Hospice services are delivered by an interdisciplinary team that seeks to provide comprehensive care to patients. The focus is on effective symptom control and patient self-determination.

Many patients who are far from dying could benefit from most services hospice programs offer. Patients facing severe loss in independence or curtailment of aspirations due to illness would benefit from a hospice provider's attentive, comprehensive care and effective symptom control. The emphasis of hospice on the emotional turmoil of dying is neither so unique (since most people faced with serious loss experience similar emotions) nor so limited to hospice (since hospitals and other settings are capable of providing adequate support) as to justify separating the endeavor and granting special funding.

Even if benefits from the coordinated program of care hospice offers are to be limited to patients reliably considered to be dying, reasons to limit benefits to cancer patients with substantial resources in home and family are even harder to discern. Instead of redressing a social inequity, this allocation serves to perpetuate or exacerbate it. The poor patient who has too few resources to comfortably die at home, or who has no home, is likely to be in greater need than the patient who will receive care under existing medical care schemes. Similarly, elderly patients, for whom the Medicare benefit is designed, are less likely to have caregivers available in the home. Thus, only the privileged elderly with a healthy spouse (or otherwise quite supportive family), and with adequate resources, will be likely to receive hospice benefits.

Poor and elderly dying patients with inadequate homes are largely cared for in hospitals and nursing homes. In hospitals, they are often considered less desirable patients and treated less assiduously than younger patients who are more emotionally appealing or elderly persons who may yet be cured. Symptom control is unlikely to be maximally effective, as staffing and practice patterns preclude rapid responses.

In nursing homes, the staff is often too small and inadequately trained to provide effectively for the patient's subjective concerns and symptoms. In addition, neither hospital nor nursing home care is likely to be paid for by Medicare once the patient's advanced disease forces the goals of treatment to be reduced to symptomatic care. Therefore, available alternatives for a patient who does not qualify for hospice care are distinctly less desirable.

Patients excluded from hospice and remanded to these other alternatives (hospitals and nursing homes) should have been excluded for better reasons than administrative convenience or political necessity. To establish policies that widen the gap between those served and those excluded is hard to justify. Laudable responses to these inequities include expanding hospice to serve all dying people or directing substantial energies and resources into those care modalities intended for dying persons who are not in hospices.

Because health care is costly and because the need for care is unpredictable, often beyond patients' control, and unevenly distributed, most people cannot provide for their health care without some mechanism for sharing costs with others. This sharing of costs is done through private insurance and through government programs. Policies that restrict access to health care financed collectively, including hospice, should not discriminate in arbitrary ways or distribute the costs of care unfairly. From the preceding discussion, it is clear that hospice care, under Medicare, will be accessible only to limited categories of patients. Yet, as a federally funded program, all citizens pay for the service. If the programs divert resources that otherwise would have gone to the underserved who rely upon Medicare in order to serve the relatively well-off, it will be difficult to justify the distribution of benefits and burdens engendered by the program.

SUMMARY

Health care is a value-rich field of human endeavor. Conflicts among values often create dilemmas for practitioners. Hospice has inherited many problems endemic elsewhere in health care, although some of the concerns become more pressing or more frequent in hospice. The Medicare benefit for hospice has created additional concerns, especially with regard to equity in the allocation of public benefits. While hospice personnel cannot resolve all of these concerns, an awareness of them and a familiarity with their importance will help to keep hospice from becoming embroiled in controversies that would best be avoided. Moreover, hospice policymakers, planners, and administrators can take a leading role in discussing and resolving those values dilemmas that have serious and persistent impacts on the hospice endeavor.

NOTES

1. Lewis Thomas, "Dying as Failure," *Annals of the American Academy of Politics and Social Science* 447 (1980): 1; John P. Callan, "The Hospice Movement," *Journal of the American Medical Association* 241 (February 9, 1979): 600; Marian Osterweis and Daphne S. Champagne, "U.S. Hospice Movement: Issues in Development," *American Journal of Public Health* 69 (May 1979): 492–496; Nina Millett, "Hospice: Challenging Society's Approach to Death," *Health and Social Work* 4 (1979): 131; Victor Zorza and Rosemary Zorza, *A Way to Die* (New York: Alfred A. Knopf, 1980).

2. Rosemary Johnson-Hurzeler, Evelyn Barnum, and John Abbott, "Hospice: The Beginning or the End? The Impact of TEFRA on Hospice Care in the United States," *University of Bridgeport Law Review* 5 (1983): 69–105.

3. The National Commission for the Protection of Human Subjects of Biomedical and Behavioral Research, *The Belmont Report* (Washington, D.C.: U.S. Department of Health, Education, and Welfare, 1978), 4-10; Tom L. Beauchamp and James F. Childress, *Principles of Biomedical Ethics*

(Oxford: Oxford University Press, 1979); The President's Commission for the Study of Ethical Problems in Medicine and Biomedical and Behavioral Research, *Summing Up* (Washington, D.C.: U.S. Government Printing Office, 1983), 66-71.

4. Talcott Parsons, "The Sick Role," in *The Social System* (New York: Free Press, 1951), 433-473; Renee Fox, "The Sting of Death in American Society" in *Social Service Review* (March 1981): 42-59; Sol Levine and Martin A. Kozloff, "The Sick Role: Assessment and Overview," *Annual Review of Sociology* 4 (1978): 317-344.

5. The President's Commission for the Study of Ethical Problems in Medicine and Biomedical and Behavioral Research, *Making Health Care Decisions* (Washington, D.C.: U.S. Government Printing Office, 1982).

6. The President's Commission for the Study of Ethical Problems in Medicine and Biomedical and Behavioral Research, *Deciding To Forego Life-Sustaining Treatment* (Washington, D.C.: U.S. Government Printing Office, 1983) (hereafter, *Deciding To Forego Treatment*), 132-133.

7. National Hospice Organization, *Standards of a Hospice Program of Care* (Arlington, Va.: National Hospice Organization, 1981); Melvin J. Krant, "Hospice Philosophy in Late-Stage Cancer Care," *Journal of the American Medical Association* 245 (March 13, 1981): 1061-1062.

8. Department of Health and Human Services, Health Care Financing Administration, "Medicare Program, Hospice Care, Final Rule," *Federal Register* 48 (December 16,1983): 56008-56036, at 56008 (hereafter, HHS, "Final Rule").

9. HHS, "Final Rule," 56027.

10. Howard Brody and Joanne Lynn, "The Physician's Responsibility under the the New Medicare Reimbursement for Hospice Care," *New England Journal of Medicine* 310 (April 5,1984): 920-922.

11. R. A. Pearlman, T. S. Inui, and W. B. Carter, "Variability in Physician Bioethical Decision-Making: A Case Study of Euthanasia," *Annals of Internal Medicine* 97 (1982): 420-425; J. E. Dunphy, "Annual Discourse: On Caring for the Patient with Cancer," *New England Journal of Medicine* 295 (1976): 313-319; Jerome W. Yates, F. Patrick McKegney, and Larry E. Kun, "A Comparative Study of Home Nursing Care of Patients with Advanced Cancer," *Proceedings of the American Cancer Society*, Third National Conference on Human Values and Cancer (1982), 207-218.

12. Sidney H. Wanzer, S. James Adelstein, Ronald E. Cranford et al., "The Physician's Responsibility toward Hopelessly Ill Patients," *New England Journal of Medicine* 310 (April 12, 1984): 955-959; *Deciding To Forego Treatment*, 24-26; Joanne Lynn, letter to the editor, "Physicians' Responsibility toward the Hopelessly Ill" in *New England Journal of Medicine* 311 (1984): 334-335.

13. *Deciding To Forego Treatment*, 82-89.

14. Note, "The California Natural Death Act: An Empirical Study of Physician's Practices," *Stanford Law Review* 31 (1979) 913.

15. John F. Potter, "A Challenge for the Hospice Movement," *New England Journal of Medicine* 302 (January 3, 1980) 53-55.

16. Ibid.

17. Peter Mudd, "High Ideals and Hard Cases: The Evolution of a Hospice," *Hastings Center Report* 12 (1982): 11-14.

18. Larry Churchill, "The Ethics of Hospice Care," in *Hospice: Development and Administration*, ed. Glen Davidson (Washington, D.C.: Hemisphere, 1984).

19. Potter, "A Challenge for the Hospice Movement."

20. HHS, "Final Rule," 56029.

21. *Deciding To Forego Treatment*; Appendix E, "Statutes and Proposals to Empower Appointment of Proxies," 390-437.

22. HHS, "Final Rule," 56010, 56027.

23. George A. Oakes, "A Prosecutor's View of Treatment Decisions," in A. Edward Doudera and J. Douglas Peters, eds., *Legal and Ethical Aspects of Treating Critically and Terminally Ill Patients* (Ann Arbor, Mich.: AUPHA Press, 1982); Abigail L. Kuzma, "Hospice: The Legal Ramifications of a Place to Die," *Indiana Law Journal* 56 (1981): 673-702; *Deciding To Forego Treatment*, 32-39.

24. Ibid., 32-39, 63-73.

25. Ibid., 68-70.

26. Mary J. Baines, "Control of Other Symptoms," in Cicely M. Saunders, *The Management of Terminal Disease* (London: Edward Arnold, 1978), 102-103.

27. Joyce V. Zerwekh, "The Dehydration Question," *Nursing 83*, 1983, 47-49; Joanne Lynn and James F. Childress, "Must a Patient Always Be Given Food and Water?" *Hastings Center Report* 13 (October 1983): 17-19.

28. The President's Commission for the Study of Ethical Problems in Medicine and Biomedical and Behavioral Research, *Securing Access to Health Care* (Washington, D.C.: U.S. Government Printing Office, 1983), 4.

29. The Tax Equity and Fiscal Responsibility Act of 1982, Sect. 122; Public Law 97-248 (U.S.C.A. Sections 1395c-1395f (West 1982)).

30. Ellen A. Pryga and Henry Bachofer, "Hospice Care under Medicare" (Chicago: American Hospital Association, Office of Public Policy Analysis, Working Paper, June 24, 1983), 13-18.

31. Ibid., 3-6.

32. HHS, "Final Rule," 56033-56034.

Chapter 13

Concepts and Applications of Bereavement Programming

David M. Dush

The hospice concept has always incorporated consideration of the family as well as the patient. The formalized bereavement service within the hospice's organizational structure is therefore a natural extension. Indeed, the provision of bereavement care is a mandated (but not reimbursed) component under current Medicare legislation in the United States and has become an integral part of the definition of hospice.[1]

This chapter examines various clinical models of bereavement care, as well as the basic elements of bereavement programming. Attention is also given to staff training, supervision, continuity of care, and liability concerns. These points are illustrated in a discussion of a case example, the bereavement services of Hospice of Central Iowa. The chapter is designed to provide an outline of major concerns for individuals developing or revising a bereavement program and to serve as a guide to selected references for further study.

BEREAVEMENT CARE: IN SEARCH OF A MODEL

Providing support to those in grief is part of hospice care, from the first family contact to the last. Even at the time of admission the family is aware of the impending death, and in most cases a complex process of "anticipatory grief" has begun in the family's accommodation to the loss.[2] The patients, too, must grieve their own death; there is a striking parallel between the components of coping with one's own death[3] and the components of grieving over the loss of a loved one.[4] Thus, while a hospice bereavement program generally deals with support of the family after the patient's death, the *process of bereavement* itself is not so sharply segmented; many of the same services and goals pertain to patient and family care prior to the death as well.

The objective of a bereavement program is to provide support for the survivors in the family and to ease their transition toward adjustment to life without the deceased. While on the surface this seems straightforward, the question of effective bereavement care is complex: what kind(s) of care, at what intensity, in what combination, for how long, should be provided to which clients, with which needs, by whom, under what circumstances, with what intended effect? The question applies whether a program is based upon neighborly volunteerism or professional models of intervention. The conceptualization of grief from which a program operates provides the basic blueprint for development and prioritization of services, and this warrants explicit attention.

Normal and Abnormal Grief

Program administrators and planners should recognize that there are *two subgroups* of the population to be served—those experiencing *normal* grief and those experiencing *pathological* grief. The boundary between these is elusive and may change over time, but the distinction is important to both supportive care and program development.

Normal grief carries no implication of psychiatric disorder. The diagnostic manual of the American Psychiatric Association notes that "A full depressive syndrome frequently is a normal reaction to such a loss, with feelings of depression and such associated symptoms as poor appetite, weight loss, and insomnia."[5] There is marked variability in the intensity, duration, and fluctuation of these symptoms, some of which may be accounted for by cultural differences.

It is useful to group the symptoms of grief into these three spheres: feelings, behaviors, and thoughts. Common feelings are sadness, disbelief, emotional pain of loss, emptiness, anger, guilt, or anxiety. Grief behaviors frequently observed include crying, panic or loss of control, withdrawal and disruption of social relationships, physical illness or distress, disruption of ability to function, overactivity, or fatigue. In the realm of thoughts and cognitive functioning one commonly finds extensive preoccupation with thoughts of the deceased and the death, disbelief, confusion, distractibility, disruptive dreams, and even hallucinations or a sense of presence of the deceased.[6] All or none of these may appear. They may come and go cyclically, they may appear after a delay, and they may last (but generally decrease) over two years or more.[7]

Under other circumstances, even a handful of severe symptoms of this type might easily suggest psychopathology. But as a response to a significant loss, all can fall within the normal process of adjustment. For most persons, this is the case. For others, the process takes on the qualities of "pathological grief," resulting in more extended debilitation and often a need for professional intervention. Current diagnostic guidelines from the American Psychiatric Association[8] suggest that there are several indications that bereavement is no longer uncomplicated:

1. Morbid or unusual preoccupation with worthlessness
2. Prolonged and severe impairment of functioning
3. Notable slowing of motoric functions
4. Guilt that goes beyond the typical concerns about what should or shouldn't have been done during the illness and the time of death
5. Suicidal ideation beyond the common questioning such as "Why not me?" or "Wouldn't I be better off dead?"

In addition to the above indicators, Worden delineates four patterns of grief that are viewed as abnormal grief reactions:[9]

1. Chronic grief reactions: bereavement is excessive in duration with little or no progress toward its resolution.
2. Delayed grief reactions: excessive grieving or emotional response occurs to a loss that happens some time after the death, perhaps even to witnessing the loss experienced by another person.
3. Exaggerated grief reactions: bereavement entails excessive intensity of emotional and functional disruption, such as suicidal ideation that poses lethal levels of risk.
4. Masked grief reactions: grief is expressed indirectly, without awareness, in forms such as physical symptoms or unusual behaviors.

A common example of masked grief is the disruptive behavior adolescents sometimes display after a parent's death, making no conscious connection between their grief and their behavior. For instance, a child may remain quite aloof from the family as death of a parent approaches, and aloof from efforts of the hospice team trying to provide support. In some cases this is accompanied by unusual increases in problem behavior or decreased performance at school of a magnitude that may warrant active intervention by the family, the hospice team, or professional back-up caregivers.

A classic example of physical expression of grief was a man whose wife had died of throat cancer after a long series of treatments and disfiguring surgeries and many changes of physicians. Aside from indications that the man felt compelled to find a cure for his wife beyond the point that was clearly the terminal phase of the illness, he appeared to cope quite well with the eventual death of his wife. However, within two weeks he lost his voice and could only whisper. He began a long series of consultations with physicians who could find no medical basis for the problem. He reluctantly complied with a psychiatric examination requested by one of the early physicians and an informal meeting with the hospice psychologist at the suggestion of his bereavement caregiver. However, he remained convinced that his disorder was physical and not at all psychological, and thus refused to participate in psychological treatments for the problem.

The three spheres of grief—feelings, behaviors, and thoughts—are closely intertwined. However, the thoughts associated with grief can be especially potent and may be pivotal in the progression from normal grief to abnormal grief. Indeed, Abrahms notes that distortions and twists of thinking are the distinctive features of pathological grief, signaled by "erroneous and overgeneralized meaning that the person ascribes to the loss."[10] In pathological grief the mourner continues to dwell on the thoughts of the deceased, but the boundaries of grief extend beyond the deceased, ultimately incorporating loss of self-worth, meaning, gratification, and hope. Abrahms characterizes normal, reality-based grief with thoughts such as "I am deeply and painfully saddened," while pathological grief becomes dominated with distorted thoughts such as "I will never be happy again." He further argues that "Time alone does not heal such ruminative and destructive thoughts. In fact, if mistaken beliefs are left unchallenged, an undesirable self-fulfilling prophecy may ensue, and the person's condition may worsen."[11]

Program Implications

The distinction between normal and pathological grief has two essential implications for administrators planning bereavement services. First, the bereaved, as a group, are "at risk" for complicated bereavement. Therefore, bereavement staff need to be trained to recognize the signs of pathological grief and have a mechanism to respond to them in a timely and effective manner. Second, bereavement program design should reflect whether direct services will be offered to those in normal grief, abnormal grief, or both.

It is probably most common for hospices to develop supportive services to be offered to all bereaved families. A typical example is Hospice of Columbus (Ohio). In this hospice, all families receive at least one follow-up visit by the team nurse, are invited to regular social/supportive suppers, and are contacted on the first anniversary date of death.[12] Persons in need of more intensive services can be referred to consulting mental health professionals or community mental health resources.

An alternative to the above approach used by many hospice administrators facing resource concerns is the provision of services to those considered to be in greatest need—that is, those at greatest risk of unfavorable adjustment. This approach is utilized at St. Christopher's Hospice, where the high volume of services (over 600 deaths per year) makes it difficult to attend to all bereaved families. Parkes has employed a "Bereavement Risk Index" to screen families at highest risk and to offer these persons intensive help by specially trained volunteer counselors.[13] Parkes and Weiss argue that this strategy may have more to offer than efficiency:

> The evidence available at this time seems to indicate that bereavement services that focus their counseling on bereaved people at special risk do succeed in their aim of reducing risk, but unselective services may be without overall beneficial effects.[14]

It is quite reasonable, of course, to blend both routine supportive services for all survivors and intensive care for those who require additional attention. There are two cautions that managers and planners should bear in mind. First, there is little empirical research that demonstrates the impact of specific types of bereavement care or combinations of interventions in hospice settings. It is necessary to rely heavily upon observation and evaluation of local program impact in building and refining the program. Second, the objectives and interventions of different types of bereavement care vary, and programming and evaluations of effectiveness must reflect these differences. Indeed, it may not be practical to measure two programs against the same standards. For example, we might expect *general* support services to show some impact on feelings of alienation, anxiety level, or perhaps perceived quality of life. On the other hand, measures of social withdrawal, morbid distortions of thinking, or level of cognitive functioning may be more appropriate outcome indices for *intensive* grief therapy interventions.

THE OBJECTIVES OF BEREAVEMENT CARE

Hospice providers must know and understand the objectives of their program's bereavement services. Worden suggests that there are four "tasks" or objectives of grief and these should be reflected in bereavement counseling:[15]

1. To accept the reality of loss
2. To experience the pain of grief
3. To adjust to an environment without the deceased
4. To re-invest emotional energy into other relationships

There is little empirical evidence that regular stages of widowhood can be identified.[16] However, Worden argues that all four of the above tasks must be negotiated in some form before grief is resolved and individual growth occurs.[17] This view closely parallels that of Parkes and Weiss, who suggest that:

> Three distinct tasks in recovery are: first, that the loss be accepted intellectually; second, that the loss be accepted emotionally; and third,

that the individual's model of self and outer world change to match the new reality.[18]

Worden provides a very useful clinical guide to the therapeutic skills and interventions needed to work with the bereaved. He distinguishes between grief "counseling" and grief "therapy," referring to work with uncomplicated versus complicated grief, respectively.[19] The goals of *grief counseling* follow directly from efforts to enhance the person's ability to complete each of the tasks of grief. Worden elaborates this into ten principles of grief counseling,[20] each of which warrants consideration by the program planner:

1. Help the survivor deal with the reality of the loss: telling and retelling the story of the death and its details (which is often discouraged by friends and family) can help one to come to grips with the finality of the loss.
2. Help the survivor express and cope with emotions: anger, guilt, anxiety, and helplessness are common feelings that are especially hard for many survivors to recognize and express.
3. Assist in the task of living without the deceased: new skills often need to be learned and many decisions and adjustments made for the survivor to reach a new stable lifestyle.
4. Help the survivor emotionally withdraw from the deceased, yet not jump too quickly into new relationships: this is a difficult area for many persons where encouragement and counseling are helpful.
5. Allow the survivor time to grieve, especially at critical times such as anniversaries and holidays.
6. Provide reassurance about the survivor's symptoms that may seem abnormal to them but in fact are normal.
7. Allow a great deal of flexibility for individual differences in the pattern and progression of grieving.
8. Provide continuing support, with especially flexible availability in critical periods, for at least a year.
9. When possible, help the survivor recognize coping styles and work toward modifications of those that are ineffective.
10. Identify warning signs of pathological grief and refer for more intensive services.

It may also be useful to explore expanded cognitive interventions as part of not only grief therapy, but grief counseling as well. Cognitive therapies have proven to be effective with depression.[21] They have yet to be adequately tested for the various levels of bereavement care, but field experience to date is encouraging. Abrahms provides several examples of application of these principles to pathological grief.[22] This entails helping persons become aware of their self-statements and patterns of thinking, assessing these cognitions and the impact that they have, and learning ways of changing or replacing thoughts that prove to be maladaptive.[23]

For example, one woman who obsessed at length about endless "ifs" relating to her husband's death repeatedly said to herself, "If I had only called the doctor sooner . . . If I had only forced him to get a check-up . . . If I had only been able to spend some time with him at home before he died," and so forth. Among other things, these thoughts kept her reliving the death in a state of unreality. Playing out the events around the death in different ways helped her to avoid her present situation. Consequently, the first task of grieving, and accepting the reality of the loss, had not been adequately resolved. She was not really aware of the frequency or pattern of these thoughts until she was instructed to deliberately monitor them. Once recognized, unwanted thoughts may still be persistent. In this woman's case, and generally for those in uncomplicated grief, recognition of these patterns helps to effectively focus efforts toward modifying them.

These principles of grief counseling are widely applicable to bereavement programming. They should be addressed in training programs for bereavement helpers and volunteers, whether they provide general support to all families or intensive care for those at high risk. Furthermore, the principles provide useful guidance in ongoing case consultation, supervision, and quality assurance review.

Worden suggests that *grief therapy*, for survivors experiencing pathological grief, requires highly skilled professionals with specialized training.[24] Pathological grief typically entails complications of preexisting problems or personality traits of the survivor, difficult circumstances of the death, inadequate social support or coping resources, and perhaps most frequently, unresolved areas of deep-rooted conflict in some aspect of the relationship with the deceased. It follows from this framework that the goals of grief therapy lie within the context of intensive psychotherapy. Clearly, the bereavement program manager must anticipate that both uncomplicated and complicated bereavement will be encountered in the survivors served. Therefore, even a hospice that elects to provide general support or grief counseling needs to have a mechanism for identification and referral of more difficult cases. If the hospice does not have its own mental health staff or consultants, referral relationships can be developed with community mental health agencies, many of which are obligated to provide free or low-cost consultation and care.

It is not always clear when the problems of a survivor have reached a level of severity that requires professional intervention. Much rests upon the adequacy of the communication and back-up systems within the bereavement program so that observations and concerns of the volunteer helper can be voiced as they arise and timely support can be provided. There is some research support for the notion than lay counselors with modest training can achieve good therapeutic results, in some cases better than professionals.[25] Effectiveness is probably enhanced when the problems are circumscribed rather than diffuse, and adequate back-up support is provided.[26] Dush, Conley and Thompson provide a training manual that may be helpful in this range of service delivery.[27] It is designed as an introductory guide for inexperienced lay counselors, with back-up of professionals. The manual operates from the hypothesis that a basic level of supportive interpersonal interaction can be helpful. At present, however, there remains a critical void of research and evaluation addressing these questions directly.

A CASE STUDY OF BEREAVEMENT CARE: HOSPICE OF CENTRAL IOWA

The developer of a bereavement program is faced with a wide range of interventions and program elements that can be used to assemble the program structure. A case illustration of a hospice program is discussed below in order to provide a context for viewing these elements.

Hospice of Central Iowa (HCI) is a home-based hospice that is a self-governing, nonprofit organization. It began as an entirely volunteer program and remains heavily volunteer staffed. Each patient care team is staffed by a part-time staff nurse and four volunteers. The volunteers spend an average of ten hours weekly in direct care. HCI is also certified as a home health agency, certified for Medicare reimbursement, and accredited by the Joint Commission on Accreditation of Hospitals. The average census is about 30. As in most such hospices, half of the patients typically die within a few weeks after admission.

There are three types of bereavement service staffing: the bereavement coordinator, the volunteers, and the professional back-up staff. The program is coordinated by a 3/4-time staff person with extensive experience in self-help grief support programs. The coordinator also has at least two direct contacts with each family served. The bulk of the direct support of survivors is provided by bereavement volunteers. Most of the volunteers have experience with direct patient care teams; many currently serve on patient care teams. All bereavement volunteers attend the standard training program for patient care volunteers and continue with specialized training in bereavement care. Volunteers and program administration also have the benefits of professional back-up. A consulting psychologist, a consulting chaplain, the medical director, a staff social worker, and the nursing staff are available as needed. Consultants meet with the coordinator weekly to review problem cases. The psychologist, social worker, and chaplain assist with in-service training programs, staffing monthly bereavement volunteer meetings and seeing clients as needed for interventions or assessment.

The coordinator attends weekly interdisciplinary meetings where all hospice patients are staffed, and thus has a basic familiarity with families at the time of the patient's death. Special problems of families, such as parent-child conflicts, generally surface during these meetings.

After notification of a patient's death, the coordinator begins planning for assignment to bereavement care. The first contact with the family does not normally occur for two or three weeks. This allows time for the family to deal with the confusion and turmoil of the death. The patient care team and the staff nurse are available to the family during this period. They may assist with arrangements, attend the funeral, address special needs, and begin to make the transition away from the family. The level of involvement at this stage varies considerably as a function of family need and preference. Many families desire a great deal of privacy immediately following the death and want little outside assistance. Others require an increased level of attention.

Typically, the first contact of the bereavement program is through a letter conveying sympathy, reminding the survivor about the availability of bereavement support and announcing that a bereavement worker will call. The second contact is by telephone. Both the letter and phone call are used to help the survivor feel more comfortable in the initial contacts and thus more likely to continue in the program. The coordinator makes the first call. The objectives of the call are to provide a supportive intervention, reaffirming concern for the survivor and availability of assistance, assessing receptivity to bereavement care, assessing clinical status and intensity of need, and informing the survivor that a volunteer will call. Few persons are highly resistant at this contact: most talk quite openly, often for an hour or more.

The next contact, within a few days, is a telephone call from the volunteer. The caller spends time getting acquainted, inquires about how things are going, assesses the survivor's receptivity to continued contact, and attempts to plan for continued contact. This can be a delicate process, and we encourage volunteers to approach the situation sensitively but within their natural style. Unless the coordinator has made some specific recommendations to the volunteer ahead of time (the coordinator should have already discussed the case and likely needs or problems with the volunteer), the method and frequency of contacts is left to emerge from this first call by the volunteer. Some clients indicate they want no further help, and this wish is respected. Volunteers are trained to try to separate this from instances where clients are simply ambivalent or reluctant to impose or ask for help. In the latter case, the volunteer will at least suggest that "I'll call again next week," rather than leaving the more tenuous status of "call me if you need me." Most often some regular pattern of contact evolves, such as occasional phone calls, home visits, or social meetings such as lunch.

Survivors are also invited to attend monthly "pot-luck" dinners. These meetings are important social events, often the only social events attended by the widowed in the first few months after the death. The agenda includes some sort of program that is either entertainment oriented or educationally oriented. Ed-

ucational topics include financial planning, presentations on community resources, or presentations on psychosocial topics such as stress management or
coping with anger. It is common for volunteers to pick up their clients and attend
these events together.

A common difficulty voiced by bereavement volunteers has to do with managing the excessive dependency that the survivor may exhibit. Two common
signs of this are the volunteer's feelings of resentment of the demands being
placed upon him or her and difficulty in bringing the helping relationship to a
close. These pitfalls warrant attention, since they can undermine the effectiveness
of the helping relationship and contribute to increased turnover of volunteers
and reduced satisfaction of the volunteer with the work. An essential counter-
measure is adequacy of assertiveness skills; this merits inclusion in volunteer
training, and further attention in supervision of volunteers who have difficult
cases or persisting areas of assertiveness skill deficits. Also emphasized with
the volunteers is the fact that the process of termination of the helping relationship
begins at the outset of the relationship. In some cases, informal friendships
continue, but the counseling contacts are expected to begin to taper in frequency,
moving toward cessation in most cases within one year. Survivors are also
provided appropriate expectations of the bereavement program's timeframe and
other limitations of the bereavement services at the initial orientation of the
family to hospice and, as needed, throughout the time of bereavement support.

The last official bereavement contact is the anniversary call one year after the
death. This serves a closure function as well as a supportive one at a time that
is difficult for most persons. Calls are made by the coordinator, providing an
opportunity for a final clinical assessment and informal evaluation of the bereavement care. The transition back to talking with the coordinator does not
seem to pose a problem for the bereaved; most of these conversations last an
hour or more.

A few exceptions occur to the above progression. In rare cases, the bereavement staff may begin contact before the death has occurred. One case in point
was a very angry spouse who was disruptively furious at the physicians, hospitals,
neighbors, and nearly everyone else over what he perceived as inept care of his
wife. It also appeared that this anger ran deeper, reflecting his own difficulties
in accepting the death of his wife, his feelings of abandonment and resentment,
his powerlessness to prevent the death, and his fear of facing life alone. Recognizing a high risk for complicated grief, a supportive relationship with a highly
experienced bereavement worker was established. This provided a symbolic link
to the bereavement ahead and initiated the building of a working relationship
for what was expected (and proved) to be a difficult negotiation of the tasks of
grief.

A second exception occurs when the bereavement helper is also part of the
patient care team. Normally, a new person is assigned. In rare instances where

there seems to be a clear clinical advantage to keeping up one of the relationships already established, an exception is made. An example might be a family where a child is having difficulty accepting the parent's death and has been able to relate openly only with difficulty and only to one member of the team.

The third type of exception is when intervention by the coordinator or the back-up staff alters the course of the progression. At HCI, all families are offered bereavement support, and ordinarily there is no direct contact with the backup staff. There are, however, mechanisms to allow the level of supportive care to be responsive to the survivor's level of difficulty in grieving. Volunteers call the coordinator if problems arise and routinely discuss their cases monthly. Regular supervision is encouraged, requiring those who miss two consecutive meetings to resume regular attendance before new cases are assigned. Problems with cases are discussed with back-up staff. From these sources, suggestions may emerge to increase or decrease the intensity of support, to discontinue some intervention, to try some new one, or to refer the client for assessment or care of the back-up staff or other professionals. Much of this constitutes an ongoing screening, from the first contact to the last. This ensures that appropriate measures can be taken to intercept problems as they develop.

Elements of Bereavement Programming

The HCI model illustrates the minimal "core elements" that administrators should address in any hospice bereavement program, regardless of whether support services are provided to all survivors or only to those at risk:

1. Direct personal contact with the survivor, with an opportunity to develop an individual supportive or therapeutic relationship
2. Flexible frequency and intensity of contacts in response to an individualized assessment of survivor needs
3. A clinically experienced coordinator, to provide volunteer support and supervision
4. A risk assessment at entry to try to predict those likely to cope poorly, using a risk index (see, for example, Parkes and Weiss[28]) or a clinical evaluation of risk indicators (see Lindstrom[29])
5. A multidisciplinary back-up team with regular involvement in training and case consultation
6. Mechanisms for review, case follow-up, and program evaluation

There is much flexibility in the way a program can be structured around these core elements. At HCI there are four principal levels of supportive care that are routinely applied:

1. Support of the patient care team around the time of death
2. Assessment, support, and follow-up contacts by the coordinator
3. Individual support by the assigned volunteer
4. Group functions such as pot-luck dinners

There are crucial advantages in having multiple levels of intervention. Foremost, people will respond quite differently to the various interventions. Many persons who respond well to one intervention, such as group functions, may want no part of other services. Second, each level of intervention provides unique effects. For example, the special bond that develops in individual sessions may be difficult to produce in group meetings or social events. The converse is equally true. Finally, multilevel programming allows for built-in responsiveness to level of need. Those patients who need and want more intensive contact have an array of support available, while others may elect more modest levels of contact.

Group support is a popular component—sometimes the only component—of hospice bereavement programs.[30] This may be partly due to the efficiency of intervening with groups rather than individuals. The potential time savings is not a trivial matter. If the average length of stay of a patient in a hospice is three months and the survivors are followed for a year, it becomes clear that the caseload for the hospice bereavement program can swell to staggering numbers. Add this to the lack of fiscal reimbursement for providing bereavement care and the allocation of resources quickly becomes a challenge.

There are also clinical factors that make group support an attractive option. For example, the HCI pot-luck dinners provide a form of support with many advantages:

1. They allow the survivor to meet with other persons in similar circumstances.
2. They allow survivors to learn of others' progress and tell their own story.
3. They encourage survivors to compare their progress to that of others.
4. They demonstrate that the survivor can still relate effectively in a social group.
5. They promote maintenance of social contacts and new friendships at a time when forces pull toward social withdrawal and isolation.
6. They provide a form of support that may be less awkward or intrusive, since it carries no stigma of "mental health treatment."
7. They provide an opportunity to slowly permit oneself to have fun again (negotiating the fears that this can't happen or that it shouldn't out of loyalty to the deceased).
8. They provide a context for a new identity to be formed in the group and assist in forming a new identity in general.

There are a number of types of group functions bereavement coordinators consider:

1. Autonomous self-help groups that are initiated by the hospice
2. Regular dinners or social gatherings
3. Field trips to social events
4. Educational presentations on topics such as nutrition, exercise, or financial planning
5. Grief-oriented educational presentations (stress management, spiritual aspects of grief, etc.)
6. Specialized support groups
7. Group psychotherapy

A continuum runs through these functions with varied hospice or professional involvement. At one extreme is the pure self-help support group that manages itself and its events without formal hospice control. These may be worthwhile groups for hospices to assist in setting up, but administrators should not rely upon them to "constitute" the bereavement program. It is, however, helpful to encourage survivors to play a large role in helping to run the groups, establishing phone networks or car pools and prioritizing the goals of the group. At the other extreme are group therapy or other highly structured group functions that are professionally staffed. Group therapy can be very helpful, but it is not appropriate for most survivors. Hospices that elect to follow the model described by Parkes and Weiss,[31] where resources are directed to those at highest risk, may find group counseling to be an effective medium for intensive supportive care.

A hybrid of group functions seems to have worked well at HCI and elsewhere.[32] At HCI the pot-luck dinners combine survivor input, entertainment and social functions, and periodic educational presentations. Specialized groups for adolescents or for relatives and friends of the deceased have proven helpful at HCI. Boulder County Hospice has similarly developed special groups for bereaved parents.[33]

ORGANIZATIONAL ISSUES FOR THE BEREAVEMENT PROGRAM

Staff Recruitment & Training

The complexity of the treatment issues in grief support and counseling lead to challenging issues in organizing a bereavement program and training staff. HCI has drawn heavily from the ranks of former bereavement clients for its bereavement volunteers. This rich resource provides managers with a reservoir of individuals who have relevant skills and experience. It is important that prospective volunteers wait at least a year after their own loss before beginning as a grief counselor. Grief counseling has a strong tendency to stir up one's own grief, even grief that seemed long since resolved. A year is minimal, but may not be sufficient; the coordinator should carefully evaluate the readiness of recruits in a face-to-face interview. The assessment should include information about the volunteer's motives, level of interpersonal social skills, openness to learning and constructive criticism, suitability for direct care versus other alternatives, and tolerance toward divergent personal values. It is useful to have some balance of volunteer characteristics such as race, age, and gender. It may be necessary to recruit specifically to fill the gaps, such as giving a presentation to local clubs and organizations.

At HCI, all bereavement volunteers go through the standard 30-hour volunteer training series. It covers broad medical, psychosocial, and pastoral aspects of hospice care. About half of the training is devoted to helping skills, death and dying, and bereavement. Ongoing special training in bereavement occurs at special seminars, at monthly meetings with the back-up staff, and in at least one all-day workshop per year. It is advisable to include generous portions of role-playing and experiential practice exercises in the training activities as well as didactic presentations.

Mantell and Ell provide a thorough curriculum for selection and training of hospice volunteers.[34] Several topics bear emphasis for bereavement care training:

1. Basic listening and empathy skills
2. Values clarification (being able to be helpful without imposing one's values)
3 Distinguishing pathological and normal grief
4. Identification of the problems of special populations such as the elderly, children, or adolescents[35]
5. Handling difficult symptoms (anger, guilt, dependency, etc.)
6. Planning for termination of the helping relationship
7. Determining how and when to consult and refer
8. Defining the helping role

The volunteer's understanding of the nature of the helping role is often over looked, but it is a cornerstone of a solid bereavement program. Volunteers are quite naturally inclined to define themselves as concerned friends of the survivors. This is a useful frame of reference. Volunteers will frequently begin to speak up during training to question "How on earth are we going to remember all these things and figure out the right thing to say?" At this point it is useful to suggest that the notion of being a good friend provides a useful, familiar "model" to guide one's decisions and responses to situations in the field. It also reassures them that it is fine to be themselves and apply their helping skills in a natural way.[36]

It is equally important for administrators to discuss with the volunteers the ways in which they are "not friends." That is, the volunteer is distinguishable from a friend in several crucial respects:

1. The volunteer's role is to help more than to be helped.
2. The volunteer is part of a service, with requirements for documentation, protection of confidentiality, and consultation among staff.
3. The volunteer's primary task is to give support and constructive feedback, not advice or answers.
4. The helping role is, from the start, designed to become obsolete.[37]

Bereavement coordinators should address professionalism and limit setting throughout the training. Those new to the helping field tend to take on the burdens of those they help. It is useful to point out that one cannot take responsibility for another's problems unless one also takes away the other's right to choose, which fosters dependency and does them no true service. In addition, the notion that, because of accountability requirements, they would be expected to pass on clinically vital information to their supervisor even if the client asked them not to do so (e.g., "Don't tell anyone, but I'm getting more and more suicidal") is typically unanticipated. It is also common that volunteers will go to considerable length, out of good intentions, to avoid actions that might lead to having their client referred for professional help. This seems to arise out of their own attachment of stigma to mental health treatment; some reassurance that persons do not need to be crazy to see a therapist helps to circumvent these obstacles.

Community organizations are valuable as training resources as well as referral resources. Agencies such as mental health centers, crisis lines, or hospitals often have extensive volunteer programs of their own. They may be very helpful in conducting part of the training, ongoing consultation, or perhaps a training program for trainers.

Continuity of Care

In the HCI model, a volunteer new to the family unit is almost always assigned at the time of the patient's death to become the bereavement caregiver. It seems at first blush that continuity of care would be better served by keeping a member of the patient care team as the bereavement worker. Experiences of hospices taking the latter route indicate frequent problems of dependency of the survivors and increased strain on the counseling and termination process for helpers as well. Assigning a new worker has the additional advantage of providing a new person to listen to the survivor's story, a support person of one's own. This individual is less strongly reminiscent of the deceased and thus less a stimulus for resurgent grief. Furthermore, the worker has a fresh perspective of the situation and is not also coping with grief over the same loss.

Continuity of care can be preserved, even when new bereavement workers are assigned, by careful attention to the interface of bereavement care and the initial patient care teams. At HCI, for example, the patient care team normally has a final team meeting after the patient's death. This helps to bring about closure and to provide mutual support for the team's grief. The bereavement coordinator or assigned worker can attend this meeting to review and assess the family's circumstances and special problems or assets of the survivors. As noted, the HCI coordinator also attends weekly staffings to keep informed about current cases. Finally, chart documentation is made available to the coordinator, including a closing summary by the team nurse and any recommendations for bereavement care. When problems arise, additional extended consultation with the team nurse is also secured.

Documentation and Liability

Hospice has entered a period of visibility as a new health care service. With this visibility and with licensure and reimbursement, hospices will be required to devote greater attention to matters of liability and documentation. In fact, the issue of liability has always been present in hospices that are not entirely volunteer. The ethical standards of psychologists, for example, assign responsibility for proper treatment to the psychologist even if the actual care was provided by a volunteer under his or her supervision. One might reasonably expect some latitude in dealing with volunteer counseling services, but this latitude is not well defined. Moreover, the professional or the program may be held liable if the structure of the system did not provide adequate safeguards for its recipients. Thus, not "knowing" about a survivor's lethal suicidal intent may not constitute any protection. These issues are discussed fully in Chapter 9.

All of this argues for competent documentation in the bereavement program. Adequate documentation also provides clinically useful data, enhances continuity of care, augments quality of care and utilization review functions, and provides a data base for evaluation and reporting requirements. In spite of the importance of documentation, many managers have yet to develop adequate systems. Miller surveyed 200 hospices and found that 34 percent of respondents had a formal bereavement assessment form, 18 percent had no assessment documented at all, and 10 percent did not even document progress.[38]

Details for developing a bereavement documentation system are suggested by the requirements of the Joint Commission on Accreditation of Hospitals. Minimally, the hospice record should contain:

1. Names and addresses of the surviving family members
2. Date of the patient's death (date of bereavement admission)

3. Date(s) of assessment
4. Documentation of the initial clinical needs assessment, including a checklist of critical symptoms (e.g., angry, sleepless, suicidal, confused, unable to stop crying) and some format to indicate an overall judgment of risk and coping adequacy
5. Staff assignment and additional service or referral recommendations (i.e., a plan of care)
6. Progress notes documenting all contacts and their dates
7. A closing form or other documentation of follow-up contacts and termination status

It is also advisable to consider data that may be needed for reporting or program evaluation that would need to be collected by the record system.

SUMMARY

This chapter examined clinical and management issues in hospice care for the bereaved. Discussions about bereavement care were premised on the notion that bereavement programs should be designed around careful, explicit clinical models of intervention. This imposes a degree of complexity that may be cumbersome to the administrator and planner, but it mirrors a complexity inherent in grief and grief counseling. Little hospice research and evaluation has appeared that clarifies the paths toward optimally effective and efficient bereavement care. Nonetheless, there is much to be learned from the experiences of hospices that have evolved reputable bereavement programs. In addition to studying HCI and the other program examples, hospice managers should consult and visit existing programs to gain first-hand observations and insights.

A final point concerns the importance of program evaluation to the bereavement program. Various models for hospice evaluation and the technology required have been discussed elsewhere.[39] The need is nowhere greater than for bereavement care; we have almost no solid research upon which to draw and little basis on which to base the effectiveness of services or the ways in which they could be enhanced. In addition, if bereavement care hopes to attain the status of "funded" as well as "mandated," refinements and empirical demonstrations of its effectiveness may well be decisive. Laboratory research cannot be expected to adequately capture the essence of hospice bereavement care. Advancement hinges upon careful field research and evaluation. Hospice managers and administrators need to consider methods for tracking patients, assessing their progress, and training volunteers in a systematic manner. They must also create incentives for internal audits that identify staff problems and point out situations of personal and organizational stress. Bereavement counseling is an integral part of hospice care. As preventive care for families it warrants the same degree of attention that pain and symptom control for patients has received.

NOTES

1. S. Stoddard,*The Hospice Movement* (New York: Vintage, 1978).

2. C. N. Aldrich, "Some Dynamics of Anticipatory Grief," in *Anticipatory Grief*, eds. B. Schoenberg, A. C. Carr, A. H. Kutscher, D. Peretz, and I. K. Goldberg (New York: Columbia University Press, 1974).

3. E. Kubler-Ross, *On Death and Dying* (New York: Macmillan, 1969).

4. M. Imaru, "Growing Through Grief," in *Hospice Care: Principles and Practice*, eds. C. A. Corr and D. M. Corr (New York: Springer, 1983).

5. American Psychiatric Association, *Diagnostic and Statistical Manual of Mental Disorders*, 3rd ed. (Washington, D.C.: American Psychiatric Association, 1980), 333.

6. I. Ainsworth-Smith and P. Speck, *Letting Go: Caring for the Dying and Bereaved* (London: Anchor Press, 1982); B. Raphael, *The Anatomy of Bereavement* (New York: Basic Books, 1983); M. L. S. Vachon, "Grief and Bereavement: The Family's Experience before and after Death," in *Care for the Dying and the Bereaved*, ed. I. Gentles (Toronto: Anglican Book Center, 1982); J. W. Worden, *Grief Counseling and Grief Therapy: A Handbook for the Mental Health Practitioner* (New York: Springer, 1982).

7. C. J. Barrett and K. M. Schneweis, "An Empirical Search for the Stages of Widowhood," *Omega* 11, 1980-81: 97-104; Imaru, "Growing through Grief."

8. American Psychiatric Association, *Diagnostic and Statistical Manual of Mental Disorders*.

9. Worden, *Grief Counseling and Grief Therapy*.

10. J. L. Abrahms, "Depression versus Normal Grief Following the Death of a Significant Other," in *New Directions in Cognitive Therapy: A Casebook*, eds. G. Emery, S. D. Hollon, and R. C. Bedrosian (New York: Guilford, 1981).

11. Ibid., 257.

12. L. Vande Creek, "A Homecare Hospice Profile: Description, Evaluation, and Cost Analysis," *Journal of Family Practice* 14 (1982): 53-58.

13. C. M. Parkes and R. S. Weiss, *Recovery from Bereavement* (New York: Basic Books, 1983).

14. Ibid., 217.

15. Worden, *Grief Counseling and Grief Therapy*.

16. Barrett and Schneweis, "An Empirical Search for the Stages of Widowhood."

17. Worden, *Grief Counseling and Grief Therapy*.

18. Parkes and Weiss, *Recovery from Bereavement*, 156.

19. Worden, *Grief Counseling and Grief Therapy*.

20. Ibid.

21. D. M. Dush, M. L. Hirt, and H. Schroeder, "Self-Statement Modification with Adults: A Meta-Analysis," *Psychological Bulletin* 94 (1983): 408-422; R. C. Miller and J. S. Berman, "The Efficacy of Cognitive-Behavior Therapies: A Quantitative Review of the Research Evidence," *Psychological Bulletin* 94 (1983): 39-53.

22. Abrahms, "Depression versus Normal Grief."

23. A. T. Beck, *Cognitive Therapy and the Emotional Disorders* (New York: International Universities Press, 1976); D. Meichenbaum, *Cognitive Behavior Modification* (New York: Plenum Press, 1977).

24. Worden, *Grief Counseling and Grief Therapy*.

25. J. A. Durlak, "Comparative Effectiveness of Paraprofessional and Professional Helpers," *Psychological Bulletin* 86 (1979): 80-92; J. A. Durlak, "Evaluating Comparative Studies of Paraprofessional and Professional Helpers: A Reply to Nietzel and Fisher," *Psychological Bulletin* 89 (1981): 566-569; J. A. Haltie, C. F. Sharpley, and H. J. Rogers, "Comparative Effectiveness of Professional and Paraprofessional Helpers," *Psychological Bulletin* 95 (1984): 534-541.

26. N. T. Nietzel and S. G. Fisher, "Effectiveness of Professional and Paraprofessional Helpers: A comment on Durlak," *Psychological Bulletin* 89 (1981): 555-565.

27. David M. Dush, G. Conley, and E. D. Thompson, *The Bereavement Helper: An Introductory Guide* (Des Moines: Hospice of Central Iowa, 1983).

28. Parkes and Weiss, *Recovery from Bereavement*.

29. B. Lindstrom, "Operating a Hospice Bereavement Program," in *Hospice Care: Principles and Practice*, eds. C. A. Corr and D. M. Corr (New York: Springer, 1983).

30. Vande Creek, "A Homecare Hospice Profile"; M. Lattanzi and D. Coffelt, *Bereavement Care Manual* (Boulder, Colo.: Boulder County Hospice, 1979); Lindstrom, "Operating a Hospice Bereavement Program."

31. Parkes and Weiss, *Recovery from Bereavement*.

32. Lindstrom, "Operating a Hospice Bereavement Program."

33. Lattanzi and Coffelt, *Bereavement Care Manual*.

34. J. E. Mantell and K. O. Ell, "Hospice Volunteer Programs: A Proposed Agenda," *The Hospice Journal: Physical, Psychological, and Pastoral Care of the Dying* 1 (1985), in press.

35. B. Conley, "Interdisciplinary Care in Adolescent Bereavement," in *Death and Grief in the Family*, eds. J. C. Hansen and T. T. Frantz (Rockville, Md.: Aspen Systems, 1984); J. D. Schumacher, "Helping Children Cope with a Sibling's Death," in *Death and Grief in the Family*, eds. J. C. Hansen and T. T. Frantz (Rockville, Md.: Aspen Systems, 1984).

36. Dush et al., *The Bereavement Helper*.

37. Ibid.

38. S. C. Miller, "Documentation in the Hospice Medical Record—Survey Results," *Journal of the American Medical Records Association*, 1983, 17-24.

39. David M. Dush and Barrie Cassileth, "Program Evaluation in Terminal Care," *The Hospice Journal: Physical, Psychological, and Pastoral Care of the Dying* 1 (1985) in press.

Chapter 14

Providing Hospice Care: The Changing Role and Status of Physicians

Paul T. Werner

As shown in the earlier chapters, the bulk of hospice care is provided by an interdisciplinary team consisting predominantly of nurses and lay volunteers. While nonphysician providers perform most hospice services, hospice movement organizers have lobbied to have programs legitimized by placing the clinical component under the direction of a physician. The exact phrase used in hospice rhetoric, as well as state and national rules, is "physician directed services." By emphasizing the physician as the "director" of services, the hospice seems to conform to the medical model of patient care, where doctors order others to carry out treatments and patient services.

In operation, however, most hospices do not duplicate the medical model. Care is provided by a team of professional and lay caregivers, all of whom have skills, knowledge, and experiences to contribute to patient care and decision making surrounding the treatment program. Furthermore, the patient and family are vital components of the caregiving team and the decision-making process. For physicians, steeped in the tradition of medicine, which expects doctors to dictate care plan decisions, the hospice represents a change in the routine conceptualization of patient care. For some physicians, hospice also represents an invasion of the physician's heretofore inviolate domain. Physicians choosing to work with a hospice team and program, either as a full-time employee or an occasional supporter, must adjust to this variation in perspective in order to be a contributing team member and a satisfied practitioner in the care of dying patients and survivors.

This chapter is designed to help decision makers understand the forces and conditions influencing physicians caring for terminally ill patients. It also explores changing roles and responsibilities of the physician in hospice settings, as well as the forces operating in physician-patient and physician-team interactions. The impact of new reimbursement legislation, selection of hospice team physicians, and benefits of physician involvement are explored.

THE HOSPICE PHILOSOPHY

The hospice philosophy of care stresses that patients are treated with respect and retain maximum control over their remaining lives. The emphasis is on allowing the patient to "live until it is time to die." This philosophy is akin to the wellness philosophy of prevention and prospective care. The hospice program of care encourages that healthy portion of the patient's life to express itself fully. This requires support to ameliorate physical symptoms of dying and pain so that the individual's emotional, spiritual, and social dimensions are fully expressed and enjoyed, even while the physical entity is failing.

What is health in the hospice context, where the focus is on death and dying? What is the physician's role when the patient's impending death seems to indict the medical profession for failing to complete its designated role as curer of disease? How do physicians change their beliefs in a philosophy focusing on the struggle against disease, with cure as the goal, to one acknowledging death, with pain and symptom control as the goal?

These questions identify major themes converging on the relationship between dying patients and their physicians. Discussing these themes facilitates partial understanding of terminal care situations and explains how physician-patient relationships become dysfunctional when the patient is dying. It also aids the physician in caring for the dying and their families.

HEALTH AND WELLNESS

The concept of health or wellness describes a disease-free status and positive attitudes concerning that status. The patient feels and is free of disease. In our culture, health status is defined through a transactional process between physicians and patients. The physician determines the presence or absence of disease, the patient decides if he or she feels "well." Wellness involves a set of beliefs about health that the patient brings to the relationship. The patient seeks a physician's help because a symptom has some ominous or negative meaning to the patient. The physician's input is needed to assist the patient in determining its real meaning and understanding the potential consequences.

Whether a specific symptom or problem is brought to the physician's attention depends on learning, cultural, social, and economic factors. Some feel comfortable bringing emotional difficulties to their physician and can afford to do so; others cannot. Unless the patient has a sense of urgency—a feeling that something has gone awry—and believes that medical attention can alleviate the symptoms, a solution in the health care system is not sought.

Beliefs about wellness also determine the patient's acceptance and compliance with the physician's advice. It is one thing for the physician to certify the patient as being free of disease; it is another to convince the patient of wellness. The possible outcomes of physician-patient interactions are fourfold:

1. The physician says there is no disease and the patient agrees. Such patients are considered "well."
2. The physician says there is no disease but the patient is not convinced. The patient might be called "worried well" and makes a number of visits to the family doctor to be reassured through regular checkups.
3. The physician says there is a problem but the patient feels there is no need for concern. The patient is considered "sick, but denying." Individuals who do not believe that they need to take their high blood pressure medications fall in this group.
4. The physician says there is a problem and the patient is worried or negative about the situation. Such a person suffers from "illness."

These four situations can be placed in a matrix, as follows:

PHYSICIAN INPUT

		No disease	Disease
PATIENT INPUT	Positive	"Well"	"Sick/Denying"
	Negative	"Worried Well"	"Ill"

The distinctions that have been described are important to physicians. Patients do not seek a physician just to know they are free of disease; they also seek reinforcement of wellness that coincides with their belief system. The physician must understand cultural beliefs, even those that seem to interfere with care. The physician who limits his or her role to disease certification will fail to restore persons to a sense of wellness. In hospice, this becomes important because, while physical deterioration takes place, the physician is a powerful force and can support and encourage a patient's beliefs and aspirations, enriching life until death.

PUBLIC AMBIVALENCE ABOUT PHYSICIANS

Everybody trusts their own physicians. The medical profession, as a whole, however, is losing stature and esteem. In our society physicians have achieved wealth, status, and power. These features of a physician's life are goals that most Americans seek and envy. The practice of medicine is embedded in a highly specialized vocabulary and occurs in places producing high stress. This stressful environment creates social distance between patients and physicians and mimics parent-child relationships: a combination of wanting to be accepted and approved with concern regarding rejection and pain. The physician tells the patient, "Take this medication and you should be better in a few days. If not, call me." The patient is given little or no information about the condition being treated, its consequences, and the possible outcomes if therapy fails. The patient is not told the name, actions, and side effects of the drug, and, more important, the patient is not given an opportunity to discuss the options for treatment or to ask questions. If failure occurs, the patient has no alternatives to follow; he or she must rely on the physician to reanalyze the situation and possibly change the therapy.

Today, patients are better informed and have great expectations of medicine, via exposure to medical information in the media. Many patients use this better understanding to achieve an adult relationship with their physicians. In such cases the physician explains the diagnosis and details available treatment options. He or she identifies the best option along with the possible factors—such as rates of success, pain, hospitalization, side effects, and costs—that might affect the patient's choice. Throughout this exchange, the physician is open to questions and is willing to repeat information. The physician may offer the patient an opportunity to read about the problem and decide at leisure or to consult another doctor for a second opinion. In the end, the patient decides on the treatment. The joint process allows both patient and physician to claim ownership for the choice.

Physicians may see this search for equality in the physician-patient relationship as an unwelcome change. It requires attitude changes and additional time during patient encounters to explore options for care and to share information. Patient requests for information and involvement in the choice of treatment options— even requests for second opinions—can be seen as threatening by some physicians.

Other changes in the practice of medicine have occurred. For example, increased numbers of malpractice lawsuits put physicians on guard and contribute to escalated social distancing. The supply of practitioners and their tendency to specialize increase the likelihood that patients have more than one physician, each of whom is concerned with less than the entire individual. This accounts, in part, for the public cry for family doctors like the ones "who knew the whole family and made house calls." The medical education system has responded by training more family physicians, but many of the new graduates merely replaced those who retired or died. Only recently has the actual supply of family doctors begun to grow. While the trend toward the return of personal or family doctors evolved in the past two decades, an equally strong trend developed toward "convenience medicine"—walk-in clinics with no-waiting policies—where patients see the next available doctor.

With a growing physician supply, greater demands for services, and newer technology, the cost of medical services rises. National policy is directed toward lowering the cost of medical care in the total economy with solutions that are likely to place a larger share of the cost on the patient. In combination, these changes in health care delivery and the physician-patient relationship contribute to an uncertainty in patients about their physicians.

Not every patient desires an adult relationship with the physician. The alert physician must understand when the patient can interact comfortably and use this discovery constructively. The patient may need different types of interactions depending on the situation. There are times when the patient wants the physician to be parental, making decisions and nurturing the patient. At other times the patient demands adult treatment. "Tell me, Doc, what are my chances?" "What are my options?" "What is this going to cost me?"

Although the patient may want the physician to take responsibility for deciding what the patient should do, in reality the physician cannot. Ideally, the patient incorporates the physician's advice and participates in treatment decisions. This requires the physician to fully disclose clinical information to the patient in an understandable format.

Unfortunately, the ideal state is rarely reached. The vast discrepancy in knowledge and decision-making experience between the patient and physician along with tongue-tying medical vocabulary are distancing. The physician who fails to use understandable vocabulary, who takes too little time to explain a problem and its consequences, and who fails to listen to the patient's worries relinquishes an opportunity to develop an adult relationship. By agreeing to make decisions for the patient, the physician assumes responsibility for treatment and attempted cure, denying the patient an opportunity to participate fully in his or her care. In hospice care, where control over one's remaining days is the central element of the program, the physician must be sensitive to shifting public attitudes about the medical profession and changing role relationships between physicians and patients.

At the center of hospice philosophy is maximization of symptom control and patients' mental clarity to enable participation in care as well as personal life decisions. The hospice provides care for patients wherever they wish—at home, in the hospital or nursing home, or in an inpatient hospice facility. Medication levels are adjusted and given reliably to suit the patient's subjective need for symptom control. This eliminates the typical acute hospital situation where pain medication is under another's uncertain control. Meals are selected carefully, visitors and pets are allowed, and spiritual, social, and emotional needs are met.

PHYSICIAN COMPETENCY

The following is a good short exercise to use when training groups of lay volunteers for hospice involvement. Participants are asked to recall the last time they visited physicians with problems about which they were worried and where the outcome was uncertain. Each is asked to think about what the physician did during the visit and to characterize the elements that made the visit "good" or "bad." Most people identify concepts denoting caring: "He talked to me." "She explained things." "He seemed interested in solving the problem." "She took enough time." Rarely will someone mention the physician's correct diagnosis or skills to handle the problem. The patient assumes and believes the physician is adequately trained. The patient would not have come to see the physician unless he or she had already decided that this man or woman was capable of dealing with the complaint. From the patient's point of view, competence relates more to the physician's conduct and demonstrated concern than to actual skills in practicing medicine.

Unfortunately, in professional peer assessment of a physician's competence, caring has little impact on whether colleagues judge another doctor as competent. This judgment is based on whether the physician makes correct diagnoses, correctly eliminates alternative explanations for the problem, and manages the patient correctly. Other factors used to assess competence include appropriateness and timeliness of referrals, length of hospital stay, and average resources consumed by the physician's treatments. These are the types of issues that colleagues, licensure agencies, and specialty boards explore.

The hospice physician's definition of personal competence should bridge the gap. Input from the profession is necessary but patient and team member input is equally important. Too often, the average physician has not been taught to value patient feedback or to consider it as important as a personal definition of competence.

In hospice, the physician often behaves in ways that may be called countercultural to those of his or her professional peers. The hospice physician is most competent when he or she stops seeking cure of the disease as a goal and substitutes skills in easing the approach of death, meets basic needs of daily comfort and support, assists in training of staff, and works cooperatively with the hospice team. In these efforts, the physician is often not the principal caregiver or team director. These behaviors may appear foreign to nonhospice physicians, who may not consider such actions within the purview of "real medicine." The hospice physician learns to internalize a reward system, recognizing that care for a dying person well done is a form of high competence. The hospice physician also learns to accept the kudos of his or her fellow team members as indicative of success, becoming less dependent on physician colleagues for such feedback. Positive feedback from patients and families also tells the physician that the treatment is accepted and appreciated. This form of success is an important part of the reward system of the hospice physician.

CANCER AS A DISEASE

Growth in the elder population has led to a shift in the causes of death. As Fox writes, certain chronic illnesses that have not yielded to the progress of medicine are now the primary causes of mortality, among them cancer, heart disease, and stroke.[1] A considerable portion of the American preoccupation with death and dying is concerned, directly or indirectly, with chronic illness and the care of the chronically ill. The disease most dreaded and feared in this connection is cancer. It has become the archetypical metaphor of "insidious, malevolent, uncontrollable, ugly, and pain-filled aspects of these chronic illness associated problems. . . ."[2]

Although other chronic illnesses may be the cause of the patient's admission to a hospice, cancer is the one disease that hospice deals with most frequently. Other diseases are important but much more rare than cancer in the hospice setting. Cancer is imbued with a group of special and frightening meanings in a manner that is shared by no other disease. While the physician must understand the special needs of hospice patients dying of stroke, heart disease, and progressive neurological deterioration, when caring for a cancer patient the fear and special meanings peculiar to cancer must also be considered. This discussion focuses on this unique feature of cancer and omits broader discussion of other disease entities in order to explore the impact of cancer's image on the physician's work with the most common problem in hospice.

Cancer evokes a unique dread in both physicians and patients. In a bizarre and, to this date, unknown fashion, the tissues of the human body have turned from functional to self-destructive. The process of cell division and growth knows no limits. It follows no rules. There are no treatment programs that reliably work for all patients. Treatment is a wait-and-see proposition. Cancer appears randomly and often is present for a long time before discovery. It is as if the body were invaded and infiltrated by a terrorist network, clandestinely working to undermine health and overthrow the well-ordered economy of the human organism.

Susan Sontag points out in *Illness As Metaphor* that, in our culture, cancer has inherited a metaphoric meaning from tuberculosis: the cancer of a previous era.[3] In the past, people died of TB by the thousands, often with the bacillus destroying tissue for a great while before becoming evident. The results were wasted tissue and death with no reliable cures. People's reactions toward TB were similar to those expressed today toward cancer. For instance, cancer and TB are both considered contagious even though it is quite difficult to catch TB and, it is believed, impossible to catch cancer. Nevertheless, the population considers cancer to be at least morally contagious. There seems to be something about cancer that, if one has it, one must have "caught it" for some reason, perhaps an event or sin in earlier life that is being punished. Cancer is often linked to characterological problems; "Why did she get cancer; she's been a good person all her life?" The implication is that there is something dark and hidden about the patient now revealed.

There is a passage in Job (33:19) that describes the picture of the cancer patient that most people fear. "He is chastened also with pain upon his bed, and the multitude of his bones with strong pain: So that his life abhorreth bread and his soul dainty meat. His flesh is consumed away so that it cannot be seen, and his bones that were not seen stick out. Yea, his soul draweth unto the grave and his life to the destroyer."

Others believe that cancer is uniformly painful and highly mutilating and that everyone who has cancer will die. The word "cancer" is synonymous with dying and death. Cancer produces a sense of utter helplessness. Even if the patient is fully cooperative, follows all the regimens, takes all the medications, there really is no guarantee of cure. In fact, in spite of the very best cooperation, cancer may kill anyway.

The physician must remember that these underlying attitudes about cancer come with the patient and the family to the hospice and prevail throughout the community. The physician must work to undermine these beliefs and to replace them with accurate facts about cancer and the likely prognosis for the individual.

Because these beliefs and attitudes are prevalent, the patient dreads hearing the word "cancer" and often confuses the messenger with the message. Anger about the diagnosis and hatred of the disease may be projected onto the physician by the patient or family, severely testing the relationship. The patient may deny the diagnosis, display anger toward the physician, and request other opinions and tests in an effort to bargain away the dreaded diagnosis. The physician must realize this is a normal response and support the patient. Too often, the physician may react in anger, out of a sense of personal failure or in reaction to the patient's projected feelings, thus destroying the relationship upon which future care depends.

When the physician teaches the patient and family about the disease, it is important to understand that information may not be heard the first time. When a patient hears "cancer" as a diagnosis the first time, whatever comes after is probably not heard. Repetitions over several encounters are needed. The physician must retain a sense of optimism on behalf of the patient until this information can be processed. Only then will the patient put "cancer" into perspective and consider necessary changes in lifestyle, vocation, beliefs, and family interactions.

The physician must resist the common medical practice of "hanging crepe."[4] This is the habit of informing the patient about his or her condition in such a way as to lead the patient to expect poor outcomes so that if something better happens, the physician will be given the credit. On the other hand, if the worst happens, the physician is not blamed for failing to warn the patient. This method of sharing prognostications with patients relieves physician anxiety while creating hopelessness or anxiety in the patient. The physician gains by seeming to be powerful in the treatment against long odds or wise in foresight about the course of the disease. While the art of prognosticating is notoriously unsuccessful in dealing with terminally ill patients, an intelligent attempt to predict outcomes and to plan likely contingencies helps the patient maintain morale and deal with reality. It may expose the physician to situations where winning will not occur, but any efforts to guarantee a "no-lose" situation run counter to the philosophy of hospice.

THE NATURE OF DEATH AND DYING

The physician-patient relationship may suffer from the handling of death and dying in our culture. Until recently, death was a normative process. It occurred in the context of the family—usually at home in one's own bed. It was considered the normal ending of life. There is a passage in Ecclesiastes (1:4 and 2:1-4) that states: "One generation passeth away, and another generation cometh. . . To every thing there is a season, a time to every purpose under heaven. A time to be born, a time to die. . . ." Death was a public happening. The community insisted that the family wear black; rapid return to public life by the deceased's spouse was not expected, to allow time for grieving. Religion had a role to play in death, with ceremonies and rites to mark it.

Today, death is a medicalized event. Though most patients want to die at home, the majority die in hospitals. They incur heavy medical debts, are isolated from family and friends, and are placed away from other patients, heavily sedated and barely recognizable behind a myriad of tubes and technologies. Now, death is an interloper, not a part of life's continuum. It is private, hidden, and denied. Grief is supposed to be temporary and discreet. "You need to buck up; get over it; get on with living."

Change in previously normative behavior surrounding death and care for the dying patient occurred in the last generation. Many older persons remember when the body was "laid out" at home, for family and friends to visit. Recent changes in dying customs create problems for the patient and family. The medicalization of death thwarts communication among family members, and bereavement is often incomplete in the period after the loss. The hospice physician must watch for isolation of the patient and family, helping to lessen the social pain of dying. The physician can use simple interventions, including referral of the patient to an available hospice. In addition, the physician can choose to assemble "ad hoc" hospice services by involving the social services, pastoral care, and nursing personnel at the hospital or in the community. Meeting with the patient and family as a group can open lines of communication when the physician has information to share. These actions show the family that the physician favors their involvement and values open discussion of treatment and prognosis. A holistic approach is adopted when the physician inquires about the patient's emotional status, need for financial or situational support, and spiritual status.

The physician can serve as a "broker" to involve the patient's family, friends, clergy, and neighbors in the care program. Home calls, for patients in that setting, are the single best method to accomplish these steps. They provide time to obtain insights not available in the more limited office or hospital setting. The home call serves as a nonverbal message of concern and respect for the patient and family.

CARE OF THE FAMILY

Death is a family disease. Nobody dies in isolation, in spite of the current trends to keep the dying patient remote. Death occurs in a context, and the most immediate context is that of the family. The family "dies" along with the patient and no longer continues in its previous form. The family context must be re-negotiated, redefined, and must reemerge, using a new set of givens that do not include, except for memories, the deceased.

Dying and death can impose drastic change, disrupt the homeostasis of the family, and unsettle a lifetime of operating rules. If a parent dies, it may upset the entire power structure of the family. Death often reopens forgotten files of "unfinished business." Things that the family thought were swept under the rug erupt at funeral time, if for no other reason than the "gathering of the clan." Physicians can learn a great deal by attending the "wake" or the funeral home showing of the deceased. The family's reactions, the appropriateness of the grief response by family members, and the number of supportive family and neighbors who are present may be assessed. In addition, the physician may form firmer bonds with the survivors through this simple act. This is an opportunity to meet and shake hands with the survivors, offer a few words of condolence, and perhaps recall a pleasant memory of the patient. Attending the funeral services, without this visit to the funeral home, does not allow for personal interaction. The physician's signature in the visitor's register is a permanent reminder to the family of the concern demonstrated.

Following the public events of the funeral, family members may find them-selves alone. It takes time for friends and neighbors to resume regular interactions with survivors. Concern that the visit might precipitate overt grief or prove uncomfortable or embarrassing makes friends withdraw. These well-intentioned sentiments mask the uneasiness that nonfamily members feel in helping the family reintegrate into the community. The result—delayed contact with the family—

may be interpreted as a lack of concern. The longer this endures, the more difficult the first contact becomes. The situation seems worse when there is a sole survivor. For these reasons hospice remains concerned with survivors for months following the patient's death. Helping survivors reconstitute their family and reenter society are goals of hospice bereavement follow-up programs.

The physician, aware of the impact of death on the family, can participate with the team to assist in the normal redefinition and reemergence of the family, while being watchful for abnormal patterns of grief or depression. If the physician is the family doctor, continued involvement with the survivors is predictable. Having insight concerning the patient's dying and the funeral assists the physician in dealing with symptoms, which may be nonphysical in cause, that occur later.

Reorganization of the family must be encouraged through exploration of feelings and interpersonal relationships. The hospice exists with this as one of its principal goals. The physician must encourage the family to seek help in addressing its problems. The hospice team looks to its physician as a leader in care planning, and the physician may inadvertently direct the team from care of the family by focusing on symptom control and physical problems. If the physician gets involved in the bereavement care as well, he or she signals support for this aspect of hospice care.

Family involvement in the care of the dying influences symptom control. In fact, if pain control suddenly fails in a patient for whom it had been controlled, the physician should look to family relationships as one area where problems may be occurring.

One report shows that male spouses have a 40 percent greater chance for death than female spouses when left a widower.[5] This sobering fact should motivate physicians to pay special attention to widowers in the period following the wife's death. The experience of many physicians confirms that the incidence of functional and emotional problems also is greater following a loss. As noted in Chapter 13, closer follow-up of family members after the death of a loved one may prevent temporary problems from becoming chronic ways for dealing with life and stress.

For all the above reasons, several authors have stated that the family physician is a natural choice to serve in a hospice program.[6] Training family physicians in hospice care has been suggested as a natural component of their curriculum. Many of the concerns echoed in the philosophy of the hospice movement also are identified by the specialty of family medicine. Since the late sixties, graduates of family practice residencies have been trained using a medical care model that treats the patient in the context of the family and community. The emphasis is on continuity of care.

Today, the family physician is trained in counseling and along with forms of psychotherapy he or she is encouraged to consider the patient from the social, spiritual, emotional, and physical perspectives. Most recently trained family physicians have worked in team-care contexts with the other types of caregivers commonly found on hospice teams. This biopsychosocial orientation is coupled with three years of training in all the various medical specialties. Such a foundation provides the family physician with appropriate attitudes and skills to cooperate with other caregivers and to attend to the spectrum of patient needs and concerns.

THE COST OF CARE

There is a myth in medical care that the patient is the consumer of medical goods and services. The reality is that the physician is the real consumer, after the patient initiates the process. The physician decides what service will be made available or used, what the cost will be, when and where it will be provided. The physician also decides whether the service is of value, that is, whether it accomplished its intended purpose. The patient rarely controls any aspect of the cost of medical care.

In our society, neither the patient nor the physician directly pays for services used. Third-party payers cover most medical care costs. At the time of utilization, the service appears as a free commodity, in that patients rarely see or pay more than a portion of the total charges. Increasingly, in instances of chronic and terminal care, cost becomes a major side effect. Insurance and other third-party payers do not provide benefits that match the costs. The physician, as the consumer of medical services, must be aware of these economic circumstances and strive for the best cost-benefit ratio.

Since 1982, Medicare benefits have been expanded to cover hospice care, but, as several authors have indicated, this has created some unique problems for physicians who work in hospices.[7] Medicare benefits have a cap of $6,500 for total expenditures on any given patient. This cap has varied, with attempts to both increase and decrease the level. There is also a variable limit on the percentage of the total funds that can be spent in a hospital setting while the patient is enrolled in a hospice program. As described in Chapter 8, daily rates have been established for respite, inpatient, and home care. Many hospice organizations claim these rates are too low and will not allow them to provide adequate care.

Hospices are prohibited by law from discontinuing care due to exhaustion of benefits. The patient is entitled to care as long as he or she lives. No extra reimbursement is given for shorter enrollments to offset those that may exceed the allotted cap. Although the Medicare hospice benefit has been likened to the first of the new diagnosis related groups (DRGs) for reimbursement by the federal government, it is not truly a DRG in that reimbursement is not independent of length of stay.

As we have seen, patients choosing the hospice benefit do so in lieu of their usual Medicare benefit. In exchange, the patient gets a broader group of benefits. To qualify for the benefit, the patient must be "certified" as terminal—having less than six months to live—by both the attending physician and the hospice physician. If the patient has no attending physician, the hospice physician may certify alone. The hospice the patient chooses must be Medicare-certified. Coverage of two 90-day periods and one 30-day period may be chosen by the patient. This allows, yet minimizes, opportunities for the patient to use hospice benefits. The hospice gambles that the patient will need only a modicum of inpatient care when electing to use the hospice benefit. The effect of this regulation is to ration hospice services to those whose needs are within the limits of the law and who can locate a Medicare-approved hospice.

Physicians are faced with challenges in complying with the Medicare hospice law. Potential conflicts may occur between the attending physician and the hospice physician in certifying the patient as terminal and in trying to preserve the fiscal resources of the hospice program. The decision as to whether the attending physician continues to see the patient, with consultative help from the hospice physician, or the hospice physician assumes full care is a potential source of disruption in physician-to-physician relationships. This will be especially true if the hospice physician must act to limit the drain on resources.

Once a hospice assumes care of an individual, it is responsible for the cost of all the patient's health care services. In addition to palliation, the hospice physician must be prepared to take over all care of the referred patient.

It may be that these conflicts in the Medicare hospice regulations could be the undoing of the hospice programs meant to be the beneficiaries.[8] Because there is no scientific basis on which to predict when a patient is six months from death, physicians are caught in a double bind. Medical judgment errors resulting in excessively lengthy hospice care could lead to dire financial consequences for hospice programs. On the other hand, preventing access to hospice benefits is detrimental to deserving patients and families.

UNIQUE PROBLEMS OF DYING PATIENTS

Terminally ill patients, especially those with cancer, have unique problems. The loss of their personal role or role relationships within the context of their daily lives is especially troubling. The patient is no longer the breadwinner, teacher, mother, father, homemaker, or parent. Pain and other physical symptoms develop that have no protective value for the patient.

Cancer pain does not protect in the same way that pain from a broken bone protects the patient from further damage and ensures medical attention. Once cancer is detected, having more pain is absolutely meaningless. The pain magnifies other themes about punishment, abandonment, guilt, and isolation. Many patients experience fear during their dying—fear of pain, fear of what may happen next, fear of losing control, and fear for the safety and welfare of survivors. Legal stresses occur surrounding writing a will and paying increasing debts. Financial burdens may overwhelm the resources of a family, placing a great deal of worry on the dying individual. The patient loses control over life, becoming increasingly dependent upon others.

The hospice physician must realize this dependence and plan to maximize the patient and family control over the environment and the symptoms. This means that the hospice physician must be comfortable receiving the feedback of the patient, the family, and other members of the hospice care team to "fine tune" the therapy. Taking great care with details is indicated, for often a change of just a few milligrams in a medication may be the difference between pain control or excess sedation.

PHYSICIAN PROBLEMS WITH DEATH AND CANCER

Physicians, as a professional group, have greater difficulty handling their own personal mortality than do other professionals.[9] Physicians seek a greater level of control over death. There is a persistent, habituating belief about death that physicians replay daily as they meet patients. It is reassuring to think that if someone is going to do some dying today, it is more likely to be the patient. The issue of personal mortality must be faced by the hospice physician in order to be effective in dealing with dying patients. Unable to cure, many physicians experience feelings of guilt, impotence, and rage when facing a dying patient. This is the ultimate proof that the physician, even with the best biomedical technology, is powerless to cure. The patient, like a mirror, shows the physician his or her own human frailty and finite life span. Other members of the hospice team, especially those with counseling skills, can be helpful to the physician in coming to terms with personal mortality.

Physicians who have not openly discussed fear of death and examined their feelings of uncertainty are likely to participate with the patient in death denial by postponing or preventing discussion of dying. Actions constituting physician dysfunction include skipping the room because the patient has his or her eyes closed, skipping rounds, refusing to sit down near the patient, or talking about nothing but the weather. The emphasis may turn to maximizing the quantity, not the quality, of the patient's remaining life.

Unwillingness to acknowledge the terminal state—pursuing new tests and treatments, asking for just one more referral—prevents the patient from exercising the option of hospice care as an alternative. The physician often justifies this behavior as an attempt to maintain hope in the patient. Yet, experience shows that although the things hoped for change as the patient faces his or her condition, hope is alive and refocused on more immediate desires: seeing a loved one, staying pain free, dying peacefully, being brave. These latter hopes are not destroyed by speaking honestly with the patient; rather the patient is given an opportunity to entertain these hopes, to enjoy them, and to take strength and comfort from them. Worby and associates, in a review article on the hospice movement, state: "Perhaps most important to the future of hospice care will be the capacity of health care personnel to confront and alter their own deeply felt aversion to the process of dying, to the moment of death, to the process of grieving, and to the underlying generic issue of loss as it is experienced across the life span."[10]

The hospice physician must do the necessary internal accounting and arrive at some peace with the concept of his or her own mortality. As an authority figure in the hospice environment, the hospice physician must be comfortable giving the patient, through actions and words, permission to deal openly with the social, emotional, and spiritual issues surrounding death. This physician must focus on more than the details of physical care, or the very essence of hospice care is undermined.

WHO HELPS THE HELPER?

The training of physicians is highly competitive and physically exhausting.[11] For many years, students and residents work for top grades in difficult courses. The learner is mixed with other high achievers and virtually all other interests, problems, and family and personal growth are set aside in favor of long hours of exacting work. Sleep deprivation and stress form a backdrop on this scene. The student learns that survival depends on having the right answers, decreasing the degree of ambiguity, and maintaining a very ordered lifestyle of study and work. He or she is reminded daily of inadequacy and shortcomings in knowledge or performance. The resulting lesson is to work harder and harder to personally conquer these deficiencies, while striving to keep them private. Throughout this educational process, personal and family concerns are tabled in favor of the compelling urgency of doing and learning medicine. The new physician learns to suppress personal fears, ethical quandaries, and evidence of personal or family stress. The physician tends not to confide in colleagues or teachers. Seeking professional counseling is seen as a sign of weakness that may blemish an otherwise perfect record. Because of this orientation, physicians pay a terrible price as evidenced by the incidence of psychopathology, depression, stress, divorce, drug abuse, and suicide.

Given eleven to fifteen years of education and rigorous training, in which a premium is placed on performance and a penalty placed on activities of personal growth, there is little wonder that many physicians have problems recognizing and dealing with the issues in this chapter. Yet, a sizable number of physicians do manage to complete the journey to their practices with experiences of personal growth. These physicians are knowledgeable about patient issues and are skilled in dealing with all aspects of care, including preventive medicine. These are the physicians that the hospice programs should seek and employ. These are the individuals who will support the activities of the hospice, whether as full-time hospice physician or supportive referring colleague. The hospice program represents a fertile environment where these individuals can find a home and from which they and the hospice team can support other colleagues.

PUTTING IT ALL TOGETHER

Who then is the hospice program seeking for a hospice physician? The answer has to be those practitioners who recognize the issues in this chapter and have adopted personal skills to manage not only biological but social and emotional concerns in the care of patients and families. The exact background or field of specialization is less important than the nature of the person.

The hospice physician needs the ability to promote a level of wellness in the patient, even if terminally ill, by supporting the patient's belief systems and basic hope and optimism. The example of Norman Cousins, as described in *Anatomy of an Illness*,[12] illustrates this point. Cousins developed a mysterious illness that defied diagnosis and would not relent under the full armamentarium of a modern medical center. He was dying. He worked with a cooperative physician to design a self-care program that emphasized a good diet, rest, massage, vitamins, and plenty of laughter, induced by watching funny films. Cousins moved from a hospital to a fine New York hotel, reducing his costs and increasing his control over events. His physician, although doubting the program, respected Cousins' decisions, offering advice when Cousins suggested very unsafe methods. Gradually, Cousins recovered fully. Cousins himself probably does not know if the treatment program or his faith in it was what cured him.

The hospice physician needs the humility to recognize that competence is caring, not curing. The risk for the physician is loss and pain when the patient dies; yet, the experience allows personal growth, pleasure from the relationship, and a sense of worth.

The physician in hospice should avoid language and/or behavior that can evoke or reinforce the metaphoric meanings of cancer and death. He or she may have to abandon a repertoire of nonverbal behaviors that may remind the patient, on a subconscious basis, of an unclean, shunned metaphoric disease image. The physician also has the power to reverse these nonverbal messages through simple actions—by visiting the patient daily, sitting down on the edge of the bed, holding the patient's hand, crying, and doing whatever else needs to be done to indicate caring. The physician who can do this is the one the hospice needs.

The hospice physician must remember the family as part of the unit of care. The patient benefits if the family is cared for properly. The hospice physician assists the patient and family to maintain control by minimizing dependency and by maintaining previous roles in life. Patients can be involved in decisions about all aspects of their care, including cost, kinds of services, timing of procedures, and other such issues. Often a decision involves something for which there is no obvious best answer or where the answer is immaterial to all but the patient. These are the times that the patient must be granted control.

The hospice physician should help the family, the patient, and the care team refocus and maintain appropriate levels of hope. One can acknowledge to the patient that certain hopes have passed—the hope of cure, the hope of no pain—without removing hope for control and comfort.

Patients and hospice programs need caring physicians to provide leadership and patient care. Yet the forces outlined in this chapter present real impediments to physician effectiveness. The long-term goal is to change the medical education system to one where the student-teacher relationship models the same warmth, respect, empathy, and trust that is expected in the ideal physician-patient relationship. Meanwhile, the short-term goal is to understand these forces and to provide a supportive environment for the physicians who choose to help the hospice team.

NOTES

1. Renee Fox, "The Sting of Death in American Society," *Social Science Review* 37 (March 1981): 42–59; Renee Fox, "The Social Meaning of Death—Preface," *The Annals* 447 (January 1980): vii–xi.

2. Fox, "The Social Meaning of Death—Preface."

3. Susan Sontag, *Illness As Metaphor* (New York: Farrar, Straus and Giroux, 1978).

4. Mark Seigler, "Pascal's Wager and the Hanging of Crepe," *New England Journal of Medicine* 293 (1975): 853–857.

5. M. Young, B. Benjamin, and C. Walker, "Mortality of Widowers," *Lancet* 2 (1976): 454.

6. Paul T. Werner, "Family Medicine and Hospice Programs: A Natural Alliance," *Journal of Family Practice* 12 (1981): 367–368; Ira R. Byock, "Hospice and the Family Physician," *Journal of Family Practice* 18 (1984): 781–784.

7. Curtis D. Keller and Howard K. Bell, "The New Hospice Medicare Benefit: A Brief and Somewhat Irreverent History," *Postgraduate Medicine* 75 (1984): 71–82; Lenora Finn Paradis, "Hospice: the First DRG—Changing Physician Roles and Reimbursement," *Health Matrix*; Howard Brody and J. Lynn, "The Physician's Responsibility Under the New Medicare Reimbursement for Hospice Care," *New England Journal of Medicine* 310 (1984): 920–922.

8. Paul T. Werner, "Managing Pain in the Terminally Ill," *Family Practice Recertification* 2 (1980): 50–56.

9. Laurens P. White, "Death and the Physician: Mortuis Vivos Docent," in *New Meanings of Death*, ed. Herman Feifel (New York: McGraw-Hill, 1977).

10. Cyril Worby, Karen Blackman, and John Schneider, "Hospice Care: Current Status and Future Prospects," *Patient Counseling and Health Education* 1 (1978): 61–64.

11. Eric Schaff and Robert A. Hoekelman, "Medical Education: At What Expense?" *Journal of Medical Education* 56 (1981): 433–435; "Physicians' Emotional Ills Linked to Medical Training," *Family Practice News* 11 (June 15, 1981): 12.

12. Norman Cousins, *Anatomy of an Illness As Perceived by the Patient: Reflections on Healing and Regeneration* (New York: Norton, 1979).

Chapter 15

The Future of Hospice

Lenora Finn Paradis

Hospice development is controlled by multiple social and political forces; therefore program managers and planners should view the long-range growth and development of hospices with guarded optimism. The future of hospice in the United States rests in the hands of federal and state policymakers. These lawmakers will determine the continued efficacy of funding hospice care as well as the level and type of funding hospice providers can expect. This concluding chapter examines changes in the status of hospice today, key issues in hospice growth, and provides policymakers, planners, and managers with an agenda for the future.

It is no surprise that the concept and organization of hospice in America has changed dramatically over the past two decades. Initially a volunteer-dominated, community-based support service, hospice has evolved into a highly professionalized industry. It contains detailed rules and regulations, requires licensure in many states, and identifies specialized skills and training for both volunteer and paid staff.

The single, most dramatic event impacting the widespread change in the organization and structure of hospices in this country was the passage of Medicare reimbursement. More than any other event, the Medicare benefit has shaped and determined a course for hospice that warrants examination by program developers in all types of settings. Passed after months of intense debate, Medicare reimbursement appealed to legislators for three primary reasons. First, it provided consumers with an allegedly new series of health care options at a substantial cost savings to taxpayers. Second, it "guaranteed" increased competition in health care delivery—a concept widely promoted by the Reagan Administration. Third, hospice was a politically safe issue appealing to the hearts and minds of millions of Americans; after all, who wants to have someone in their family die alone and in pain. Legislators, therefore, garnered favorable press and publicity by supporting the passage of the benefit and thus also have a political stake in ensuring that hospice can and does deliver the savings and competition it was purported to provide.

Medicare reimbursement assured hospice program managers of survival. If approved for participation they would not have to rely solely on donations from community supporters and local philanthropy. However, the benefits have significant social and administrative costs. They will escalate the trend toward hospice professionalization, encourage the development of mergers with existing health care providers, create fierce competition among providers, require increased standardization, and demand strong attention to the costs of providing patient care. Accompanying professionalization and specialization is greater reliance on paid staff. Out of necessity, care will become constrained and less individualized. Volunteers will no longer provide patient care but instead will be relegated to administrative or nonreimbursable services such as bereavement counseling. Increased professionalization may exclude nontrained persons, primarily volunteers, from operating all-volunteer programs. The early concept of care for the dying that involved the entire community may be altered so that dying is viewed as a time when the family must call on hospice specialists to monitor the final days of life. Further, as hospice becomes part of the traditional health care system, it will be hard to distinguish hospice from more conventional care.

Increased professionalization and standardization, the Medicare benefit, and the policies of the Reagan Administration, such as the utilization of Diagnostic Related Groups (DRGs), will force hospice providers to compete with other providers to contain cost. These requisites may prove difficult for hospice caregivers. Competition among hospice and other providers already exists. Hospitals and home health agency representatives opposed the Medicare reimbursement claiming that it would create duplicative systems of care, result in higher costs, fragment existing provider relationships, and cut into their own profit margins. Home health agency representatives further argued that hospice programs were originally designed to provide cooperative working arrangements with area home health agency providers. Instead, hospice program representatives have sought home health certification and competed with area agencies for home care patients. According to both hospital and home health agency spokespersons, hospice care was not really unique and could be easily provided within existing organizational structures with the aid of volunteers and educational programming.[1]

The cost of hospice care has been particularly controversial. Medicare expenditures under the new hospice benefit (which took effect November 1, 1983) are expected to be $22 million in fiscal year 1984 and $104 million in fiscal year 1985.[2] Other insurers are looking at potential costs for this new benefit. As the cost of providing hospice care becomes more apparent, policymakers are asking if hospice is really different from other forms of health care.

Furthermore, the Medicare benefit requires hospice programs to assume responsibility for all facets of patient care and to provide a variety of services for which they receive no reimbursement. The concept behind this extended service and limited reimbursement arrangement is consistent not only with cost-containment philosophies but also with the emphasis on self-help and increased reliance on the family rather than the state for social services. The hospice concept considers the family as part of a care team. The primary care provider is expected to provide the bulk of the hospice care and, as such, to save the cost of institutionalized services. This philosophy has interesting ramifications throughout the health care delivery system and may become extended to other areas of patient care.

ECONOMIC CONSIDERATIONS: PREDICTIONS FOR THE FUTURE

Considering the political nature of hospice growth and development, the future for the American hospice movement will depend on five primary factors: (1) consumer demand, (2) hospice supply, (3) hospice professionalization, (4) resource allocation, and (5) market penetration. Each of these variables operates together with the others and, depending on the strengths or weaknesses of any one, will impact the continuation of hospice.

Consumer Demand

Health care consumers, or more specifically those sick or dying, have heard about and often expect hospice or hospicelike care. Criticisms of the medical profession's treatment of the dying escalated during the past two decades beginning in the 1960s with the work of Glazer and Strauss[3] and Elisabeth Kubler-Ross.[4] The decade from mid-1960 through mid-1970 "witnessed a great deal of collective bustle in the United States (and other parts of the industrial world) over death and dying."[5] Articles in *Newsweek*, *Time*, the *New York Times*, the *Chicago Tribune*, and other major publications across the country ran articles on "living with death" or "new concepts in care for the dying." In 1976 the *New York Times* reported that "each year since its paperback publication in 1970, *On Death and Dying* by Elisabeth Kubler-Ross has sold a greater number of copies and has now reached a total of 1,032,000."[6] In a recent bibliography of literature related to hospice, Foster and Finn Paradis catalogued over 1,000 articles, excluding those appearing in newspapers and magazines, and listed several dozen other bibliographies available in specialized topics, such as pediatric hospice care and bereavement counseling.[7]

In short, public awareness of issues related to death and dying is at its peak. Heightened awareness is due, in part, to the increased incidence of cancer, improved longevity, and growing concerns over rising health care costs. These reasons aside, public pressure on established practitioners and institutions has risen and consumers demand more and different types of medical care. They want to be "treated as a person," made "comfortable," "relieved of discomfort," and "coherent until the end." "Take me off the respirator " is an increasingly voiced cry. "Let me die at home. I want to be somewhere familiar."

The hospice philosophy has been widely sold to the American public as a way of making the dying process more comfortable. Death is a natural state and, as such, should not be prolonged solely by sophisticated technology. The hospice movement promises the dying patient a painless home death, surrounded by his or her family, in a comfortable position. For many, fearing the dread of cancer and other insidious disease, this idyllic vision has widespread appeal. Hospice, like a new consumer good, promises a great deal. But can it deliver? As one hospice administrator wrote in confidence, "Sometimes I think things are a bit out of hand. We in the hospice movement make ourselves out to be demigods and promise bliss. Patients and families come to expect more than we are really able to give. . . . Sometimes I feel frightened. I'm not sure I can meet everyone's expectations. Other times I'm angry at the demands."

In spite of the concern over unkept promises, many hospice patients and families are satisfied with the service they received and have expressed their feelings to friends and relatives.[8] As consumer knowledge, expectation, and demand for hospice care increase, it will be difficult, if not impossible, for traditional health care providers as well as hospice providers to discontinue hospice care or hospicelike services. Hospice services will continue as long as demand escalates.

Hospice Supply and Professionalization

According to a recent survey by the National Hospice Organization, the number of hospice programs increased from a handful in 1978 to more than 1,500 today.[9] Many of the new hospice programs are institutionally affiliated, that is, associated with a home health agency, hospital, or nursing home. Increased availability of third-party funds and the use of volunteers make it possible for traditional providers to begin offering this service.

The emergence and expansion of hospice organizations combined with rapidly escalating public support and legal mandates resulted in a professional hospice industry. Within a few years after the movement began (the opening of the Connecticut Hospice is used as the movement's benchmark), a cadre of professional hospice nurses, social workers, lay volunteers, and administrators developed. Throughout the country, workshops, courses, and programs for specialized hospice training are advertised. Nursing schools, for example, offer specialized training in cancer, oncology, and hospice care. Hospital administration programs offer seminars in alternative forms of health care and include hospice in classroom discussions. Social workers and psychologists now have specialized programs and courses in death and dying and grief and loss.

Books, manuals, and journals describing varied aspects of hospice care have appeared across the country. National and international meetings, training programs in nursing skills, patient recordkeeping, grief counseling, and bereavement therapy are offered for costs ranging from hundreds to several thousand dollars. Colleges and universities have announced the availability of specialty degrees in hospice patient care management and administration. In October 1984 the National Hospice Organization began a hospice careers service for members advertising hospice career openings.

As the supply of hospice services grows, systems are being created to train individuals in specialized hospice skills. The increased supply in hospice care is directly proportional to the increased growth of professionals to deliver necessary services. Ads for hospice administrators are appearing in newspapers across the country and many positions require prior experience. Two recent journals, *The Hospice Journal* and the *American Journal of Hospice Care*, offer information to hospice professionals. Moreover, millions of dollars have been invested by the U.S. Government as well as large public foundations, such as the W.K. Kellogg, John A. Hartford, and Robert Wood Johnson Foundations, to study the hospice movement and to develop care standards.

As hospice is increasingly integrated into the traditional health care system, licensed health professionals will undoubtedly play a major role in patient care. Volunteers' roles will lessen as they are replaced in favor of paid employees held accountable for potential care problems. As this happens, costs will necessarily rise. The old adage if you want quality you have to pay for it may not hold true in the hospice area, especially if the volunteers who worked so hard to realize an ideal are asked to step aside in favor of licensed professionals.

Government policies to decrease federal and state involvement in health care programming may alter the structure of hospice. By mandating the use and training of hospice professionals, federal funding will ensure that hospice programming refers to the larger health care delivery systems. This ironic twist may drive up hospice costs and force legislators to take a long hard look at existing hospice policies.

Resource Allocation

Hospice programs receive direct financial support as well as in-kind contributions from varied sources. Many of these sources have shifted over time and some cease to exist as a resource. Contributions to programs are influenced by the community's involvement in the program, the model of care, the location of the hospice, and the ability of the hospice to involve individuals who can garner funds through grants and contracts.

Early hospice programs (pre-Medicare funding) obtained most of their support from individual donations, memorials, philanthropic contributions, and grants to local service organizations. These programs also received resources from the organizations that would later become competitors, such as hospitals, home health agencies, and nursing homes. Once Medicare and other third-party benefits, such as Blue Cross-Blue Shield, became available, community resources and organization donations dwindled. Moreover, much of the seed money provided for initial hospice development and research by major foundations such as the Robert Wood Johnson Foundation and the W.K. Kellogg Foundation are no longer available. The Robert Wood Johnson Foundation allocated thousands of dollars to Brown University for hospice research. The W.K. Kellogg Foundation provided funds for the creation of hospice standards by the Joint Commission on Accreditation of Hospitals and for the development of an "ideal type" hospice program in Battle Creek, Michigan.

In addition to fiscal and organizational supports, hospice program administrators have generated additional resources through volunteer efforts. Volunteers provide surplus labor that subsidizes organizational profit. They lower labor costs and reduce state investments in social services. In the past few years, with incentives for social programs to increase reliance on unpaid labor and reduce the need for paid staff, significant social service spending cuts have encouraged numerous welfare and health-oriented agencies to replace paid staff with volunteers. This policy will most likely continue as high spending deficits continue to plague the U.S. economy.

Volunteers provide other resources for hospice programs. They provide a mechanism for testing new product lines and services. New concepts in human service delivery, such as hospice, have often depended on the efforts of volunteers to prove their value before being formally adopted by government agencies or health and social service institutions. In this way, voluntary efforts in the area of hospice development play an important role in assessing whether a market for hospice services exists.

Volunteers have assisted hospice organizations in fund-raising activities, encouraged public affirmation of the legitimacy of hospice, and enhanced the image of many institutions initiating hospice programs. In a sense, voluntary time and resource contributions corroborate the idea that the hospice exists to serve beneficial outcomes.[10]

The shifting resource base of hospice programs, from predominately voluntary commitments to stabilized third-party arrangements, and the widespread use of volunteers to cover many of the nonreimbursable items, has enabled hospice programs to further penetrate the traditional marketplace and become likely targets for acquisition by existing health care organizations. This takeover has positive and negative attributes. On the positive side it ensures the continuation of the hospice concept, which is both reimbursable and marketable to health care consumers. Major drawbacks to this shifting resource base include increased reporting requirements and the decreased uniqueness and individualized care that early program developers purported was a primary advantage of hospice care.

Market Penetration

Market penetration has two aspects: first, the degree to which hospice care is adopted by the existing health care system, and second, the degree to which individual programs expand their market area and increase their patient or client population. Few will disagree that the concept of hospice care has been widely adopted by traditional health care professionals. Now, with the availability of federal resources, this adoption process has increased. Hospitals and home health agencies have begun advertising their "hospicelike" service for both terminal and nonterminally ill patients. Recent data from the Health Care Financing Administration (HCFA) on Medicare certification showed that the majority of applicants (68 percent, or 99 programs) are home health agency or hospital-based programs. The figure increases to 73 percent if long-term care facilities are included.[11] Moreover, hospitals and other types of institutions are considering the potential benefits of hospice program linkages. Nurses are learning about palliative care and the difference between palliation and cure. Volunteers are available to assist patients throughout the hospital, and, with this linkage, physicians can become more sensitive to holistic care and family needs. Counseling and therapy services can be sold and marketed to an increased number of consumers. Health care administrators see the advantage of advertising a homelike atmosphere in the hospital and for relaxing rules regarding visiting hours. Hospice strategies can be used to reduce patient stays, an economic benefit rewarded through DRGs.

Widespread market penetration of hospice offers a mixed blessing. As the hospice philosophy penetrates the traditional medical marketplace, individual hospice programs may be at a disadvantage. Larger, established health care institutions that adopt the hospice concept have a distinct advantage over newly developed freestanding, community-based models. Most existing health care institutions have a highly developed infrastructure allowing them to use personnel in designing and implementing programs, keeping client records, soliciting funds, billing third-party insurers, and obtaining other community resources. New developing hospice programs do not have these advantages. They must begin from scratch, designing recordkeeping techniques, recruiting, hiring, and training paid and volunteer staff, designing inventory controls, and the like. Existing organizations can easily expand services to include hospice or consider mergers and takeovers of local hospice programs. In fact, merger or acquisition strategies have been used by home health agencies and hospitals across the country to more efficiently incorporate hospice services as part of their established practice options.[12]

Institutionally affiliated hospice programs have the distinct advantages in the area of market penetration. They can use existing personnel and resources to develop marketing strategies and to efficiently and effectively recruit and train volunteers. Moreover, these organizations do not have to rely on outside funding to provide hospice or hospicelike services. Many hospitals advertise palliative care or hospicelike service availability in cancer wards. Staff training in hospice philosophy varies, as does the range of services available, from such items as pain and symptom control to more elaborate options including planning for patient and family support services. Increasingly, existing institutional structures are using the development of affiliated hospice programs to drive out smaller free-standing programs that compete for home health patient populations.

Like large businesses with a strong competitive edge, institutionally affiliated hospice programs have strong advantages over nonaffiliated programs and have a greater ability to penetrate and to hold an expanding hospice population. As hospice programs become increasingly integrated, their ability to penetrate and to hold potential markets depends not only on available resources but also on size, intraorganizational structure, and community support. The small, all-volunteer programs will have the greatest competitive disadvantage.

The interaction among hospice demand, supply, professionalization, resource allocation, and market penetration are important and must be considered by hospice planners, administrators, and managers. The future and fate of hospice depends on its ability to balance these five areas and to use them in planning and developing both research and legislative agendas.

DEVELOPING AGENDAS: RESEARCH AND LEGISLATIVE

In 1986, Congress will evaluate the efficacy of continued hospice financing. At issue will be the Medicare benefit, as well as the continuation of hospice in general. To ensure long-term hospice survival advocates must initiate research endeavors and social policy that strengthen the position of hospice in America. This section explores national issues in hospice research and policy development.

There are varied approaches to research that can be undertaken to evaluate models of patient care, to assess volunteer recruitment and retention strategies, and to measure the effectiveness of bereavement and related hospice programs. Earlier chapters on evaluation point to diverse research endeavors undertaken by hospice program managers and administrators. Central to any research agenda is the ability of the results to influence public policy and to guarantee the continuation of hospice care. From this perspective, managers and planners should concentrate their efforts on investigations directed at assessing the social benefits of hospice care for patients who are not terminal, the cost savings that accrue from hospice care, and the widespread demand for hospice.

At the same time, the investigations that are used to promote and maintain hospice financing may also uncover problem areas and may, in fact, show duplicative service delivery, increased care costs, and inappropriate service delivery. Negative findings could be used to improve hospice, illustrate differences in care patterns or, in some areas, to illustrate the need for a better traditional delivery system rather than the initiation of a hospice alternative.

Questions regarding different models of hospice care, reimbursement for hospice programming, and medical and nursing involvement in patient care constitute critical research issues. They should be framed in a way that provides useful and practical application to policymakers. For example, understanding the importance of the nursing aspect of hospice is essential. However, it is necessary to move further and relate the importance of the nursing function to patient care in general and to underscore differences between nursing and medical care. If nurses are really the principal hospice caregivers, then public policy should be directed toward allowing them to perform their function in the most efficient and effective manner. This may mean increased independence from the medical professional.

Just as the use of certain professionals, such as nurses, provides a basis for analysis, so do other aspects of hospice programming. Pain and symptom control, bereavement, respite care, and spiritual counseling are all relatively new areas. They are largely unexplored and remain peripheral functions of hospice. Yet these functions also contribute to the uniqueness of hospice. If hospice managers are to continue to receive or to gain financial remuneration for performing these functions, they need documentation regarding the cost and usefulness of these areas to patient care.

Use of volunteers and the family for health care provision is another area in which investigations are needed. The use of volunteers and family members as surplus labor in hospice care is an important policy issue. Should social service funding be based on the amount of voluntary or family assistance available? Should volunteer assistance and family support be a mandated part of all health care policies? Should family members be financially compensated for their time or to provide for health care of a spouse or child? Should worker benefits and labor laws be revised to provide sick leave for family members caring for an ill relative? Researchers need to study more than the gender, age, and income level of hospice volunteers, patients, and families. Investigations should focus on the use of alternative labor throughout the health and social service sector and the public policies requiring organizations to use volunteers or community support to receive federal and state monies. This will lead to broader debates regarding the social service funding philosophy in the U.S.

Research of all types, particularly evaluation research, is directly related to social policy. Since the Nixon Administration, program evaluation has played a key role in continued health and social service funding. The question of whether a program or service really makes an impact sufficient enough to warrant continuation has been asked over and over again by lawmakers. Results from well-designed research will be crucial in determining the continuation of hospice and related social policies. Administrators should be concerned with patient and family confidentiality, but not overly concerned so as to prevent important program assessments. Managers and planners will be required to examine the uniqueness of hospice care and the dramatic social policy shifts brought about by hospice financing. The need for volunteers, spiritual counseling, and bereavement care also requires examination. For continued appropriations, the doors to research and policy exploration need to remain open. Hospice administrations would be wise to encourage widespread public analysis.

In terms of effective public policy development, the hospice industry has a national organization, the National Hospice Organization, which serves as a trade organization. Much like the American Medical Association, the American Nursing Association, and the American Hospital Association, the National Hospice Organization has spearheaded efforts in hospice development, financing, and public policy formation. Incorporated in 1979, the NHO has grown in size and power and, through its staff and members, effectively lobbied for the creation of the Medicare hospice benefit.

The NHO's changing budget, staff, leadership, and organizational focus has reflected membership changes and philosophical differences among advocates. The organization must identify differences among members and develop goals for the future. Criticized for its "overconcern" for the needs of larger, institutionally affiliated programs, the NHO has been challenged by members to coalesce differences. At the 1984 annual meeting in Hartford, Connecticut, members of rural and volunteer intensive programs voiced concern over existing policies to NHO leadership at a public meeting. Claiming that the NHO had long given up on the needs of the smaller programs that have neither the rights nor the voice of larger programs, critics demanded that leadership consider their needs in upcoming public policy. Yet it is questionable whether the direction taken by NHO leadership will, in fact, benefit the small volunteer-dominated programs. Some contend that it will not and point to recently passed bylaw revisions as an example of their position. The NHO bylaws committee proposed an amendment, passed by membership, allowing board officers to elect three other members to the board, without general membership, vote from business, private philanthropy, labor, and public sectors.

The rationale behind the amendment, as argued by NHO President Carolyn Fitzpatrick, is to allow foundation chairmen, such as the president of the W.K. Kellogg Foundation, to be a member of the NHO board without the embarrassment of running for that office against other foundation representatives. The inclusion of leaders from these organizations would provide the NHO with increased financial support. However, their participation may also result in further industry changes. For example, as we have noted, the Kellogg Foundation provided funding for development of hospice accreditation standards by the JCAH. These standards have received widespread criticism, especially among smaller, all-volunteer hospice groups, because they encourage standardization and professionalization among hospice providers and decrease the unique nature of hospice care. Inclusion of labor, business, and philanthropic leadership such as Kellogg representatives may move hospice to align with more traditional providers and potentially dilute the original hospice care principles.

As the NHO develops its goals and policies for the future, activities that ensure greater market penetration, increased consumer demand, professionalization, and supply and resource acquisition will ensure hospice survival. Service to a broad member base, along with visible promotion of hospice and the use of hospicelike practices throughout the traditional health care system, will expand NHO influence. Sales of NHO services to nonhospice providers who wish to adopt some aspect of hospice programming and care are other expansion strategies. Patients who are not dying can benefit from the social and emotional support services available to terminal patients. In short, the hospice philosophy can be expanded to a broader patient care market.

NHO's stand toward increased hospice professionalization is not without problems. Increased specialization may hurt small, all-volunteer programs or require the employment of specialists not yet available in a given geographic area. However, it has the decided advantage of allowing the NHO and hospice in general to build a vast and comprehensive industry. Specialty courses, training sessions, and certification all require the development of elaborate systems and structures. Once these structures are in place it is very difficult to eliminate them. The expansion of hospice into the traditional health care system and the use of the NHO to assist in further development will increase hospices' scope of power and support. Alliances with traditional providers, particularly home health agencies and hospitals, can increase NHO's political strength. Coalitions or cooperative working relationships with existing providers can provide a base for NHO and individual hospice programs from which to expand and market services.

Increased demand for hospice care has opened the door for coalition building. However, to build coalitions and form working alliances, exchange relationships must be established. Hospices often stand to benefit more in terms of financial and other resources than do hospitals or home health agencies from these affiliations. However, hospitals and home health agencies can and have accrued benefits from allegiances to local hospices, particularly in the way of increased voluntary contributions and public support. At national, state, and local levels, the need for and importance of interinstitutional relationships warrants careful consideration, especially in light of required public evaluation for continued hospice servicing without a primary care provider and without a terminal diagnosis.

SUMMARY

No future is forged without struggle. The hospice approach presents a unique option of care for terminally ill patients and has obtained considerable support in health circles throughout the nation. Nonetheless, concerns have been lodged by a number of early advocates that some of the original idealism accompanying the introduction of hospice programs has faded. As hospice programs sought greater integration into the medical mainstream, tradeoffs were made. Program goals were altered, leadership changed, and organizational structures were revised. In the struggle for reimbursement, program managers needed to assure others that their orientation was competitive, professionalized, and marketable to a broader segment of society. To survive in a western medical system some compromise was needed.

Hospice administrators and planners have a strong source of supply, demand, and resource allocation. Professionalization and market penetration are still in their early stages and warrant improvements. Research and policy endeavors need to be specific and directed at ensuring survival. If hospice is to continue to receive third-party reimbursement, it must not create a parallel system of patient care. The National Hospice Organization, state and local lobbying groups, and other trade and professional organizations must form liaisons to examine existing Administration policy and determine the impact on the future of hospice.

Hospice administrators, managers, planners, and policymakers can ensure that the future of hospice is filled with promise. The essential ingredients for success are available and can be obtained if hospice advocates work toward consensus building and establish compatible relationships with the existing medical industrial complex. With good, strong leadership and a sound sense of public policy and patient needs, hospice developers can look forward to a rewarding future.

NOTES

1. Lenora Finn Paradis, Jill Schultz, Kay Hollers, and Keith Markstrom, "Home Health Agency and Hospice Mergers: Will the Marriage Bells Ever Sound?" *Nursing and Health Care*, forthcoming.

2. "Washington News Briefs," *American Journal of Hospice Care* 1 (Summer 1984): 11.

3. Barney Glaser and Anseln Strauss, *Awareness of Dying* (Chicago, Ill.: Aldine), 1965.

4. Elisabeth Kubler-Ross, *On Death and Dying* (New York: Macmillan), 1969.

5. Lyn H. Lofland, *The Craft of Dying* (Beverly Hills, Calif.: Sage, 1978).

6. Ibid., 11.

7. Finn Paradis et al., "Home Health Agency and Hospice Mergers.'

8. David S. Greer, Vincent Mor, Howard Burnbaum, Sylvia Sherwood, and John N. Morris, *National Hospice Study Preliminary Final Report*, Extended Executive Summary (Providence, R.I.: Brown University, 1983).

9. National Hospice Organization, *Delivery and Payment of Hospice Services: Investigative Study*, Final Report (Arlington, Va.: National Hospice Organization, 1979).

10. Burton A. Weisbrod, "The Private Nonprofit Section: What Is It?" Discussion paper no. 416–77 (Madison, Wisc.: University of Wisconsin, Institute for Research on Poverty, May 1977).

11. Health Care Financing Administration, phone discussion with analyst Mary Hoffmann, Rockville, Md. November 21, 1984.

12. Lenora Finn Paradis and Jill Schultz, "Hospice and Home Health Together in Harmony or Discord," *Caring*, forthcoming.

13. Finn Paradis et al., "Home Health Agency and Hospice Mergers."

BIBLIOGRAPHY

Bass, David M. "Response Bias in Studying Hospice Client Needs," *Omega* 4 (1982): 305–318.

Bucher, Rue, and Stilling, Joan. *Becoming Professional*. Beverly Hills, Calif.: Sage, 1977.

Burns, Nancy, and Carney, Kim. "Hospice: Economic and Nursing Insights," Unpublished paper, University of Texas at Arlington, April, 1983.

Finn Paradis, Lenora. "The Integration of Hospice Programs into the Traditional Health Care System," Unpublished dissertation, Michigan State University, East Lansing, Michigan, 1983.

Finn Paradis, Lenora. "The Integration of Hospice into the Traditional Health Care System," *Death Education* 8 (1984): 383–398.

Foster, Larry, and Finn Paradis, Lenora. *Hospice and Death Education: A Resource Bibliography*. Allendale, Mich.: Grand Valley State College, 1985.

Fox, Renee. "The Social Meaning of Death—Preface," *The Annals* 447 (January 1980): vii–xi. "The Sting of Death in American Society," *Social Science Review* 37 (March 1981): 42–59.

Geogolopous, Basil, and Mann, Floyd. "The Hospital as an Organization." In *The Community General Hospital* (New York: Macmillan 1962), 5–15.

Mechanic, David. *Medical Sociology*. New York: The Free Press, 1978.

Perlstadt, Harry, and Finn Paradis, Lenora. "Cooptation and Cooperation Between Hospices and Home Health Agencies." *The Hospice Journal*. forthcoming.

Rossman, P. *Creating New Models of Care for the Terminally Ill*. New York: Association Press, 1971.

Vicker, Richard. "The Hospice Movement in the United States." *Long Term Care and Health Services Administration Quarterly* 3 (1979): 253–283.

Index

Note: Pages appearing in italics indicate entries found in art work.

Blue Cross-Blue Shield, 14, 46, 47
199, 200, 202, 220, 220-221, 368
Blumer, Herbert, 9, 16
Boulder County Hospice, 337
Bourque, Dan, 209
Breindel, Charles L., 36
Brown University, 8, 45, 198, 211, 368
Budget, 51, *52-54*, 58, 183-184
See also Costs
Butterfield-Picardo, Helen, 94

C

Cairns, Nancy U., 165
Califano, Joseph, 7, *20*, 198
Cancer, 32, 46, 89, 175, *179*,
195, 269-270, 351-353
mortality statistics, 11, 33, 35, *36*,
150, 196
Caring aspects, 96-97, 142-143, *251*,
256, *257, 260, 261, 263, 265, 267,
268, 272-275*, 339-340, 354-355,
356-357
See also SW study
Caseload, 175
Certificate of need (CON), 38, 185,
224
See also Regulations
Certification of Home Care Agency,
185
Certification of hospices, 42, 43, 50,
187, 211, 212, 216, 219-220, 275,
369
Chart forms, 135, 136
Children. *See* Pediatric programs
Chiles, Lawton, 204
Christoffell, J.D., 77
Chronic obstructive pulmonary
diseases, 33
Church Hospital (Baltimore,
Maryland), 35
Cohen, Kenneth P., 27, 48
Committees, *27*
Communication, 58, 88, 163
Community needs assessment, 174-176
See also Home care program,

Community support, 25, *26*, 27-28, 66,
69, 71, 73, 74
centralized effort, 28-30
decentralized approach, 30-31
defined, 26
Competency of physicians. *See*
Physicians
Competition, 188-189, 364, 370
Concepts, hospice, 3-4, 16, 84, 90,
110-111, 120, 124, 173, 194, 311,
355
See also Philosophy
Congressional Budget Office (CBO),
196-197, 203, 211
Continuous Medicare History File, 199
Continuous home care, 50
Core/non-core services, 213, 216, 217,
219, 237
Corporate liability, 235-239
Corporate negligence, 240-242
Costs, 12-14, 46-48, 78, 123-124,
136-137, 185, 193-194, 196, 202,
269, 356-357, 364
CBO study, 196-197, 203, 206
comparison of studies, 195, 196,
200-201
concepts, 194-195, 281-282
containment, 299
conventional care studies, 199-200
demand in health sector, 283-284
demand for hospice care, 196,
284-285, 290, 299
economic analysis, 290
Hospice Council of Northern Ohio
study, 47, 197-198
law of demand, 283
reimbursement, 196
starting, 38, 51, 54
supply and prices, 285-286, *287*
See also Fiscal planning
Cousins, Norman, 36

D

Data collection, 252-253, 277
encounters, 290, 292, *294*

About the Editor

LENORA FINN PARADIS,PH.D., is an assistant professor in the department of Allied Health Education and Research, College of Allied Health Professions, A. B. Chandler Medical Center, University of Kentucky. She is a member of the National Hospice Organization's Research and Evaluation Committee. In addition, she has developed a statewide hospice data base for the State of Michigan, has authored many articles on hospice program development in the United States, and is currently involved in new hospice research activities in Kentucky.

About the Contributors

DAVID M. BASS, PH.D., is a research associate at the Margaret Blenkner Research Center of the Benjamin Rose Institute in Cleveland, Ohio. He has published numerous research articles on hospice care and serves as an advisory member of the Research and Evaluation Committee of the National Hospice Organization.

JOHN BLUM, J.D., is an associate professor in health planning and administration at Pennsylvania State University. As a health care legal specialist, he has written many articles in the area of health care financing and legislation. He recently co-authored a comprehensive review of hospice licensure across the United States.

NANCY BURNS, R.N., PH.D., is an associate professor in the School of Nursing, The University of Texas at Arlington. She has served on various advisory boards including the American Cancer Society area advisory committee and has worked nationally as a consultant in the area of oncology nursing and nursing management. She has initiated extensive research in the area of hospice and nursing care.

KIM CARNEY, PH.D., is Professor of Economics, University of Texas at Arlington. She has received national and local research grants in the hospice field, and is well known for applying economic models to study hospice care.

DAVID DUSH, PH.D., is an assistant professor at Central Michigan University and an evaluation research psychologist for the Midland-Gladwin Community Mental Health Board. He is the former coordinator of psychosocial services at the Hospice of Central Iowa and has been very active in the hospice field. Dr. Dush is the editor of *The Hospice Journal* and has published widely in the area of hospice bereavement.

T. NEAL GARLAND, PH.D., is an associate professor of sociology at the University of Akron, Ohio, specializing in medical sociology and the family. He has worked extensively in the area of patient and satisfaction research for chronically ill and dying patients.

CATHERINE LAMB, R.N., M.P.H., is the Director and Administrator of Amicare Home Health Services in Ann Arbor, Michigan. She has served as a hospice board member and has a long-standing interest and involvement in hospice and home health care.

KENNETH LAZARUS, M.D., is Chief of Pediatric Hematology at Wilford Hall USAF Medical Center in San Antonio, Texas. He is the founder and director of the Wilford Hall Pediatric Hospice. Dr. Lazarus' specialty is pediatric hematology/oncology.

JOANNE LYNN, M.D., is Assistant Clinical Professor of Health Care Sciences and Medicine, Division of Geriatric Medicine, George Washington University. She also serves as Medical Director of the Washington Home Hospice. As former Assistant Director of the President's Commission for the Study of Ethical Problems in Medicine and Biomedical and Behavioral Research, she has made significant contributions to the Commission's reports on the subject of defining death and decisions to forego life-sustaining treatment.

KAREN MCARDLE, R.N., M.A., has been Director of the STAR Hospice program at St. Therese Hospital since its inception in 1980. The STAR Hospice program provides inpatient and home care services directly.

GREG OWEN, PH.D., is a Senior Research Scientist at the Amherst H. Wilder Foundation in St. Paul, Minnesota. He is also an adjunct associate professor at St. Navy's College, Winoma, Minnesota. Dr. Owen has spent time at St. Christopher's Hospice in England and is co-editor of the book *Death and Dying: Challenge and Change.*

LINDA PROFFITT, M.B.A., M.S.S.A., is a health care consultant for Zunt and Associates in Cleveland, Ohio. Former Executive Director of the Hospice Council for Northern Ohio, Proffitt co-authored research on the cost and financing of hospice care. The research was sponsored by Blue Cross/Blue Shield of Northern Ohio.

MICHAEL ROSEN, M.H.A., is director of the Methodist Hospital Hospice Program. He was a founder and board member of the National Hospice Organization and chaired the NHO Licensure and Reimbursement Committee during the time the organization lobbied for Medicare reimbursement. He is considered one of the early hospice founders in the United States.

PAUL WERNER, M.D., is Director of the Family Practice Residency Program at Pontiac General Hospital in Pontiac, Michigan. From 1978–81 he served as Care Team Director for the Bay de Noc Hospice in Escabana, Michigan—the first operating hospice in Michigan. Later, he assisted in establishing hospices in Macon, Georgia, and Tuscaloosa, Alabama. He currently serves on the board of the Michigan Hospice Organization.